OBSTETRICS & GYNECOLOGY MORNING REPORT
Beyond the Pearls

Book Editors

JOEY ENGLAND, MD
Assistant Professor
Department of Obstetrics, Gynecology and Reproductive Sciences
Division of Maternal Fetal Medicine
McGovern Medical School
University of Texas Health Science Center at Houston (UTHealth)
Houston, Texas, United States

KATE V. MERIWETHER, MD
Assistant Professor
Associate Fellowship Program Director
Department of Obstetrics and Gynecology
Division of Female Pelvic Medicine and Reconstructive Surgery
University of Louisville
Louisville, Kentucky, United States

Series Editors

RAJ DASGUPTA, MD, FACP, FCCP, FAASM
Assistant Professor of Clinical Medicine
Assistant Program Director of Internal Medicine Residency
Associate Program Director of Sleep Medicine Fellowship
Department of Internal Medicine
Divisions of Pulmonary / Critical Care / Sleep Medicine
Keck School of Medicine of University of Southern California
Los Angeles, California, United States

R. MICHELLE KOOLAEE, DO, CCD
Assistant Professor of Clinical Medicine
Department of Internal Medicine
Division of Rheumatology
Keck School of Medicine of University of Southern California
Los Angeles, California, United States

ELSEVIER

ELSEVIER

1600 John F. Kennedy Blvd.
Ste 1800
Philadelphia, PA 19103-2899

Notices

Knowledge and best practice in this field are constantly changing. As new research and experience broaden our understanding, changes in research methods, professional practices, or medical treatment may become necessary.

Practitioners and researchers must always rely on their own experience and knowledge in evaluating and using any information, methods, compounds, or experiments described herein. In using such information or methods they should be mindful of their own safety and the safety of others, including parties for whom they have a professional responsibility.

With respect to any drug or pharmaceutical products identified, readers are advised to check the most current information provided (i) on procedures featured or (ii) by the manufacturer of each product to be administered, to verify the recommended dose or formula, the method and duration of administration, and contraindications. It is the responsibility of practitioners, relying on their own experience and knowledge of their patients, to make diagnoses, to determine dosages and the best treatment for each individual patient, and to take all appropriate safety precautions.

To the fullest extent of the law, neither the Publisher nor the authors, contributors, or editors, assume any liability for any injury and/or damage to persons or property as a matter of products liability, negligence or otherwise, or from any use or operation of any methods, products, instructions, or ideas contained in the material herein.

Content Strategist: James Merritt
Content Development Specialist: Meghan Andress
Project Manager: Srividhya Vidhyashankar
Design Direction: Ashley Miner

Printed in China.

Last digit is the print number: 9 8 7 6 5 4 3 2 1

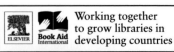

Working together
to grow libraries in
developing countries

www.elsevier.com • www.bookaid.org

To my husband, Stephen, and my parents and grandparents, who always offer me love and wisdom...no matter what. Lastly, I would like to dedicate these chapters to my patients and mentors, who continue to teach me what doctoring is all about.
Kate V. Meriwether

To my parents Les and Sung England and brother Joe England for their unending encouragement and strength. In memory of Lina Bolanos and Richard Field for their beauty and dedication to medicine.
Joey England

We would like to dedicate this book to my parents Arabinda and Tita Dasgupta, for all their hard work and sacrifices they have made for our family throughout their life to make sure all our dreams come true. Even now they help my wife and me by being the best grandparents to our two beautiful children, Mina and Aiden.
Raj Dasgupta & R. Michelle Koolaee

Anubhav Agrawal, MD
Attending Urogynecologist
Department of Obstetrics and Gynecology
University of California San Francisco - Fresno
Fresno, California, United States

Frances M. Alba, MD
Assistant Professor
Department of Surgery
Division of Urology
University of New Mexico School of Medicine
Albuquerque, New Mexico, United States

Ahmet Baydur, MD
Professor
Department of Clinical Medicine
Keck School of Medicine of the University of
Southern California [USC]
Los Angeles, California, United States

Ashlee Bergin, MD, MPH
Assistant Clinical Professor, Assistant Ryan
Program Director
Department of Obstetrics, Gynecology, and
Women's Health
University of Louisville
Louisville, Kentucky, United States

Shan Biscette, MD, MSc
Assistant Professor
Obstetrics & Gynecology
University of Louisville
Louisville, Kentucky, United States

Braden Barnett, MD
Clinical Assistant Professor
Department of Medicine
Division of Endocrinology
Keck School of Medicine of the University of
Southern California [USC]
Los Angeles, California, United States

John David Carmichael, MD
Associate Professor
Co-Director USC Pituitary Center
Department of Medicine
Keck School of Medicine of University of
Southern California
Los Angeles, California, United States

Sara Cichowski, MD
Assistant Professor
Assistant Fellowship Director
Department of Obstetrics & Gynecology
Division of Female Pelvic Medicine and
Reconstructive Surgery
University of New Mexico
New Mexico VA Health Care System
Albuquerque, New Mexico, United States

Shannon Clark, MD
Associate Physician
Department of Obstetrics and Gynecology
Division of Maternal Fetal Medicine
UC Davis Children's Hospital
Sacramento, California, United States

Jean Cox, MS, RD, BS, MS
Patient Educator
Maternity and Family Planning Program
Volunteer Faculty
Department of Obstetrics and Gynecology
University of New Mexico
Albuquerque, New Mexico, United States

Lauren F. Damle, MD, FACOG
Assistant Professor of Clinical Obstetrics and
Gynecology
Department of Women's and Infants'
Services
Division of Pediatric and Adolescent
Gynecology
Georgetown University School of Medicine;
Department of Surgery
MedStar Washington Hospital Center
Children's National Medical Center
Washington, DC, United States

Raj Dasgupta, MD, FACP, FCCP, FAASM
Assistant Professor of Clinical Medicine
Assistant Program Director of Internal
Medicine Residency
Associate Program Director of Sleep
Medicine Fellowship
Department of Internal Medicine
Divisions of Pulmonary / Critical Care /
Sleep Medicine
Keck School of Medicine of University of
Southern California
Los Angeles, California, United States

Mark Dassel, MD
Cleveland Clinic
Cleveland, Ohio, United States

Kimberly DeQuattro, MD, MM
Fellow, Division of Rheumatology
Department of Medicine
University of California
San Francisco, California, United States

Nita Desai, MD, MBA
University of Arizona College of Medicine
St. Joseph's Hospital and Medical Center
Phoenix, Arizona, United States

Yelena Dondik, MD
Department of Obstetrics and Gynecology
Division of Reproductive Endocrinology and
Infertility
University of Louisville
Louisville, Kentucky, United States

Gena Dunivan, MD
Associate Professor
FPMRS Fellowship Director
Department of Obstetrics and Gynecology
Division of Female Pelvic Medicine and
Reconstructive Surgery
University of New Mexico
Albuquerque, New Mexico, United States

Holly E. Dunn, MD
University of Texas
Galveston, Texas, United States

Shaina R. Eckhouse, MD
Section of Minimally Invasive Surgery
Department of Surgery
Washington University School of Medicine
Saint Louis, Missouri, United States

Kara A. Ehlers, MD, FACOG
University of Louisville
Louisville, Kentucky, United States

Joey England, MD
Department of Obstetrics, Gynecology and
Reproductive Sciences
Division of Maternal Fetal Medicine
McGovern Medical School at The University
of Texas Health Science Center at Houston
(UTHealth)
Houston, Texas, United States

Kylie G. Fowler, MD
Fellow, Pediatric and Adolescent Gynecology
Department of Pediatric and Adolescent
Gynecology
Medstar Washington Hospital Center and
Children's National Medical Center
Washington, DC, United States

Tanya Ellis Franklin, MD, MSPH, FACOG
Assistant Professor
Department of Obstetrics and Gynecology
University of Louisville
Louisville, Kentucky, United States

Adrienne L. Gentry, DO, MS
Reproductive Endocrinology and Infertility
Fellow
Department of Obstetrics and Gynecology
and Women's Health
University of Louisville School of Medicine
Louisville, Kentucky, United States

Katherine K. Green, MD MS
Medical Director
Sleep Center at the University of Colorado
Hospital
Assistant Professor and Director of Sleep
Surgery
Department of Otolaryngology
Head and Neck Surgery University of
Colorado School of Medicine

Robin Hardwicke, PhD, FNP-C, AACRN
Professor
Department of Obstetrics Gynecology and
Reproductive Sciences
McGovern Medical School
University of Texas Health Science Center at
Houston
Houston, Texas, United States

Sandra Herrera, MD
University of Texas Medical Branch
Galveston, Texas, United States

Alexandria J. Hill, MD
Perinatologist
Maternal Fetal Medicine
High Risk Pregnancy Center
Las Vegas;
Clinical Assistant Professor
Texas A&M College of Medicine
College Station
Texas;
Clinical Assistant Professor
University of Arizona
Phoenix, Arizona, United States

Deslyn T.G. Hobson, MD, FACOG
Division of Female Pelvic Medicine &
Reconstructive Surgery
University of Louisville
Louisville, Kentucky, United States

Alexis N. Hokenstad, MD
Fellow, Gynecologic Oncology
Mayo Clinic
Rochester, Minnesota, United States

Bradly Holbrook, MD
Resident Physician
Department of Obstetrics and Gynecology
University of New Mexico
Albuquerque, New Mexico, United States

Traci E. Ito, MD
Department of Obstetrics and Gynecology
Division of Minimally Invasive Gynecology
University of Louisville
Louisville, Kentucky, United States

Luis A. Izquierdo, MD, MBA
Associate Professor
Department of Obstetrics and Gynecology
University of New Mexico School of Medicine
Albuquerque, New Mexico, United States

Joses Abhishek Jain, MD
Clinical Fellow
Department of Obstetrics and Gynecology
Division of Maternal Fetal Medicine
Columbia University Medical Center
New York, New York, United States

Sangeeta Jain, MD
Associate Professor
University of Texas Medical Branch at
Galveston
Galveston, Texas, United States

Ambareen Jan, MD
Division of Minimally Invasive Gynecology
Department of Obstetrics and Gynecology
University of Louisville
Louisville, Kentucky, United States

Jason Jarin, MD
Assistant Professor
Department of Obstetrics and Gynecology
Pediatric and Adolescent Gynecology
UTSW Medical Center
Childrens Health
Dallas, Texas, United States

Gregory Kanter, MD, MS, FACOG
Attending Physician
Urogynecology-Salinas Valley Memorial
Healthcare System
Salinas, California, United States

Beatrice Kenol, MD
Assistant Professor of Medicine
Clinical Rheumatologist
Department of Internal Medicine
Division of Rheumatology and Immunology
The Ohio State University Wexner Medical
Center
Columbus, Ohio, United States

Casey Kinman, MD
Female Pelvic Medicine & Reconstructive
Surgery
Baylor Scott & White
Irving, Texas, United States

R. Michelle Koolaee, DO, CCD
Assistant Professor of Clinical Medicine
Department of Internal Medicine
Division of Rheumatology
Keck School of Medicine of University of
Southern California
Los Angeles, California, United States

Nevena Krstic, MS, CGC
McGovern Medical School
University of Texas Health Science Center at
Houston
Houston, Texas, United States

Amanika Kumar, MD
Assistant Professor
Division of Gynecologic Surgery
Division of Medical Oncology
Mayo Clinic
Rochester, Minnesota, United States

Beverly Jean Long, MD
Gynecologic Oncology Fellow
Department of Obstetrics and Gynecology
Division of Gynecologic Surgery
Mayo Clinic
Rochester, Minnesota, United States

Virginia Mensah, MD
Reproductive Endocrinology and Infertility
Specialist
Reproductive Science Center of New Jersey
Eatontown, New Jersey, United States

Kate Vellenga Meriwether, MD
Assistant Professor
Associate Fellowship Program Director
Department of Obstetrics and Gynecology
Division of Female Pelvic Medicine and
Reconstructive Surgery
University of Louisville
Louisville, Kentucky, United States

Laura Anne Mihalko, MD
Urology Resident
Department of Surgery
University of New Mexico
Albuquerque, New Mexico, United States

Ruth Minkin, MD
Pulmonologist
New York-Presbyterian/Brooklyn
Methodist Hospital
New York, New York, United States

Andrew Morado, MD
Keck School of Medicine of the University of
Southern California
Los Angeles, California, United States

Kathy Morris, MSSW, LCGC
Department of Obstetrics and Gynecology,
Maternal Fetal Medicine
University of New Mexico Health Sciences
Center
Albuquerque, New Mexico, United States

Hind N. Moussa, MD
University of Cincinnati
Cincinnati, Ohio, United States

Ellen Mozurkewich, MD
Department of Obstetrics and Gynecology
University of New Mexico
Albuquerque, New Mexico, United States

Noelle Niemand, MD, FACOG
Faculty
Department of Obstetrics and Gynecology
Medical City Arlington
Arlington, Texas, United States

Kelly Pagidas, MD, FACOG, FRCSC
Professor, Division Director
Program Director, REI Fellowship
Department of Obstetrics, Gynecology and
Women's Health
Division of Reproductive Endocrinology and
Infertility
University of Louisville School of Medicine
Louisville, Kentucky, United States

Jennifer Deaver Peterson, MD
Cosmetic Dermatologist
Suzanne Bruce & Associates
Texas Tech University Health Sciences Center
School of Medicine
Houston, Texas, United States

Sara Petruska, MD
Associate Professor
Medical Student
Clerkship Director
Department of Obstetrics, Gynecology and
Women's Health
Generalist Division
University of Louisville School of Medicine
Louisville, Kentucky, United States

Aarti Ramdaney, MS, CGC
McGovern Medical School
University of Texas Health Science Center at
Houston
Houston, Texas, United States

Rebecca G. Rogers, MD
Professor
Vice Chair for Clinical Integration and
Operations
Department of Women's Health
The University of Texas Austin Dell Medical
School
Austin, Texas, United States

Antonio F. Saad, MD, FACOG, FCCM
Assistant Professor
Associate MFM Fellowship Program Director
The University of Texas Medical Branch
Galveston, Texas, United States

Jessica A. Shepherd, MD, MBA, FACOG
Assistant Professor
Director of Minimally Invasive Gynecology
Department of Obstetrics and Gynecology
University of Illinois at Chicago
Chicago, Illinois, United States

Linda-Dalal J. Shiber, MD, FACOG
Assistant Professor
Department of Obstetrics & Gynecology
Division of Advanced Gynecologic Surgery
Metrohealth Hospital/Case Western Reserve
University
Cleveland, Ohio, United States

Eva E. Szabo, MD
Department of Anesthesiology and Critical
Care Medicine
University of New Mexico
School of Medicine
Albuquerque, New Mexico, United States

Jeff R. Temple, PhD
Associate Professor
Department of Obstetrics and Gynecology
UTMB Health
Galveston, Texas, United States

Lauren Thaxton, MD, MD, MBA
Instructor
Department of Obstetrics and Gynecology
University of New Mexico
Albuquerque, New Mexico, United States

Jennifer C. Thompson, MD
Fellow
Urogynecology
University of New Mexico
Albuquerque, New Mexico, United States

Valerie Valant, BA
University of Illinois at Chicago
Chicago, Illinois, United States

Maria I. Villegas Kastner, MD
SBH Health System
Bronx, New York, United States

Oscar A. Viteri, MD
McGovern Medical School
The University of Texas Health Science
Center at Houston (UTHealth)
Texas, Houston, United States

Vera von Bergen, MD
Assistant Professor
McGovern Medical School
University of Texas Health Science Center at
Houston
Houston, Texas, United States

Sumer K. Wallace, MD
Assistant Professor
Division of Gynecologic Oncology
University of Wisconsin
Madison, Wisconsin, United States

Alan Waxman, MD, MPH
Professor
Department of Obstetrics and Gynecology
University of New Mexico
Albuquerque, New Mexico, United States

Christy Williams, BS
University of Illinois at Chicago
College of Medicine
Chicago, Illinois, United States

It is with great pleasure once again that we present our second book, the 1st edition of "Obstetrics and Gynecology Morning Report: Beyond the Pearls". Dr. Koolaee and I envisioned a series of books that incorporates United States Medical Licensing Examination (USMLE) Steps 1, 2, and 3 along with up-to-date evidence based clinical medicine. We wanted the platform of the text to be drawn from a traditional theme, such as the "morning report" format that many of us are familiar with from residency. Just as our first book "Medicine Morning Report: Beyond the Pearls", this book is geared toward a wide audience, from medical students to attending physicians practicing in general Obstetrics and Gynecology. Each case has been carefully chosen and covers scenarios and questions frequently encountered on the Obstetrics and Gynecology boards, shelf exams and clinical practice; integrating both basic science and clinical pearls.

We would like to sincerely thank all of the many contributors who have helped to create this text. Your insightful work will be a valuable tool for medical students and physicians in order to gain an in-depth understanding of Obstetrics and Gynecology. It should be noted that while a variety of clinical cases in Obstetrics and Gynecology were selected for this book, it is not meant to substitute a comprehensive Obstetrics and Gynecology reference.

Dr. Koolaee and I would like to thank our volume editors Dr. Merriweather and Dr. England for all their hard work and dedication to this book. It was truly a pleasure to work with both of you and we look forward to our next project together.

Drs. Dasgupta and Koolaee are to be congratulated for developing the new and much needed series of case-based books for in-training and practicing medical professionals, Morning Report: Beyond the Pearls. With Ob-Gyn volume editors, Drs. Kate Meriwether and Joey England, the team has succeeded in delivering what every Ob-Gyn can use: in-depth, user-friendly clinical cases with practical take-home facts. Whether for the medical student, the resident, or the clinician in practice for decades, this Morning Report keeps us fresh, current and sharp. After knowing Dr. Dasgupta for years since doing our training at the same hospital, I am not surprised that he has executed this magnum opus. He's a true 'doctor's doctor': loves learning, loves practicing, and loves teaching. Thank you, Raj.

Jennifer Ashton, MD
Hygeia Gynecology, Englewood, NJ
Chief Women's Health Correspondent for ABC News
Chief Women's Health Contributor, Dr. Oz Show
Columnist, Cosmopolitan

CONTENTS

Obstetrics

Gynecology

General gynecology

Female Pelvic Medicine and Pelvic Surgery

Lauren Thaxton, MD, MBA ▪ Alan Waxman, MD, MPH

A 34-Year-Old Woman With Cervical Dysplasia in Pregnancy

A 34-year-old G2P1 female presents for initial prenatal care at 11 weeks gestational age. As you review her past history, you note that she has not been screened for cervical cancer since the birth of her last child, 8 years ago.

What is the etiology of cervical cancer?

According to the National Cancer Institute (NCI) Surveillance, Epidemiology, and End Results (SEER) Program, 12,990 new cases of cervical cancer will be diagnosed in 2016 and 4,120 women will die of cervical cancer in that same year. Rates of new diagnosis of this disease have fallen dramatically since the 1950s in the United States; however, mortality has not significantly decreased.

Cervical cancer continues to be the second most common cancer in women worldwide, though in the United States, with its long tradition of screening, it is much less common. Deaths due to this disease should be rare because it is the only cancer wherein the primary etiologic agent is known, highly effective preventative vaccines exist, and the length of preinvasive disease is long.

Human papillomavirus (HPV) is the infective agent that causes almost all cases of cervical cancer. This virus is ubiquitous among sexually active men and women. It is estimated to be the most common sexually transmitted infection (STI), with 6.2 million new cases estimated in the United States each year. Most infections are without symptoms and resolve within a few years of incident infection. HPV specifically targets the transformation zone of the cervix, the region of normal squamous metaplasia (i.e., transition from columnar epithelium to squamous epithelium). Squamous cell carcinoma is the most common histological type; however, adenocarcinomas seem to be increasing. While the Pap test is effective in diagnosing squamous cell carcinoma, it is much less sensitive for adenocarcinomas. There are 15–18 genotypes of high-risk HPV that can cause cancer; HPV types 16 and 18 are responsible for approximately 70% of cervical cancers and 50% of preinvasive lesions, cervical intraepithelial neoplasia (CIN) 3, worldwide.

BASIC SCIENCE PEARL	STEP 1

The primary oncogenes of HPV are E6 and E7, which neutralize the p53 and retinoblastoma tumor suppressor proteins.

CLINICAL PEARL	STEP 2/3

Cervical cancer is initially asymptomatic. Late manifestations of disease can present with vaginal bleeding, a palpable mass, or pelvic pain.

What are the vaccination options for cervical cancer?
There are three vaccines for HPV approved by the U.S. Food and Drug Administration (FDA) and currently available in the United States: Gardasil 9, Gardasil 4, and Cervarix. Cervarix targets immunogenicity against HPV 16 and 18. Gardasil 4 protects against the same two oncogenic HPV types as well as the two types known to be associated with genital warts (6 and 11). Gardasil 9 protects against the same types as Gardasil 4 plus five additional high-risk oncogene types (31, 33, 45, 52, and 58). These vaccines are recommended in three injections over the course of 6 months. Ideally, the vaccine should be given prior to coital debut. The Gardasil vaccines are recommended for girls and boys aged 9 to 26 years. Cervarix is FDA approved for girls alone.

What are screening recommendations for cervical cancer?
The American Cancer Society (ACS), American Society for Colposcopy and Cervical Pathology (ASCCP), and the American Society for Clinical Pathology (ACP) released the following recommendations for cervical cancer screening in 2012. For ease of reference, these may be accessed through the ASCCP website (www.asccp.org) and were reaffirmed in the 2016 ACOG Practice Bulletin on Cervical Cancer screening and prevention (Table 1.1).

> The patient notes that she did not receive the HPV vaccine; however, she has no prior history of abnormal Pap tests. You perform a Pap and HPV test at this visit. She returns to discuss the results a few weeks later. You discuss with her that her Pap test revealed a diagnosis of a high-grade squamous intraepithelial lesion (HSIL). Additionally, her HPV screening is positive for HPV 16.

What are the recommendations for management of HSIL in the nonpregnant woman?
The combination of this Pap test result and her HPV test put her at high risk for downstream development of cervical cancer. In a cohort of women older than 30 years in a prepaid health care system, the 5-year risk of cervical cancer with HPV-positive HSIL on cytology was 6.6%. For this reason, in the nonpregnant woman, either colposcopy with assessment of the endocervical canal or proceeding directly to excisional treatment are reasonable alternatives depending on age and desire for future pregnancies.

How is a colposcopy performed?
Colposcopy is a diagnostic procedure in which the cervix, and specifically the cervical transformation zone, is visually evaluated under magnification for evidence of dysplasia and cancer. In order to complete this exam, providers require an exam table, colposcope, dilute acetic acid, and biopsy forceps. The colposcope is an operating microscope used to magnify the cervix and facilitate visualization (Fig. 1.1).

TABLE 1.1 ■ **Screening Recommendations for Cervical Cancer**

Age	Screening Recommendation
<21	No Pap test; however, anticipatory guidance on safe sex practices, contraception, and sexually transmitted infections (STIs) is indicated in this age group.
21–29	Pap test every 3 years.
30–64	Pap test plus HPV testing every 5 years. If HPV testing is not available, Pap test alone every 3 years is acceptable.
65+	Women without a history of CIN2 or greater in the past 20 years and adequate prior screening may stop cervical cancer screening at this time. Adequate screening means three consecutive negative Pap tests or two consecutive negative HPV tests within the past 10 years, with the most recent within the past 5 years.

First, the patient situates herself in the low lithotomy position. The external genitalia are inspected for concerning findings such as evidence of genital warts or other HPV-related lesions. Once the speculum is placed, the cervix is inspected for neovascularization, leukoplakia, erosion, or ulceration. Then, the cervix is washed with 3%–5% acetic acid. White table vinegar is a suitable substitute for pharmaceutical grade acetic acid. The acetic acid accentuates the demarcation of the squamocolumnar junction. It also highlights areas of dysplastic cells because cells with a high nuclear-to-cytoplasmic ratio will reflect more light. If visualized, this is called *acetowhite epithelium*. Concerning findings include dense acetowhite epithelium with straight borders or a cobblestone or punctuate vascular appearance, called *mosaicism* and *punctation*, respectively. Cervical biopsies should be taken in the most concerning areas using the biopsy forceps, taking care to incorporate the transformation zone. If the transformation zone was not fully visualized, in the nonpregnant patient, it is recommended that an endocervical curettage be performed.

Since 71% of women with HSIL cytology and positive HPV testing will have CIN 2 or worse within 5 years, it is reasonable in the nonpregnant patient to bypass colposcopy and proceed directly to an excisional treatment, such as loop excision. Because of concerns regarding premature birth in women previously treated with excision procedures, an alternative option in women wanting future fertility is colposcopy, biopsy, and awaiting biopsy results. If the biopsy results fall short of CIN 3, conservative management with semi-annual cytology and colposcopy is recommended in this group.

What additional considerations are made in pregnancy?
Some reproductively aged women may not engage in routine health maintenance outside of the setting of pregnancy. This patient's story of a new diagnosis of an abnormal Pap test in pregnancy is not uncommon and presents interesting clinical issues.

In pregnancy, the goals of cervical cancer screening are to identify invasive cervical cancer. HSIL found on biopsy (CIN 2, CIN 3) is not treated until after pregnancy is completed. This patient with a cytologic diagnosis of HSIL merits diagnostic examination with colposcopy to assure that invasive cancer is not present. Patients can be reassured that colposcopy with biopsy

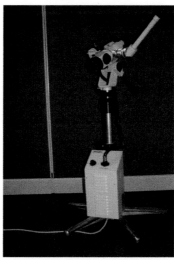

Fig. 1.1 A pedestal-mounted colposcope with teaching head attached and fiberoptic light source. *(From Newkirk G. Colposcopic examination. In Pfenninger and Fowler's procedures for primary care. 2011;919–35. https://www.clinicalkey.com/#!/content/book/3-s2.0-B9780323052672001370?scrollTo=%233-s2.0-B9780323052672001370-f137-008-9780323052672)*

will not cause miscarriage or otherwise adversely affect the pregnancy. This examination may be much more complicated for the colposcopist in pregnancy, however, due to physiologic changes such as vaginal wall redundancy, copious mucus, cervical enlargement, and neovascularization. Additionally, cervical biopsies, if not performed by a practitioner expert in colposcopy in pregnancy, can be associated with heavy vaginal bleeding, which can be troublesome to pregnant women. Bleeding may be controlled by taking fewer biopsies than in the nonpregnant state and very promptly applying Monsel's paste and pressure to biopsy sites. Endocervical curettage is contraindicated in pregnancy due to risks of hard-to-control bleeding and rupture of membranes.

> You decide to perform a colposcopy. You counsel the woman about bleeding precautions. Her colposcopic exam is adequate and shows dense acetowhite epithelium with straight borders in the upper right quadrant. You perform biopsies without complication. The patient returns a week later for biopsy results, which reveal HSIL (Fig. 1.2).

BASIC SCIENCE PEARL   STEP 1

Koilocytes are atypical cells that can be seen on biopsy or Pap test and are suggestive of HPV infection. They are identified by their increased nuclear-to-cytoplasmic ratio, darkening of the nucleus or hyperchromasia, and clearing of the area surrounding the nucleus.

How do you counsel this patient about her biopsy results?
Her histologic findings are concerning; however, the risk of progression to invasive disease over the course of pregnancy is very low. Therefore, the consensus management guidelines recommend that women with HSIL be followed without treatment in pregnancy. Repeat cytologic and colposcopic examinations may be performed but no more frequently than every 12 weeks, with repeat biopsies only recommended if the lesion appears to have worsened and there is concern for invasive cancer. Alternatively, re-evaluation with cytology and colposcopy can be deferred until 6 weeks postpartum. While postpartum follow-up is extremely important, it should be noted that regression of dysplasia postpartum is not uncommon and progression to invasive disease is unlikely.

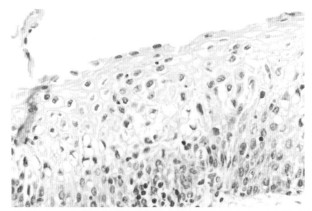

Fig. 1.2 Colposcopic biopsy of high-grade squamous intraepithelial lesion demonstrating perinuclear halos with binucleation (features of koilocytosis). In the parabasal area, nuclear crowding is present and the cells within the epithelium lack some degree of maturation. *(From Massad L. High-grade squamous intraepithelial lesions. Colposcopy. 2008; 231–60. https://www.clinicalkey.com/#!/content/book/3-s2.0-B9781416034056100137?scrollTo=%233-s2.0-B9781416034056100137-gr5)*

The patient has an uncomplicated prenatal course. She goes into labor spontaneously at 39 weeks and 2 days gestation and presents to Labor and Delivery.

How should her cervical dysplasia affect her mode of delivery?
This patient's mode of delivery (cesarean delivery vs. vaginal birth) should be guided only by obstetric factors and is not altered by her cervical dysplasia. Based on the obstetric history given, she would be an excellent candidate for a vaginal birth.

She has an uncomplicated, normal, spontaneous vaginal birth. You see her on morning rounds on postpartum day 2. She is meeting all postpartum milestones and would like to start a reliable form of contraception.

Does the patient's cervical dysplasia limit her options for postpartum contraception?
No. All postpartum methods of contraception would be available to this patient without restriction. Notably, the patient might elect the placement of an intrauterine device (IUD). While this method should be offered without restriction, the patient will need to be counseled about possible issues inherent in this plan. Specifically, if high-grade cervical dysplasia continues to exist on re-evaluation, this may prompt recommendation for an excisional treatment procedure such as a loop electrosurgical excision (LEEP/LLETZ) or cold knife conization. In the process of an excisional treatment procedure, IUD strings are vulnerable and may be inadvertently cut. When she desires ultimate removal of her IUD, this may require instrumentation or hysteroscopy.

LEEP uses an electrocautery-enabled wire loop to excise the transformation zone. It can be performed in the clinic setting with local intracervical anesthesia such as lidocaine with epinephrine or vasopressin for hemostasis. Alternatively, cold knife conization is an option for treatment. Typically, this procedure is performed in the operating room setting under general or regional anesthesia. Again, intracervical local anesthetic with a vasoconstrictor is commonly utilized. Additionally, "stay sutures" are placed with a figure-of-eight suture at the three and nine o'clock positions in order to occlude some blood supply to the cervix as well as to facilitate manipulation of the cervix. A scalpel is used to transect the transformation zone in the form of a cone. The width and depth can be modified based on preoperative assessment of the lesion. Another benefit of cold knife conization is the ability to fully evaluate the margins of the sample because the procedure avoids thermal artifact on the specimen. Complications of these procedures are rare and can include bleeding, uterine perforation, infection, or failure to cure dysplasia (Fig. 1.3).

Six weeks postpartum, she returns to see you for a postpartum check-up and follow-up of her cervical dysplasia. She continues to meet all of her postpartum milestones. She is satisfied with her IUD for contraception.

What are your options for management?
Given her findings of HSIL on biopsy during pregnancy, you have two options: immediate treatment or repeat cytology and colposcopy. If immediate treatment is chosen, colposcopic examination should be carried out to determine if the acetowhite lesion noted in pregnancy persists. If so, a loop excision procedure or ablation can be carried out. If immediate treatment is not elected, both colposcopy and cytology should be performed. If both are negative, we recommend continued close follow-up with repeat colposcopy and cytology in another 6 months. If both are again negative, we recommend co-testing in 1 year, 2 years, and 5 years. If colposcopy shows persistent HSIL, the patient would follow the management guidelines of a nonpregnant adult woman: an ablative or excisional treatment procedure.

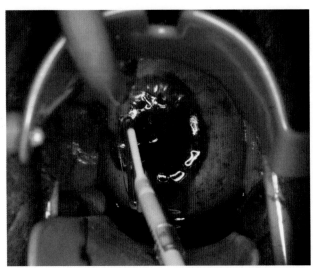

Fig. 1.3 Loop electrosurgical excision (LEEP) procedure begins by plunging the loop into the cervix just lateral to the transformation zone. *(From Spitzer M, Brotzman G, Apgar B. Practical therapeutic options for treatment of cervical intraepithelial neoplasia. Colposcopy. 2008;505–19. https://www.clinicalkey.com/#!/content/book/3-s2.0-B9781416034056100265?scrollTo=%233-s2.0-B9781416034056100265-gr2)*

The most common ablative procedures include cryotherapy and carbon dioxide laser. Ablative therapies do not produce a histological specimen and therefore should not be used if there is any question of invasive malignancy. Ablation should be performed only if the lesion involves less than 75% of the cervix, if the entire squamocolumnar junction is visualized, if endocervical sampling is negative, and, if cryosurgery is selected, that the cryoprobe completely covers the lesion.

> The patient has a LEEP without complication, and results reveal HSIL with negative margins.

What is the follow-up plan for this patient?

Following a treatment procedure the recommended follow-up is a Pap test and HPV test in 12 and 24 months. If both are normal at these two time points a third co-test 3 years later is recommended. If still negative the patient may return to routine screening. It is important to keep in mind that this patient remains at elevated risk for cervical dysplasia and cancer and therefore should continue to have routine Pap and HPV testing. After a diagnosis of HSIL, routine screening is recommended to continue for at least 20 years, even if this extends beyond age 65.

BEYOND THE PEARLS

- Cervical cancer is preventable because the primary infective agent is known, highly effective preventative vaccines exist, screening procedures are well developed, and the length of preinvasive disease is long.
- Regular screening using Pap and HPV testing allows for early detection of cervical dysplasia, a precursor of cervical cancer.
- Pregnancy may be the only time a healthy, reproductively aged woman sees a health care provider, so it is an important opportunity for cervical cancer screening.
- Management of diagnosed cervical dysplasia in pregnancy is typically deferred until after delivery.
- Treatment for high-grade dysplastic lesions is recommended using either ablative or excisional techniques.

Case Summary

- A 34-year-old G2P1 female presents for initial prenatal care at 11 weeks gestational age. She has not had cervical cancer screening in 8 years.
- You perform a Pap test and HPV screening that reveals HSIL with positive high-risk HPV.
- The patient undergoes a colposcopic examination with biopsy findings consistent with Pap test results.
- Her pregnancy continues to term with a plan for postpartum management of her cervical dysplasia.
- Six weeks after her delivery the patient has a LEEP to treat her cervical dysplasia. She remains at elevated risk of dysplasia and should be counseled about the importance of screening.

References

American College of Obstetricians and Gynecologists (2016). Cervical Cancer Screening and Prevention. Practice Bulletin No. 157. *Obstetrics and Gynecology*, *127*, e1–e20.

Bosch, F., Burchell, A., Schiffman, M., et al. (2008). Epidemiology and natural history of human papillomavirus infections and type-specific implications in cervical neoplasia. *Vaccine*, *26*(Suppl. 10), K1–K16.

Katki, H., Schiffman, M., Castle, P., et al. (2013). Five-year risks of CIN 3+ and cervical cancer among women with HPV-positive and HPV-negative high-grade Pap results. *Journal of Lower Genital Tract Disease*, *5*(Suppl. 1), S50–S55.

Massad, L., Einstein, M., Huh, W., et al. (2013). 2012 updated consensus guidelines for the management of abnormal cervical cancer screening tests and cancer precursors. *Obstetrics and Gynecology*, *121*(4), 829–846.

Rodriguez, A., Schiffman, M., Herrero, R., et al. (2010). Longitudinal study of human papillomavirus persistence and cervical intraepithelial neoplasia grade 2/3: critical role of duration of infection. *Journal of the National Cancer Institute*, *102*(5), 315–324.

Santesso, N., Schunemann, H., Blumenthal, P., et al. (2012). World Health Organization Guidelines: use of cryotherapy for cervical intraepithelial neoplasia. *International Journal of Gynaecology and Obstetrics*, *118*(2), 97–102.

Smith, H., Tiffany, M., Qualls, C., et al. (2000). The rising incidence of adenocarcinoma relative to squamous cell carcinoma of the uterine cervix in the United States–a 24-year population-based study. *Gynecologic Oncology*, *78*(2), 97–105.

Walboomers, J., Jacobs, M., Manos, M., et al. (1999). Human papillomavirus is a necessary cause of invasive cervical cancer worldwide. *The Journal of Pathology*, *189*(1), 12–19.

Wheeler, C. (2008). Natural history of human papillomavirus infections, cytologic and histologic abnormalities, and cancer. *Obstetrics and Gynecology Clinics of North America*, *35*(4), 519–536, vii.

Yost, N., Santoso, J., McIntire, D., et al. (1999). Postpartum regression rates of antepartum cervical intraepithelial neoplasia II and III lesions. *Obstetrics and Gynecology*, *93*(3), 359–362.

Shannon Clark, MD

A 23-Year-Old Woman with Hyperemesis Gravidarum

A 23-year-old G1P0 woman presents to the emergency department at 9 weeks of gestation by last menstrual period with a 1-week history of nausea and vomiting. She has not yet established prenatal care. A pelvic sonogram reveals an intrauterine pregnancy at 8 weeks 2 days gestation. She reports the inability to keep solids down but is able to tolerate some liquids. She has approximately four episodes of emesis daily and intermittent nausea throughout the day. She also reports a 2.3 kg (5-lb) weight loss. She does not report fever, chills, diarrhea, or sick contacts.

What questions should be asked when interviewing this patient?

When a pregnant female presents with nausea and vomiting in early pregnancy, it is important to ask questions about the onset, timing, and severity of symptoms, as well as any aggravating or alleviating factors. In addition, inquire about any sick contacts. Next, ask whether she has any co-existing medical problems that would cause nausea and vomiting in pregnancy (i.e., gastro-esophageal reflux disease, diabetes, and/or any other gastrointestinal conditions or prior abdominal surgeries). Finally, it is necessary to ask the patient how many episodes of nausea, vomiting, and dry-heaving she is having per day; whether she is tolerating any solid food or liquids; and if she is urinating normal volumes.

CLINICAL PEARL   **STEPS 2/3**

A thorough physical exam is necessary. There are conditions that could be life-threatening, like a ruptured ectopic pregnancy or ruptured appendix.

It is particularly important to assess the duration of nausea and vomiting and ability to tolerate liquids in order to determine the potential risk for a more severe medical condition, *Wernicke's encephalopathy*, which is due to prolonged nausea and vomiting and subsequent vitamin B_1 (thiamine) deficiency. Memory loss, apathy, decreased level of consciousness, or blurred vision are additional symptoms associated with thiamine deficiency. Deficiencies in vitamins B_6 and B_{12} may also occur and are associated with anemia and peripheral neuropathy. Finally, vitamin K deficiency and coagulopathy can cause bleeding (Fig. 2.1).

BASIC SCIENCE PEARL   **STEP 1**

A rare complication of hyperemesis gravidarum is Wernicke's encephalopathy, a severe thiamine deficiency caused by poor dietary intake, emesis, and increased metabolic demands of pregnancy. Frequency is reported at between 0.1% and 0.5% of pregnancies, with clinical features including a triad of ocular abnormalities, confusion, and ataxia.

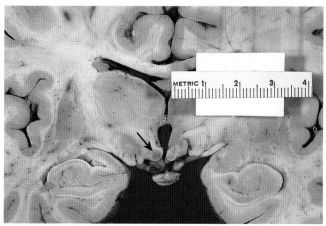

Fig. 2.1 Bilateral small mammillary bodies *(arrow)* are very suggestive of remote damage due to Wernicke's encephalopathy. *(From Connolly A, Finkbeiner W, Ursell P, et al. Atlas of gross autopsy pathology. https://www. clinicalkey.com/#!/content/book/3-s2.0-B9780323287807000160?scrollTo=%233-s2.0-B9780323287807000160-f016-326-9780323287807)*

What should the physical exam include?

When examining the patient, the abdominal and pelvic exams are particularly important. Suprapubic pain could indicate cystitis, and right lower quadrant pain on exam could indicate acute appendicitis, the most common general surgical emergency in pregnancy. The pelvic exam should include a sterile speculum exam and a bimanual exam. The cervix should be assessed for any bleeding and signs of infection, and the bimanual exam will not only reveal an enlarged, gravid uterus, but whether there are any signs of infection, as seen with pelvic inflammatory disease, or adnexal fullness, which could indicate an ectopic pregnancy or adnexal mass. Finally, the patient should be assessed for signs of dehydration (i.e., dry mucous membranes and decreased skin turgor).

On physical exam, the patient has a temperature of 36.6°C (98.0°F), a heart rate of of 80/min, and a blood pressure of 110/80 mm Hg. Her neck is normal to palpation without masses, tenderness, or lymphadenopathy. Her abdomen is soft, nontender to palpation, and without rebound or guarding. She does not have suprapubic or costovertebral angle tenderness. On pelvic exam, the patient has normal external female genitalia without lesions or pain. No vaginal discharge, bleeding, or malodor is present.

What is the differential diagnosis?

When a pregnant patient presents with nausea and vomiting, it should not be assumed that it is due to pregnancy alone. One should also look for atypical symptoms or physical exam findings that may indicate another cause for the nausea and vomiting, especially if a patient initially presents with nausea and vomiting after 10 weeks of gestation.

CLINICAL PEARL	**STEPS 2/3**

It should never be assumed that nausea and vomiting in the first trimester is due to the pregnancy alone. Pregnant women in the first trimester can have other conditions that are associated with nausea and vomiting. These should not be overlooked.

TABLE 2.1 ■ Other Causes of Nausea and Vomiting in Pregnancy

Hepatitis
Central nervous system abnormality
Pancreatitis
Helicobacter pylori infection
Hepatitis
Cholecystitis
Acute fatty liver of pregnancy
Hyperthyroidism
Peptic ulcer disease

There are some conditions that should be ruled out when any pregnant patient presents with nausea and vomiting (Table 2.1). If the patient has a fever, a source of infection should be sought. (i.e., urinary tract infection [cystitis or pyelonephritis] or gastroenteritis). If peritoneal signs exist, suspicion for acute abdomen is raised (i.e., acute appendicitis). Headache associated with nausea and vomiting can occur with dehydration, but preeclampsia should be considered, especially if there is elevated blood pressure and the patient presents after 20 weeks of pregnancy. Although epigastric pain and hematemesis are rare in pregnancy, a Mallory Weiss tear from prolonged vomiting may occur. Finally, heartburn and gastric reflux occur in a significant number of pregnant women. As a result, determining whether the patient has gastroesophageal reflux disease is important.

What is the working diagnosis?
If the patient presents at less than 10 weeks of gestation, the leading diagnosis is nausea and vomiting of pregnancy (NVP), which occurs in 50%–90% of pregnancies. NVP has been traditionally referred to as "morning sickness," but nausea can occur at any time of the day or night and occur with or without episodes of vomiting. NVP typically starts between 4 and 9 weeks gestational age, with maximal symptoms at 12–15 weeks, and resolution of symptoms by 20 weeks gestational age. Symptoms of NVP include any combination of the following: nausea, gagging, retching, dry heaving, vomiting, and odor and/or food aversion.

CLINICAL PEARL   **STEPS 2/3**

If the diagnosis of NVP or hyperemesis gravidarum (HG) is made, but there is poor response to treatment, an atypical presentation, or initial presentation after 10 weeks, another etiology of the symptoms should be sought.

CLINICAL PEARL   **STEPS 2/3**

Up to 20% of women experience symptoms well into the second trimester and possibly throughout the entire pregnancy.

What laboratory evaluation and radiologic testing should be performed on this patient?
Determining the gestational age of the pregnancy and the number of fetuses present, especially in a patient with no prenatal care, is essential. This is achieved through a pelvic sonogram.

Assessment of dehydration status can easily be done with a urine dipstick to check for urinary ketones. If the patient shows signs of dehydration and has moderate to severe ketones on urine dipstick, obtaining a blood urea nitrogen (BUN), creatinine, aspartate aminotransferase (AST) and alanine aminotransferase (ALT), and electrolytes should be considered. If there are any concerns for pancreatitis, add an amylase and lipase.

> The patient's urine dipstick is positive for ketones, and her lab evaluation is significant only for hypokalemia with a potassium level of 3 mEq/L.

It is known that human chorionic gonadotropin (hCG) cross-reacts with thyrotropin (thyroid stimulating hormone or TSH) and stimulates the thyroid gland, making TSH lower in pregnancy, especially in the first trimester. TSH and free T4 (FT4) should be checked if there is a history of thyroid disease or the patient is exhibiting other signs and clinical symptoms of thyroid disease.

CLINICAL PEARL   **STEPS 2/3**

Part of a thorough physical exam includes a thyroid exam to assess for fullness or nodules, especially if the patient has a history of thyroid disease. Symptoms of thyroid disease can mimic the symptoms of pregnancy, which can make diagnosing thyroid disease more difficult.

What is the etiology of NVP?
The hormonal changes that occur during pregnancy are known to contribute to the symptoms of NVP. Estrogen, hCG, progesterone, and thyroid hormone levels change throughout pregnancy, especially during the first trimester, triggering nausea and vomiting. Conditions like multiple gestation and molar pregnancy that are associated with increased placental mass and increased levels of hCG are associated with more severe symptoms of NVP.

However, it is the structural similarity in the biomolecular structure of hCG and TSH that plays a particularly significant role in NVP. Increased hCG in pregnancy cross-reacts with TSH thus stimulating the thyroid gland, particularly in the first trimester. As a result, patients with NVP and its more severe form, HG, may have abnormal thyroid function tests (TFTs).

Subclinical hyperthyroidism is commonly seen (low TSH and normal to high-normal thyroid hormone levels) with NVP or HG. However, TFTs should not be assessed as part of the routine assessment for NVP unless the patient has a history of thyroid disease or is showing signs or symptoms of thyroid disease. Finally, treatment for subclinical hyperthyroidism is typically not necessary as the TFTs will normalize as symptoms resolve and the pregnancy progresses.

CLINICAL PEARL   **STEPS 2/3**

Women with a history of severe NVP or HG requiring hospitalization or medical therapy may be hesitant to become pregnant again. It is reasonable to offer these women early or prophylactic treatment in the next pregnancy.

An additional contributor to NVP involves the physiologic changes in pregnancy involving the gastrointestinal (GI) tract. The GI tract is anatomically affected by the growing uterus and displacement of the abdominal organs, and its transit time is slowed by the hormonal changes of pregnancy (i.e., estrogen and progesterone). Furthermore, the gastroesophageal junction is altered, leading to reflux and/or nausea and vomiting.

What are the risk factors for NVP?

Genetics does play a role in the development and severity of NVP and HG. Not only are NVP and HG likely heritable diseases, but the severity of symptoms may also be associated with a genetic predisposition. Women are at the greatest risk for developing NVP if their mother or sister had NVP or HG, or if the patient herself had NVP or HG in a prior pregnancy. Other risk factors include multiple gestation, molar pregnancy, and young, nulliparous, obese women. Factors associated with more severe symptoms of NVP include stress, lack of sleep, chronic *Helicobacter pylori* infection, peptic or duodenal ulcers, migraines, and prenatal vitamins.

CLINICAL PEARL   **STEPS 2/3**

Because NVP is predominantly a condition of the first trimester, concerns for fetal exposure to medications arise. Trying conservative measures first for the treatment of NVP is recommended, but medical therapy should not be withheld if indicated. Progression of symptoms can lead to the more severe form of NVP, HG.

How is NVP treated?

Up to 10% of pregnant women will require medical treatment of their NVP after failure of conservative measures (Table 2.2).

A combination of oral pyridoxine hydrochloride (vitamin B_6) and doxylamine succinate (histamine-1 [H_1] receptor antagonist) is recommended as first-line treatment for NVP if pyridoxine monotherapy does not relieve symptoms. These medications are available individually over-the-counter or as a sustained-release formulation of 10 mg of pyridoxine and 10 mg doxylamine.

CLINICAL PEARL   **STEPS 2/3**

In women with HG, the values of TSH and FT4 may be similar to that seen in Graves' disease, but without the clinical signs and symptoms of Graves' disease or the presence of thyroid antibodies.

After initiating treatment with pyridoxine and doxylamine, breakthrough nausea and vomiting can be treated with a variety of medications. Examples include dimenhydrinate (H_1 receptor antagonist), promethazine (dopamine [D_2]) receptor antagonist), or metoclopramide (dopamine receptor antagonist). These agents can also be used as second-line therapy if the pyridoxine-doxylamine combination fails. Third-line therapy includes serotonin 5-hydroxytryptamine3-receptor (5-HT3) antagonists or ondansetron.

TABLE 2.2 ■ Conservative Measures for the Treatment of Nausea and Vomiting of Pregnancy (NVP)

Avoid aversive odors or foods	Get adequate rest
Eat multiple small meals a day with higher protein and carbohydrate and lower fat content	Drink smaller volumes of liquids multiple times a day: up to 2 liters of fluid per day
Try the bananas, rice, applesauce, and toast diet (BRAT)	Avoid stress

BASIC SCIENCE PEARL   STEP 1

Doxylamine inhibits the action of histamine at the H_1 receptor, acts at the vestibular system, and exhibits some inhibition of muscarinic receptors in the vomiting center. Promethazine belongs to a class of dopamine (D_2) receptor antagonists that inhibit gastric motility through the D_2 receptors of the GI tract and decrease stimulation of the chemoreceptor trigger zone. Metoclopramide is a dopamine receptor antagonist that is an antiemetic and prokinetic. It decreases gastrointestinal emptying time and decreases stimulation of the chemoreceptor trigger zone. Ondansetron works at the 5-HT3 receptors located in the small bowel, vagus nerve, and chemoreceptor trigger zone (Fig. 2.2).

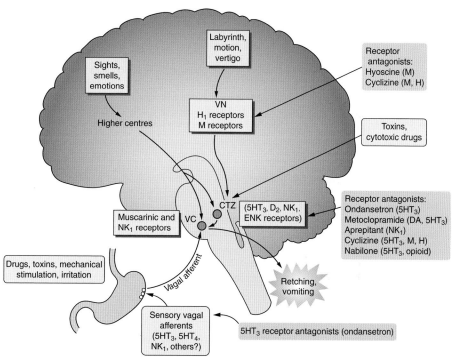

Fig. 2.2 Neuronal pathways and receptors involved in the control of nausea and vomiting. The chemoreceptor trigger zone (CTZ) has neuronal connections to the vomiting center (VC), which is a collection of nuclei including the dorsal motor nucleus of the vagus and the nucleus tractus solitarius. *5-HT3*, 5-Hydroxytryptamine type 3 receptor; *DA*, dopamine receptor; *ENK receptor*, enkephalin (opioid) receptor; *H1*, histamine type 1 receptor; *M*, muscarinic receptor (possibly M2); *NK1*, neurokinin 1 receptor; *VN*, vestibular nuclei. *(From Waller D, Sampson A. Nausea and vomiting. In* Medical pharmacology and therapeutics, *2014;391–8. https://www.clinicalkey.com/#!/content/ book/3-s2.0-B9780702051807000324?scrollTo=%233-s2.0-B9780702051807000324- f032-001-9780702051807)*

The patient is given 1 L intravenous hydration, potassium replacement, and intravenous ondansetron. As her nausea begins to improve, vitamin B_6 and doxylamine are initiated. She feels much improved after 48 hours of hospitalization, with improvement in her labs and clinical status, and is discharged to home.

What is the more severe form of NVP?

HG occurs in up to 3% of pregnancies and is characterized by severe and persistent nausea and vomiting, a loss of 5% or more of prepregnancy body weight, electrolyte abnormalities, ketonuria, dehydration, and potential vitamin or mineral deficiencies. Patients with HG may present frequently to the emergency room or Labor and Delivery for intravenous fluid hydration and antiemetics and require inpatient admission when symptoms are severe and/or prolonged. Inpatient admission is usually required if the patient is ketotic and dehydrated in order to properly treat and investigate any other potential causes for the nausea and vomiting. *Failure to diagnose and/or properly treat NVP can lead to the development of HG. As a result, asking your patient about the symptoms of NVP early in pregnancy and treating when necessary can lead to a more manageable course for the patient and potentially prevent the progression of NVP to HG.*

BEYOND THE PEARLS

- Alternative therapies including acupuncture and ginger have been studied for NVP with inconsistent results.
- Enteral tube feedings may be effective; however, some patients continue to have persistent emesis.
- Total parenteral nutrition (TPN) is reserved for patients with significant weight loss (>5% of body weight without response to antiemetic regimens and cannot be managed with enteral feedings); TPN is associated with risk of line sepsis and steatohepatitis.

Case Summary

- A 23-year-old G1P0 woman presents to the emergency department at 9 weeks of gestation with nausea and vomiting.
- History and physical examination reveal hemodynamic stability, absence of fever, and a nonsurgical abdomen. Laboratory evaluation is significant for ketonuria and hypokalemia.
- The patient receives IV fluids, electrolyte replacement, and antiemetics. She begins dietary adjustments. Her ketonuria and hypokalemia resolve, and she is able to tolerate intake by mouth. She is discharged home with antiemetics and prenatal vitamins and scheduled for a follow-up clinic appointment to establish prenatal care.

References

Badell, M. L., Ramin, S. M., & Smith, J. A. (2006). Treatment options for nausea and vomiting during pregnancy. *Pharmacotherapy, 26*(9), 1273–1287.

Bottomley, C., & Bourne, T. (2009). Management strategies for hyperemesis. *Best Practice & Research. Clinical Obstetrics & Gynaecology, 23*(4), 549–564.

Chiossi, G., Neri, I., Cavazzuti, M., et al. (2006). Hyperemesis gravidarum complicated by Wernicke encephalopathy: background, case report, and review of the literature. *Obstetrical & Gynecological Survey, 61*(4), 255–268.

Clark, S. M., Costantine, M. M., & Hankins, G. D. (2012). Review of NVP and HG and early pharmacotherapeutic intervention. *Obstetrics and Gynecology International, 2012*, 252676.

Davis, M. (2004). Nausea and vomiting of pregnancy: an evidence based review. *The Journal of Perinatal & Neonatal Nursing, 18*(4), 312–328.

Gill, S. K., & Einarson, A. (2007). The safety of drugs for the treatment of nausea and vomiting of pregnancy. *Expert Opinion on Drug Safety, 6*(6), 685–694.

Koren, G., & Bishai, R. (2000). *Nausea and vomiting of pregnancy: state of the art 2000, vol. 1 of the Motherisk Program.* Toronto: Motherisk.

Markl, G. E., Strunz-Lehner, C., Egen-Lappe, V., et al. (2008). The association of psychosocial factors with nausea and vomiting during pregnancy. *Journal of Psychosomatic Obstetrics and Gynaecology, 29*(1), 17–22.

Miller, F. (2002). Nausea and vomiting in pregnancy: the problem of perception—is it really a disease? *American Journal of Obstetrics and Gynecology, 186*, S182–S183.

Nausea and vomiting of pregnancy. (2015). Practice bulletin no. 153. American College of Obstetricians and Gynecologists. *Obstetrics and Gynecology, 126*, e12–e24.

Niebyl, J. R., & Goodwin, T. M. (2002). Overview of nausea and vomiting of pregnancy with an emphasis on vitamins and ginger. *American Journal of Obstetrics and Gynecology, 186*(5), S253–S255.

Niebyl, J. R. (2010). Nausea and vomiting in pregnancy. *The New England Journal of Medicine, 363*(16), 1544–1550.

O'Brien, B., & Zhou, Q. (1995). Variables related to nausea and vomiting during pregnancy. *Birth, 22*(2), 93–100.

Robinson, J. N., Banerjee, R., & Thiet, M. P. (1998). Coagulopathy secondary to vitamin K deficiency in hyperemesis gravidarum. *Obstetrics and Gynecology, 92*(4), 673–675.

Jennifer Deaver Peterson, MD

A 31-Year-Old Woman With Rash in Pregnancy

A 31-year-old primigravida Caucasian woman at 30 weeks' gestation presents to your outpatient obstetrics clinic complaining of blisters on her body for the past 2 weeks. She reports the blisters are very itchy, which is resulting in difficulty sleeping and resultant fatigue. She denies any recent infections, fever, chills, or myalgias. She is currently taking prenatal vitamins daily, but no other medications. All prenatal office visits and lab work have been normal thus far, and she has no significant medical history. She has no sick contacts, and her husband does not have any blisters or rashes on his skin.

When a pregnant woman develops blisters, what is important to know in her history?
Blistering rashes are not a common occurrence in pregnant patients. Some of the most critical questions to ask are timing, location where blisters first presented on the body, associated symptoms, history of a similar condition, travel history, sick contacts, and new or recent exposure to topical or systemic medications, plants, or topical skin care products. Most inflammatory blistering rashes result in pruritus, or itching. Bacterial or viral causes of blistering rashes more commonly cause pain and are often more localized.

Your patient tells you she has never had a rash like this before. She reports that the blisters first appeared 2 weeks ago and were very small on her abdomen. Then the blisters began to enlarge and become greater in number. Last week blisters appeared on her arms, legs, and buttocks. She was on vacation in Florida 1 week before the rash began, but she had taken all of her own routine cleansers, lotions, and sunscreen with her. She went to the hotel pool and spent her time reading. She did not go swimming or go to the beach. She has not been using any other oral or topical medications other than her prenatal vitamins. She has been hesitant to start any over-the-counter therapies because she doesn't want to risk harm to her growing baby. Finally, she has had very little sleep in the past week due to the severe itching she is experiencing.

Viral infections due to the herpes virus family can result in painful blistering skin disorders in pregnancy. Herpes simplex virus (HSV) type 1 can result in grouped vesicles (blisters <1 cm) on an erythematous base (Table 3.1 and 3.2).

CLINICAL PEARL   **STEPS 2/3**

While HSV type 1 commonly affects the perioral area and results in herpes labialis, it can also affect any other skin surface area such as the face, nose, neck, trunk, or extremities. In these instances the condition is known as herpes simplex.

TABLE 3.1 ▪ **Morphologic Descriptions**

Vesicle	A blister <1 cm in diameter
Bulla	A blister >1 cm in diameter
Tense bulla	A firm blister
Flaccid bulla	A blister that is fragile and easily ruptures
Papule	Elevated lesion, <1 cm in diameter
Plaque	Elevated lesion, >1 cm in diameter
Nodule	Very large, firm lesion
Macule	Flat lesion, <1 cm in diameter
Patch	Flat lesion, >1 cm in diameter

TABLE 3.2 ▪ **Dermatologic Adjectives**

Erythematous	Red
Violaceous	Light purple
Purpuric	Dark purple
Hyperpigmented	Darker than skin tone
Hypopigmented	Lighter than skin tone
Depigmented	Absence of pigment; white to porcelain color
Honey-crusted	Dried honey-colored translucent crusts. Indicative of a staphylococcal infection
Heme-crusted	Dried blood on skin surface
Excoriated	Scratched. May see linear scratches or "dug-out" appearance
Urticarial	Swollen, pink or red, hive-like papule or plaque
Targetoid	"Bull's-eye" target shape
Annular	Ring shape
Nummular	Coin-like shape and size
Reticulated	Net-like appearance
Umbilicated	Elevated lesion with central indentation
Herpetiform	Grouped vesicles on an erythematous base; herpes-like appearance
Atrophic	Thinned, indented
Hypertrophic	Thickened
Indurated	Firm
Sclerotic	Scar-like

BASIC SCIENCE PEARL **STEP 1**

The Tzanck smear is a smear of an opened skin vesicle and is used to assay for HSV; a positive test reveals multinucleated giant cells (Fig. 3.1).

HSV type 1 often has a history of recurrences in the same location. Varicella zoster virus (VZV) is also known as shingles, HSV type 3, or herpes zoster. While the typical patient with zoster is in her 60s to 80s, it can develop in pregnancy. VZV is characterized by grouped vesicles on an erythematous base in a unilateral dermatomal distribution and is due to reactivation of varicella virus (chicken pox). It is extremely rare for VZV to recur in the same location. If a patient describes a history or recurrences it is most likely HSV1. Swab cultures and direct fluorescence antibody tests can be used to differentiate between HSV1, HSV2, and VZV because the dosing schedules to treat these conditions are different.

What clues in the history point away from a diagnosis of allergic contact dermatitis?

Allergic contact dermatitis (ACD) is a type of allergic reaction due to the skin coming in contact with an external substance that causes a type IV delayed hypersensitivity reaction. One of the

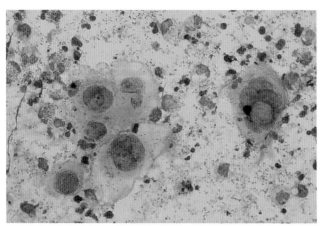

Fig. 3.1   Tzanck smear demonstrating multinucleated epithelial giant cells from a patient with herpes simplex viral infection. *(From Mendoza N, Madkan, V. Human herpesviruses. 2012;1321–43. https://www.clinicalkey. com/#!/content/book/3-s2.0-B9780723435716000804?scrollTo=%233-s2.0-B9780723435716000804-f080-011-9780723435716)*

most well known types of ACD is due to exposure to poison ivy; however, the most common allergens responsible for this type of reaction include nickel, topical neomycin, fragrances, dyes, and preservatives in skin care products. ACD due to plants typically results in linear distributions of the rash due to contact with the edges of leaves. Photoallergic contact dermatitis reactions can occur following the application of chemical-based sunscreens and sun exposure. This diagnosis is less likely in this patient's case because there has been no change in her routine skin care product usage or other environmental exposures.

What clues in the patient's history could point toward a diagnosis of an arthropod assault?
The patient has traveled recently to Florida and stayed in a hotel while on vacation. This travel history could put her at risk for an arthropod assault due to bedbugs, scabies, mosquitos, or sandflies. Some patients present with such an exuberant reaction to arthropod bites that they develop both urticarial (edematous erythematous round plaque) lesions and bullous (blistering) lesions. Bedbugs often bite in areas of skin exposed to the bed; for example, a woman sleeping in a short tank top and shorts could develop bites on the neck, chest, abdomen, and extremities (Fig. 3.2).

Scabies mites can bite anywhere on the skin but most commonly spare the face and scalp in adults. Scabies mites can burrow under the skin and form visible tracks known as *burrows*, which are most often encountered on the web spaces of the fingers, wrists, and umbilical areas in women (Fig. 3.3).

Scabies bites produce severe itching, which is often worse at night and may lead to insomnia.

Finally, mosquitos and sandflies should also be considered and can bite on any exposed skin surface. Mosquitos species from Florida can harbor multiple viruses including Zika, West Nile, Eastern equine encephalitis, and St. Louis encephalitis.

CLINICAL PEARL   **STEPS 2/3**

Don't be misled if a patient's spouse or significant other does not have a rash or itching; reactions to bedbug bites vary greatly from patient to patient. Scabies mites, eggs, and feces can be detected with a simple skin scraping followed by microscopic analysis performed in the office.

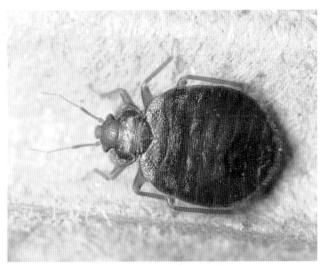

Fig. 3.2 Bedbug. *(From Williams J. Bed bugs in hospitals: more than just a nuisance.* Can Med Assoc J. *2013;183(11):E524. https://www.clinicalkey.com/#!/content/journal/1-s2.0-S0820394613604782?scrollTo=% 231-s2.0-S0820394613604782-fx1)*

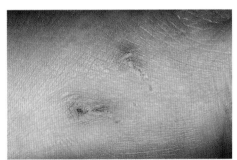

Fig. 3.3 Burrow of *Sarcoptes scabiei* on the side of a finger. *(From Ooi W, Morse S. Infestations.* Atlas of sexually transmitted diseases and AIDS. *2010;324-6. https://www.clinicalkey.com/#!/content/book/3-s2.0-B9780702040603000017X?scrollTo=%233-s2.0-B9780702040603000017X-f11)*

What clues in this patient's history might point toward pruritic urticarial papules and plaques of pregnancy (PUPPP)?

PUPPP is an inflammatory skin condition typically presenting in the third trimester or imme-diately postpartum. It has an incidence of 1 in every 200 pregnancies and most often occurs in primiparous women.

The typical lesions are urticarial papules and plaques, but bullae and targetoid (bull's eye target like shapes) lesions can also occur. These lesions first appear along the abdomen and in abdominal striae distensae (stretch marks) but spare the umbilicus. The rash may then spread to involve the extremities and trunk, but the mucous membranes, face, palms, and soles are often spared. Itching can be severe for many patients (Fig. 3.4).

This patient is primigravida, in her third trimester, and has a rash that began on her abdomen, which can favor PUPPP. However, additional information is needed.

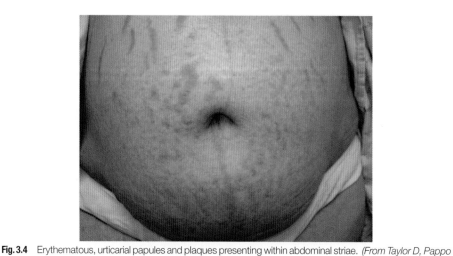

Fig. 3.4 Erythematous, urticarial papules and plaques presenting within abdominal striae. *(From Taylor D, Pappo E, Aronson I. Polymorphic eruption of pregnancy.* Clin Dermatol. *2016;34(3):383–91. https://d1niluoi1dd30v. cloudfront.net/0738081X/S0738081X16X0003X/S0738081X16300268/gr2.jpg?Expires=1480842978&Key -Pair-Id=APKAICLNFGBCWWYGVIZQ&Signature=N7Cysauh18gb4m0TVE9hhr4A-LJHG5iVhu76PGoLpCN %7ENYMqzKO0y5FKZJZOGY%7EwCJ6ClZA6iQqDYkr0mbNZLDfmMjv9aGdGKQUtbu-Ghe0ua5ljmEPazx2- igTVn2FrucAGlA8%7E2tpo3dWnPToW8mc7EY1GiVo0b803s02PhBw_)*

CLINICAL PEARL   **STEPS 2/3**

PUPPP can sometimes be very subtle, and the lesions may be faint and not as elevated. Make sure to examine the patient in bright light. Transillumination may be helpful to thoroughly examine the appearance of the striae distensae.

What clues in this patient's history might point toward gestational pemphigoid?

Gestational pemphigoid, also known as pemphigoid gestationis, is an extremely rare autoimmune skin disease with antibodies produced to a skin protein. Gestational pemphigoid most commonly develops in the periumbilical area and then spreads outward to involve the extremities and buttocks. In severe cases, the majority of the skin can be involved including the palms and soles, but the mucous membranes and face are often spared. The patients may have urticarial and/or tense bullae. Most patients complain of severe itching and may also develop malaise, chills, or subfebrile temperatures.

Gestational pemphigoid most commonly presents in the second or third trimesters but can also develop postpartum. Our patient reports a history and timeline that could also favor a diagnosis of gestational pemphigoid, so we must collect more information.

BASIC SCIENCE PEARL   **STEP 1**

Collagen XVII, also known as bullous pemphigoid antigen 2 (BPAG2), is found in the basement membrane zone of the skin and is essential for keeping the epidermis and dermis joined together. Once the antibodies are produced, there is lack of adhesion between the epidermis and dermis, and subepidermal bullae result.

CLINICAL PEARL   **STEPS 2/3**

Gestational pemphigoid has a high affinity for periumbilical skin, so this location should really clue you in to the diagnosis.

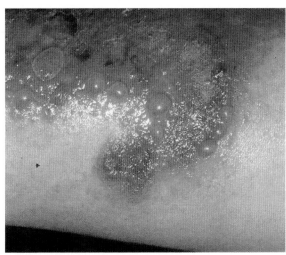

Fig. 3.5 Gestational pemphigoid. Multiple tense blisters and erosions on an erythematous base are present. *(From Korman N. Macular, papular, vesiculobullous, and pustular diseases. 2016;2671–82. https://www.clinicalkey. com/#!/content/book/3-s2.0-B9781455750177004396?scrollTo=%233-s2.0-B9781455750177004396- f439-007-9781455750177)*

Gestational pemphigoid is also known as herpes gestationis, but does this mean there is a viral etiology to this condition?

In 1872, this disease was originally named "herpes gestationis" because the clinical lesions had a "herpetiform" or "herpes-like" appearance due to the appearance of grouped blisters with a background of erythema. However, there is no association with any of the subtypes of herpes viruses; consequently, the disease was renamed "gestational pemphigoid."

On physical exam, the patient has a temperature of 37.3°C (99.2°F), a heart rate of 75/min, and a blood pressure of 118/76 mm Hg. She has extensive, large tense bullae on her abdomen, umbilicus, buttocks, lower back, arms, and legs (Fig. 3.5). Her face, web spaces, palms, soles, and mucous membranes are uninvolved. There are multiple excoriations on her abdomen, arms, and upper thighs suggesting recent scratching of the lesions. There are no honey-colored crusts present on any of her skin lesions.

Based on the exam, can we narrow this patient's differential diagnosis? What are the next steps in this patient's work-up?

The overall lesion distribution and lack of burrows and web space lesions lessens the chance of scabies infestation. Bedbugs and PUPPP could still be considerations, but the distribution along the abdomen and umbilicus is very suggestive of gestational pemphigoid. Routine blood work should be ordered including a complete blood count with differential and complete metabolic panel. Peripheral eosinophilia may be detected.

Referrals to a dermatologist and high-risk maternal–fetal physician should be placed. A dermatologist will perform a history and physical examination of the patient along with at least two punch biopsies of the skin.

CLINICAL PEARL   **STEPS 2/3**

The exact locations for the punch biopsies are critical for the diagnosis. A hematoxylin and eosin stain is taken at the edge of the blister so that the skin just adjacent to the blister can be examined.

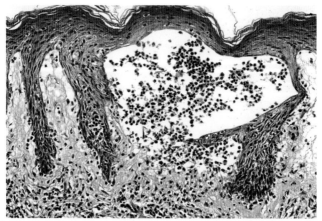

Fig. 3.6   Pemphigoid gestationis. Small subepidermal eosinophil-rich blister. *(From Brinster N, Liu V. Pemphigoid (herpes) gestationis. Dermatopathology: high-yield pathology. 2011;75–6. https://www.clinicalkey.com/#!/content-/book/3-s2.0-B9781416099765100434?scrollTo=%233-s2.0-B9781416099765100434-f43-07-9781416099765)*

This shows epidermal edema and dermal inflammation perilesionally along with the beginning edge of the subepidermal bullae and its roof and eosinophils contained inside. If this biopsy is done through the bullae, then the bullae roof is lost, eosinophil inside the bullae are lost, and perilesional skin is unaffected. Another punch biopsy will be done just adjacent to a blister on "perilesional skin" for direct immunofluorescence (DIF) stain. Tissue for DIF must be submitted in special medium called Michel's transport medium in order to preserve the presence of autoantibodies.

What treatment options can begin before the patient sees the dermatologist?

Severe and widespread arthropod assault, PUPPP, and gestational pemphigoid can all result in significant pruritus. Consider beginning a systemic, nonsedating antihistamine in the morning, such as oral cetirizine 10 mg, along with a sedating antihistamine at night to help improve the patient's sleep quality, such as diphenhydramine 25–50 mg every 4–6 hours as needed. A low- to mid-potency topical glucocorticosteroid (desonide, hydrocortisone butyrate, or fluocinolone) can be beneficial for all of these conditions to reduce pruritus and inflammation, along with gentle skin care consisting of fragrance-free cleansers and lotions. If the patient is unable to see the dermatologist in the next 24 hours, consider beginning prednisone at 0.5 to 1 mg/kg per day.

These patients have severe itching, and control of their pruritus is essential in their care. Prevention of secondary *impetiginization*, staphylococcal infection of their bullae, is also critical and can be achieved with gentle skin care and bleach baths if needed. The patient should also be advised to avoid calamine-based lotions, aloe, and diphenhydramine lotions because these can all result in ACD in a patient with an already damaged skin barrier.

BASIC SCIENCE PEARL   **STEP 1**

Prednisone produces antiinflammatory actions via inhibition of multiple inflammatory cytokines and nuclear factor–κB (NF-κB), reduction of circulating eosinophils, and reduction of neutrophils in the inflammatory site.

The pathology results are complete and show eosinophilic spongiosis, papillary dermal edema, subepidermal blister with eosinophils, and perivascular infiltrate of lymphocytes and eosinophil (Fig. 3.6). Direct immunofluorescence reveals a pattern of linear staining along the basement

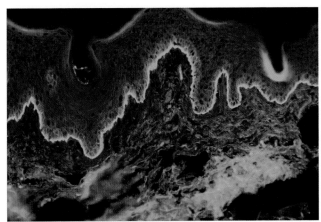

Fig. 3.7 Pemphigoid gestationis. There is striking linear C3 deposition along the dermal–epidermal junction. *(From Brinster N, Liu V. Pemphigoid (herpes) gestationis. Dermatopathology: high-yield pathology. 2011;75–6. https://www.clinicalkey.com/#!/content/book/3-s2.0-B9781416099765100434?scrollTo=%233-s2.0-B9781416099765100434-f43-07-9781416099765)*

membrane zone of IgG and C3 (Fig. 3.7). The dermatopathologist confirms that the findings are consistent with gestational pemphigoid. Of note, the patient has a slight eosinophilia detected on complete blood count. Her liver function tests and remaining laboratory tests are normal. What are the next steps for her treatment?

The patient will need to be jointly followed by the dermatologist and high-risk maternal–fetal physician. The patient should remain on systemic antihistamines for symptomatic control, gentle skin care, and systemic and topical glucocorticosteroids. The prednisone dose can be increased if needed to 1–2 mg/kg per day until the lesions begin to subside and then slowly tapered postpartum. Flares are common peripartum and immediately postpartum and therefore the prednisone dosage may have to be increased at these time points. If the patient fails to respond to prednisone, then intravenous immunoglobulin (IVIG), azathioprine, and/or cyclosporine can be added to the prednisone. Again, therapy will need to be continued and slowly tapered in the postpartum period. Abrupt discontinuation or a quick taper off glucocorticosteroids may result in a significant flare of the disease. Immunosuppressants need to be tapered slowly over a period of months. Topical glucocorticosteroids applied to the lesional skin can be very beneficial while tapering off systemic immunosuppressants.

The patient is very concerned for the safety and health of her child. What are the risks to the fetus?
Prematurity and intrauterine growth restriction may occur, and the risk is increased when the disease presents in the second trimester or is widespread. Due to the mother's need for prolonged glucocorticosteroid use in pregnancy, the newborn will need to be evaluated for the presence of adrenal insufficiency.

About 3%–5% of newborns can be born with infantile gestational pemphigoid while another 5%–10% may have erythematous papules and macules at birth. The pathogenesis of neonatal gestational pemphigoid is due to placental transfer of antibodies. These lesions resolve without scarring within weeks of delivery, and treatment beyond gentle skin care is rarely warranted.

The patient is concerned regarding the postpartum duration of the rash; will she have permanent scarring?
On average the bullae will resolve within 1 month and the urticarial lesions within 4 months. Occasionally, it can take up to a year for some patients to fully resolve. Most patients heal without

scarring; however, the patient should be discouraged from picking or manipulating the lesions as these actions can result in scarring. If the patient reports she is picking and scratching at night, then suggest that she wear gloves during sleep.

The patient undergoes a spontaneous vaginal delivery of a healthy 2500 g baby at 37 weeks' gestation with Apgar scores of 9 and 9. The newborn, although small, is otherwise healthy with normal skin. The mother's disease flared, as expected, in the peripartum period. The patient is now back in your outpatient obstetrics clinic and is 4 weeks postpartum. She is doing well, and her bullae have resolved. She still has mild urticarial lesions, and her physicians have begun to taper her prednisone, which will continue slowly over a 4-week interval. She is actively breastfeeding, and her infant is otherwise healthy and growing well.

She is curious if this condition will recur in future pregnancies; what advice can you give her?
Recurrences in subsequent pregnancies range from 50% to 90%. Often the recurrences begin earlier in pregnancy and the disease is more severe.

BEYOND THE PEARLS

- Gestational pemphigoid, also known as pemphigoid gestationis, is a rare autoimmune blistering skin reaction with an incidence of 1:200,000 to 1:500,000 pregnancies.
- Prednisone is the first-line therapy and is begun at 0.5–1 mg/kg per day. Flares are common in the peripartum and postpartum periods, and the dosage may have to be increased to 1–2 mg/kg per day.
- Up to 25% of patients can have recurrences with menstruation or oral contraceptive pills (OCPs). Patients with a history of gestational pemphigoid are also at long-term risk for other autoimmune diseases, the most common being Graves' disease.
- For patients interested in birth control measures and/or experiencing recurrences with menstruation, an intrauterine device intrauterine device (IUD) may be an appropriate option to limit menstruation and avoid the need for oral contraceptives.

Case Summary

- A 31-year-old primigravida Caucasian woman presents at 30 weeks' gestation with pruritic, periumbilical bullae extending to her abdomen and trunk.
- History, exam, and dermatopathology reveal the patient has gestational pemphigoid, and she is begun on antihistamines, gentle skin care, and oral and topical glucocorticosteroids.
- The patient's condition flares peripartum, requiring an increase in prednisone, and she undergoes spontaneous vaginal delivery at 37 weeks' gestation. Her child is born small for gestational age but shows no active clinical evidence of neonatal gestational pemphigoid.
- As her disease begins to improve 4 weeks postpartum, her prednisone therapy is slowly tapered over a period of at least 4–6 weeks in order to avoid a flare of her condition. Her infant is doing well.
- The patient is advised that the risk of recurrence is high in subsequent pregnancies, often with more severe disease. The patient is also counseled that flares are possible with menstruation and the use of oral contraceptive pills.

References

Al-Saif, F., Elisa, A., Al-Homidy, A., et al. (2016). Retrospective analysis of pemphigoid gestationis in 32 Saudi patients – cliniciopathological features and a literature review. *Journal of Reproductive Immunology, 116*, 42–45.
Danesh, M., Pomeranz, M. K., McMeniman, E., et al. (2016). Dermatoses of pregnancy: nomenclature, misnomers, and myths. *Clinics in Dermatology, 34*, 314–319.
Lehrhoff, S., & Pomeranz, M. K. (2013). Specific dermatoses of pregnancy and their treatment. *Dermatologic Therapy, 26*, 274–284.

Lipozencic, J., Ljubojevic, S., Bukvic-Mokos, Z. (2102). Pemphigoid gestationis. *Clinics in Dermatology*, *30*, 51–55.

Mehta, N., Chen, K. K., & Kroumpouzos, G. (2016). Skin disease in pregnancy: the approach of the obstetric medicine physician. *Clinics in Dermatology*, *34*, 320–326.

Rapini, R. (2005). *Practical dermatopathology*. Philadelphia, USA: Elsevier Mosby, 92–93.

Sadik, C. D., Lima, A. L., & Zillikens, D. (2016). Pemphigoid gestationis: toward a better understanding of etiopathogenesis. *Clinics in Dermatology*, *34*, 378–382.

Holly E. Dunn, MD

CASE 4

A 38-Year-Old Woman with GDM

A 38-year-old G4P3 woman presents to your office for entry to prenatal care at 27 weeks. Her physical exam is significant for obesity, and fetal well-being is reassuring by handheld Doppler. You recommend testing for gestational diabetes mellitus (GDM).

What is GDM?

GDM refers to any degree of glucose intolerance first noted with the onset of pregnancy or first recognized in pregnancy. This condition complicates approximately 5% of all pregnancies and includes some women who have undiagnosed pregestational diabetes. The hormonal changes that accompany pregnancy may expose a genetic predisposition to diabetes mellitus. Of patients diagnosed with GDM, an estimated 50% will become diabetic within 15 years. The progression to type 2 diabetes may be influenced by ethnicity and the presence of obesity. High-risk ethnic groups include Hispanic, African American, Native American, Asian, and Pacific Islander women. Women with GDM are at higher risk of development of gestational hypertension, preeclampsia, and the need for a cesarean delivery. Fetal complications associated with GDM include macrosomia, shoulder dystocia, neonatal hypoglycemia and hyperbilirubinemia, and an increased risk of stillbirth if the maternal fasting glucose is persistently higher than 105 mg/dL.

What are some relevant questions in your history that might suggest GDM?

The patient should be asked about signs or symptoms of hyperglycemia, which can include polyuria, polydipsia, excessive hunger or thirst, fatigue, headaches, blurry vision, trouble concentrating, dry mouth, dry or itchy skin, and recurrent infections such as otitis externa or vaginal yeast infections. She should also be asked about symptoms suggestive of hypoglycemic episodes, such as feeling diaphoretic, shaky or presence of tremors accompanied by dizziness, tinnitus, nausea, tunnel vision or scotoma, or presyncope or syncope.

CLINICAL PEARL   STEPS 2/3

Investigating into her obstetrical history may reveal a history of GDM with past pregnancies, prior large for gestational age (LGA) infants and/or polyhydramnios, history of shoulder dystocia with delivery, or infants requiring extended hospitalization after birth due to hypoglycemia or hyperbilirubinemia warranting phototherapy. She may also have a strong family history of diabetes.

The patient tells you she has had three vulvovaginal yeast infections this pregnancy, which she treated with over-the-counter miconazole. She notes increasing urinary frequency since early second trimester with associated increased thirst and appetite. She denies any urinary tract infections or vaginal bleeding or spotting. She reports that she was told she had glucose in her urine when she was seen in an urgent care clinic 2 weeks ago for a yeast infection. Her obstetrical history is significant for a 3.9 kg (8 lb 10 oz) infant at 38 weeks, a 4.2 kg (9 lb 8 oz) infant at 38 weeks, and 4.4 kg (9 lb 12 oz) infant at 39 weeks. Her mother and two maternal aunts have diabetes. On presentation to clinic, she has 3+ glycosuria on urine dipstick.

What risk factors does this patient have for GDM?

The patient presents with several risk factors for GDM. She is over 30 years of age, from an ethnic group at increased risk for type 2 diabetes mellitus, she is obese, and has a first-degree relative with type 2 diabetes. In addition, she has an obstetrical history significant for LGA neonates. She is currently spilling large amounts of glucose in her urine.

Who should be screened for GDM?

All pregnant patients should be screened for GDM. Patients with GDM are typically asymptomatic. There is a small cohort of pregnant women in whom routine screening for GDM is not cost-effective. These are women under age 25 who have normal body mass index (BMI <25 kg/m²), no first-degree relatives with diabetes, no risk factors (such as a history of GDM, insulin resistance or polycystic ovarian syndrome [PCOS], a prior macrosomic infant, a prior unexplained late fetal demise, and women with persistent glycosuria), and who are not members of ethnic or racial groups with a high prevalence of diabetes (such as Hispanic, Native American, Asian, or African American). As such patients are rare, most experts and organizations recommend screening for GDM in all pregnant women. The ideal time to screen for GDM is at 24–28 weeks of gestation. For women at high risk of developing GDM (just listed), early screening for GDM is recommended at the first prenatal visit. If the early screen is negative, it should be repeated at 24–28 weeks Table 4.1.

How is GDM diagnosed?

The most common screening test for GDM is the glucose challenge test (GCT), which is a nonfasting 50 g oral glucose challenge followed by a venous plasma glucose measurement at 1 hour. Most authorities consider the GCT to be positive if the 1-hour glucose measurement is greater

---

TABLE 4.1 ▪ **Screening Strategy for Detecting Gestational Diabetes Mellitus (GDM)**

GDM risk assessment should be ascertained at the first prenatal visit.

Low risk: Blood glucose testing not routinely required if all of the following characteristics are present:

- Member of an ethnic group with a low prevalence of GDM
- No known diabetes in first-degree relatives
- Age younger than 25 years
- Weight normal before pregnancy
- No history of abnormal glucose metabolism
- No history of poor obstetric outcome

Average risk: Perform blood glucose testing at 24–28 weeks using either:

- *Two-step procedure*: 50 g glucose tolerance test followed by a diagnostic oral glucose tolerance test in those meeting the threshold value in the glucose tolerance test
- *One-step procedure*: Diagnostic oral glucose tolerance test performed on all participants

High risk: Perform blood glucose testing as soon as feasible using the procedures described previously if one or more of these are present:

- Obesity (BMI ≥30)
- Strong family history of type 2 diabetes
- History of GDM, impaired glucose metabolism, or glycosuria
- *If GDM is not diagnosed, blood glucose testing should be repeated at 24–28 weeks or at any time a patient has symptoms or signs that are suggestive of hyperglycemia*

than 140 mg/dL. Use of a lower cutoff (such as >135 mg/dL) will increase the detection rate of women with GDM and thus increase the sensitivity of the test. However, a lower cutoff will also result in a substantial increase in the false-positive rate.

There is no GCT cutoff that is considered diagnostic of GDM. A definitive diagnosis of GDM necessitates a 3-hour glucose tolerance test (GTT). In pregnancy, the GTT involves a 100 g oral glucose challenge after an overnight fast. Venous plasma glucose is measured fasting and at the 1-hour, 2-hour, and 3-hour time marks. Although there is agreement that two or more abnormal values are required to confirm the diagnosis, there is disagreement about the glucose values that define the upper range of normal in pregnancy (see later discussion). Most institutions use the National Diabetes Data Group (NDDG) or Carpenter and Coustan cutoffs Table 4.2. The International Association of Diabetes and Pregnancy Study Groups proposed a single-step assessment for GDM using a 75 g glucose load. Measurement of glycated hemoglobin (HbA1c) levels is not useful in making the diagnosis of GDM, although it may be useful in the diagnosis of pregestational diabetes. Gestational and pregestational diabetes may be further classified utilizing the White classification Table 4.3.

In this patient, the findings of significant glycosuria should prompt the performance of a glucose determination before the patient leaves the clinic.

TABLE 4.2 ■ Commonly Used Criteria for Diagnosis of Gestational Diabetes Mellitus (GDM) in the United States

	NDDG		Carpenter and Coustan		Sacks et al.	
Oral GTT	mg/dL	mmol/L	mg/dL	mmol/L	mg/dL	mmol/L
Fasting	105	5.8	95	5.3	96	5.3
1-hour	190	10.6	180	10	172	9.4
2-hour	165	9.2	155	8.6	152	8.3
3-hour	145	8	140	7.8	131	7.2

GDM is diagnosed if patient has ≥2 abnormal values.
NDDG, National Diabetes Data Group.

TABLE 4.3 ■ White Classification of Diabetes

Gestational Diabetes Mellitus

A1: Diet-controlled; fasting glucose <105 mg/dL; 2 hour postprandial <120 mg/dL
A2: Requires insulin or oral medications to keep the glucose within normal limits

Pregestational Diabetes Mellitus

Class	Onset (age)	Duration (yrs)	Vascular disease
B	≥20 yrs age	<10 yrs	None
C	10–19 yrs age	10–19 yrs	None
D	<10 yrs age	≥20 yrs	Benign retinopathy
F	Any	Any	Nephropathy
H	Any	Any	Heart disease
R	Any	Any	Proliferative retinopathy
T	Any	Any	Renal transplant

TABLE 4.4 ■ International Association of Diabetes and Pregnancy Study Groups Diagnostic

| 2-hour 75 g oral GTT | Criteria for GDM and Overt DM in Pregnancy | | | |
| | Criteria for GDM | | Criteria for Overt DM | |
	mg/dL	mmol/L	mg/dL	mmol/L
Fasting	≥92 but <126	5.1	≥126	7
1-hour	≥180	10	–	–
2–hour	≥153	8.5	–	–
Hemoglobin A1C	–	–	≥6.5	
Random plasma glucose	–	–	≥200	11.1

In addition to evaluating the urine dipstick for glycosuria, what other information should be gathered from this patient on exam or initial evaluation?

This patient should have a 50 g GCT as this test can be done in the nonfasting state. If she declines the test that day due to time constraints, a random capillary glucose can be obtained; a value of greater than 200 is suggestive of pregestational diabetes Table 4.4. A full physical examination should be performed, including a pelvic exam. Her external genitalia should be inspected for edema, erythema, and satellite lesions (discrete pustulopapular lesions surrounding areas of clearly demarcated erythema), and possible excoriations and fissures. A thick, adherent, and cottage cheese–like vaginal discharge may be seen on speculum exam (Fig. 4.1). A wet mount may reveal the presence of yeast Fig. 4.2 (budding hyphae on wet mount, thick white curd-like vaginal discharge on speculum exam).

BASIC SCIENCE PEARL	STEP 1

Acanthosis nigricans (dark patches of skin within the groin, axillae, or nape of the neck with a thick velvety texture) often accompanies hyperinsulinemia and may also be significant for central obesity.

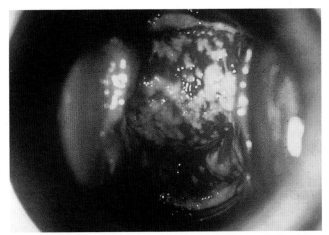

Fig. 4.1 Vaginal candidiasis has a curd-like appearance. *(From Epstein O, Perkin G. Female breasts and genitalia. Clin Exam. 2008;226–51. https://www.clinicalkey.com/#!/content/book/3-s2.0-B9780723434542500143?scrollTo=%233-s2.0-B9780723434542500143-f08-36-9780723434542)*

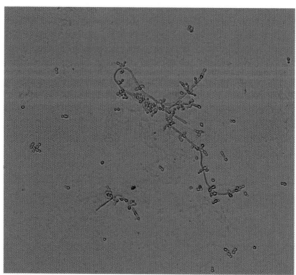

Fig. 4.2 A wet mount of *Candida albicans* shows branching hyphae and budding yeast. *(From Edwards L. Vaginitis. Obstetric and gynecologic dermatology. 2008;301–16. https://www.clinicalkey.com/#!/content/book/3-s2.0-B9780723434450100244?scrollTo=%233-s2.0-B9780723434450100244-gr3)*

On physical exam, the patient has a temperature of 36.7°C (98.2°F), a heart rate of 74/min, and a blood pressure of 127/70 mm Hg. Her abdomen is soft, with marked central obesity, and a fundal height of 30 cm. On pelvic exam, the patient has normal external female genitalia, with no lesions or discharge. Her cervix is long and closed. Her 1-hour GCT is 156. Her 3-hour oral GTT values are 130, 200, 154, 142. She is diagnosed with GDM.

Three of the four values of her 3-hour GTT are elevated and her fasting glucose level is 130 mg/dL. How should her GDM be managed?
The goal of antepartum treatment of GDM is to prevent fetal macrosomia and its resultant complications by maintaining maternal blood glucose at optimal levels throughout pregnancy, defined as a fasting glucose level of less than 95 mg/dL and a 1-hour postprandial level of less than 140 mg/dL or a 2-hour postprandial level of less than 120 mg/dL.

CLINICAL PEARL   **STEPS 2/3**

Initial recommendations should include a diabetic diet (36 kcal/kg or 15 kcal/lb of ideal body weight plus 100 kcal per trimester given as 40%–50% carbohydrate, 20% protein, and 30%–40% fat to avoid protein catabolism), moderate exercise, daily home glucose monitoring, and weekly antepartum visits to monitor glycemic control.

If diet alone does not maintain blood glucose at optimal levels, hypoglycemic therapy may be required. If initial fasting glucose levels are greater than 95 mg/dL, treatment can be started immediately.

Insulin given by injection remains the gold standard for the medical management of GDM as it does not cross the placenta. Regular and NPH insulin are most routinely used, but long-acting agents such as ultralente (Humulin), insulin glargine (Lantus), and insulin detemir (Levemir) are also likely to be safe in pregnancy Table 4.5.

CLINICAL PEARL   **STEPS 2/3**

The use of oral hypoglycemic agents has traditionally been avoided in pregnancy Table 4.6 because of concerns over fetal teratogenesis and prolonged neonatal hypoglycemia. However, recent studies suggest that second-generation hypoglycemic agents (glyburide, glipizide) do not cross the placenta in substantial amounts, are safe in pregnancy, and can achieve adequate glycemic control in 85% of pregnancies complicated by GDM.

TABLE 4.5 ■ Insulin Split-Dose Regimen

- Total daily dosing based on gestational weeks
  - <18 weeks: 0.7 units/kg
  - 18–26 weeks: 0.8 units/kg
  - 26–36 weeks: 0.9 units/kg
  - >36 weeks: 1.0 units/kg
- Administration
  - AM dose (2/3 of total daily dose): 2/3 NPH and 1/3 regular insulin before breakfast
  - PM dose (1/3 of total daily dose): 1/2 regular insulin before dinner; 1/2 NPH before bed time

---

TABLE 4.6 ■ Glyburide and Metformin Comparisons

- Glyburide
  - Class: Second-generation sulfonylurea
  - Mechanism of action: Stimulates insulin release from pancreatic β cells; can cause hypoglycemia
  - Crosses placenta; fetal glyburide level is 70% of maternal level
  - Regimen: Start with 2.5 mg in AM; increase AM dose by 2.5 mg every 3–7 days as needed; add 5 mg in PM; increase AM or PM dose by 5 mg as needed; max dose 20 mg daily
  - Predictors of failure:
    - GDM diagnosis <25 wks gestational age
    - Maternal age ≥34 yrs
    - Multiparity
    - Fasting glucose >112
- Metformin
  - Class: Biguanide
  - Mechanism of action: Enhances glucose uptake in liver and muscle, decreases gluconeogenesis; does not cause hypoglycemia or weight gain; can cause nausea, abdominal discomfort, or diarrhea
  - Crosses placenta
  - Regimen: 500 mg daily or b.i.d. and increase weekly to maximum dose 2500 mg daily
  - Failure rate higher than glyburide (35% vs. 16%)

What are the risks of untreated GDM?

GDM poses very little maternal risk. Such women are not at risk of diabetic ketoacidosis (DKA), which primarily occurs in those who are insulin deficient. However, GDM has been associated with an increase in infant birth trauma and perinatal morbidity and mortality. The risk to the neonate is directly related to its size. Fetal macrosomia is defined as an estimated fetal weight (not birthweight) of 4500 g or more in diabetic mothers. It is a single cutoff that is unrelated to gestational age, the sex of the baby, or to the actual birthweight.

Is antenatal testing indicated with GDM?

Yes, depending on her glucose control. As in patients with pregestational diabetes women with poorly controlled GDM could also be at risk of fetal demise. Such antenatal testing could include twice-weekly nonstress tests (NSTs), weekly biophysical profile (BPP) testing, and serial ultra-sounds for fetal growth assessment. Patients should also be encouraged to perform daily fetal kick counts. There is no clear consensus regarding antenatal testing in women with diet-controlled GDM.

How should labor and delivery be managed in patients with GDM?
To minimize the risk of intrapartum insults and neonatal hypoglycemia, maternal glucose levels should be maintained at 100–120 mg/dL during labor. This can be achieved with either a sliding scale insulin regimen with short-acting insulin or a continuous insulin drip. Continuous fetal monitoring is recommended throughout labor, with careful attention paid to labor progression. Neonatal blood glucose levels should be measured within 1 hour of birth and early feeding encouraged.

How should the patient be managed postpartum?
The source of the counterregulatory hyperglycemia hormones that cause GDM is effectively removed after delivery. Therefore, no further management is required in the immediate postpartum period. A 2-hour GCT should be performed at 6–8 weeks postpartum in all women with GDM to definitively rule out pregestational diabetes.

The patient was initiated on the following split-dose insulin empirically: 20 units NPH and 10 units regular insulin in the morning, 12 units regular insulin before dinner, and 12 units NPH at bedtime. This was adjusted slightly after reviewing her glucose log sheets in clinic each week. She did well on this regimen and maintained adequate control until 32 weeks' gestation, when her total insulin dose was increased by 20%.

At 28 weeks, the patient was instructed to perform twice-daily fetal movement counts for fetal well-being assessment. At 32 weeks, twice-weekly NSTs were initiated for antenatal surveillance. Serial ultrasounds at 24, 28, 32, and 36 weeks revealed appropriate interval growth. At 39 weeks, the patient experienced spontaneous labor and underwent a vaginal delivery of a 3.7 kg (8 lb, 4 oz) girl. The infant did not demonstrate hypoglycemia or respiratory morbidities at birth.

Postpartum, skin-to-skin contact was performed and breastfeeding was initiated within the first hour of life. She and the infant were discharged on postpartum day 1. Six weeks after delivery, she returned to the clinic for postpartum evaluation, Paragard intrauterine device (IUD) placement, and glucose tolerance evaluation. Her fasting glucose level was 100, and, after a 2-hour 75 g oral GCT, her 1-hour and 2-hour glucose levels were 156 and 121, respectively. Given these findings, she did not meet the diagnostic criteria for overt diabetes mellitus.

BEYOND THE PEARLS

- When patients present before 20 weeks' gestation with significant risk factors for GDM, early screening should be undertaken.
- The finding of glycosuria should prompt a random capillary glucose performed immediately and a follow-up fasting venous plasma glucose or nonfasting 1-hour GCT.
- Given an elevated fasting venous plasma glucose, such patients should be started immediately on either oral antihyperglycemic medications or insulin therapy and followed with self-monitoring of blood glucose using the criteria recommended by the Fifth International Workshop-Conference on Gestational Diabetes Mellitus.
- Patients warranting treatment with insulin are at increased risk for fetal demise, and, for that reason, antepartum fetal testing with NSTs should be performed.
- For such patients who do not enter spontaneous labor, induction of labor at 39 weeks is appropriate.

Case Summary

- A 38-year-old multiparous Hispanic woman presents for a new OB visit and has a past history of LGA infants. She is also of advanced maternal age and has glycosuria.
- History and physical reveals that the patient has glucose intolerance and obesity. She rules in for GDM based on diagnostic testing.
- The patient undergoes nutrition counseling and initiation of a split-dose insulin regimen. Antenatal testing is performed starting at 32 weeks of gestation.
- After her delivery, she warrants further glycemic testing with a 2-hour 75 g oral GTT.

Resources

The following resources are for informational purposes only. Referral to these sources and web sites does not imply the endorsement of these authors. These resources are not meant to be comprehensive. The exclusion of a source or web site does not reflect the quality of that source or web site. Please note that web sites are subject to change without notice.

National Heart, Lung, and Blood Institute. Calculate your body mass index. Available at: http://www.nhlbi support.com/bmi. Retrieved July 20, 2016.

Perinatology.com. Gestational diabetes: calculation of caloric requirements and initial insulin dose. Available at: http://www.perinatology.com/calculators/GDM.htm. Retrieved July 20, 2016.

References

Carpenter, M. W., & Coustan, D. R. (1982). Criteria for screening tests for gestational diabetes. *American Journal of Obstetrics and Gynecology, 144*, 768–773.

Gabbe, S. G., Mestman, J. H., Freeman, R. K., et al. (1977). Management and outcome of class A diabetes mellitus. *American Journal of Obstetrics and Gynecology, 127*, 465–469.

Gestational diabetes mellitus. (2013). Practice bulletin no. 137. American College of Obstetricians and Gynecologists. *Obstetrics and Gynecology, 122*, 406–416.

Landon, M. B., & Gabbe, S. G. (2011). Gestational diabetes mellitus. *Obstetrics and Gynecology, 118*, 1379–1393.

Metzger, B. E., & Coustan, D. R. (1998). Summary and recommendations of the Fourth International Workshop- Conference on Gestational Diabetes Mellitus. The Organizing Committee. *Diabetes Care, 21*(Suppl. 2), B161–B167.

U.S. Preventive Services Task Force. (2008). Screening for gestational diabetes mellitus: U.S. Preventive Services Task Force recommendation statement. *Annals of Internal Medicine, 148*, 759–765.

Joey England, MD ■ Robin Hardwicke, PhD, FNP-C

CASE 5

A 27-Year-Old Woman With Human Immunodeficiency Virus in Pregnancy

A 27-year-old G1P0 woman with human immunodeficiency virus (HIV) in pregnancy at 8 weeks of gestation presents for initial prenatal care.

Describe the pertinent history and physical examination for the patient with HIV.

A thorough history and physical exam includes history of opportunistic infections; extensive sexual history; sexually transmitted infections (STIs); medication use, both present and past, particularly antiretrovirals: immunization history: and substance abuse history. Sexual history should include age at first intercourse, number of lifetime partners, number of partners in the past year, most recent sexual encounter, and number of partners since the last known negative HIV test. It is important to elicit sexual orientation and practices, including if the patient has ever had sex with a woman, ever had anal intercourse, if she has ever been sexually abused, and if the current sex partner and/or father of the baby is aware of both her and the partner's HIV status.

Physical exam includes compete physical with focus on signs of STI, evidence of wasting, presence of thrush, and liver disease (hepatomegaly, splenomegaly, or spider angiomata).

Her medical history is obtained, which is significant for diagnosis of HIV type 1 (HIV-1) 2 years ago after undergoing testing for STIs. She is currently taking tenofovir/emtricitabine and atazanavir-ritonavir. She conceived without assisted reproductive technology. She denies current complaints with exception to mild nausea and breast tenderness today, which she attributes to her pregnancy. She has normal vital signs and a normal physical exam. The oropharynx is clear of thrush/sores and there is no lymphadenopathy on exam. Her heart is regular in rate and rhythm, and bilateral lungs are clear to auscultation without crackles or wheezes. She has a normal breast and pelvic exam. No hepatosplenomegaly is noted on abdominal exam. Her skin appears normal without lesions, dermatitis, or rash.

HIV is a single-stranded, positive-sense ribonucleic acid (RNA) virus that can cause acquired immunodeficiency syndrome (AIDS). It contains three structural genes (gag, pol, env) and six regulatory genes. There are two types, HIV-1 and HIV-2, of which HIV-1 is the more widely distributed and more pathogenic. HIV infects clusters of differentiation 4 (CD4+ T) cells and uses its reverse transcriptase to transcribe its RNA genome into double-stranded deoxyribonucleic acid (DNA), which is integrated into the host cell genome (Fig. 5.1).

HIV can be transmitted through intercourse, blood transfusions, intravenous (IV) drug needle sharing, or vertically from a mother to her fetus. In 1994, AIDS Clinical Trial 076 evaluated zidovudine prophylaxis for the prevention of perinatal transmission. Women in the intervention group had a significantly lower risk of transmitting HIV to their newborn (25% vs. 8%). Further declines in mother-to-child HIV transmission (MTCT) were additionally attributed to earlier initiation of antiretroviral therapy (ART). MTCT rates were lower among women with a viral load of less than 50 copies/mL near delivery (0.09%) compared to women who had higher viral loads between 50 and 399 copies/mL (1%).

What laboratory evaluation provides the diagnosis for HIV?
HIV screening is first performed by HIV-1/2 Ag/ Ab combination immunoassay or fourth-generation HIV test.

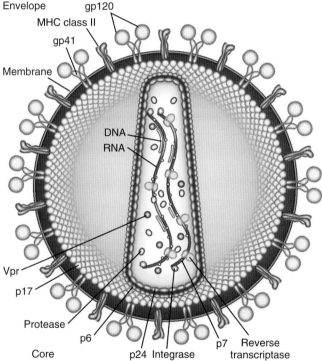

Fig. 5.1   Structure of the human immunodeficiency virus type 1 (HIV-1) virion. The viral envelope is formed from the host cell membrane, into which the HIV-1 envelope proteins gp41 and gp120 have been inserted and may include several host cell proteins, most significantly the major histocompatibility complex (MHC) class II proteins. The matrix between the envelope and the core is formed predominantly from Gag protein p17. The core contains the viral RNA, closely associated with Gag protein p7, in addition to reverse transcriptase (RT) and integrase. It has also been shown that virions contain complementary DNA, as shown, synthesized by the RT. The major structural proteins of the core are Gag proteins p24 and p6. Also present within the virion are the protease and two cleavage products from the Gag precursor protein (p1 and p2, not shown) of undetermined position within the virion. Viral protein R (Vpr) is also packaged in the virion and is thought to be localized within the core, as shown. *(From Reitz M, Gallo R. Human immunodeficiency viruses. In* Mandell, Douglas, and Bennett's Principles and Practice of Infectious Diseases, *updated edition. 2015:2054-65. e3.* https://www.clinicalkey.com/#!/search/HIV/%7B%22facetquery%22:%5B%22+contenttype:IM%22,%22+contenttype:VD%22%5D%7D?page=3)

BASIC SCIENCE PEARL	STEP 1

Enzyme-linked immunosorbent assay (ELISA) detects presence of a protein or antigen (Ag) and is utilized to screen for HIV. Specifically, the HIV Ag is coated on a plate, test serum is added, and if antibodies (Ab) are present they will bind to the Ag. The plate is washed, leaving only bound antibodies. Anti–human gammaglobulin Ab is added with bound color-producing enzyme, and the substrate for the enzyme is added. If HIV antibodies are present in the serum, there will be a color change for detection.

Recently, previous screening for HIV was third-generation testing and included a two-tiered approach: ELISA with confirmatory Western blot. Current recommendations from the Centers for Disease Control and Prevention (CDC) now recommend fourth-generation testing: HIV Ag/Ab combination immunoassay followed by a confirmatory immunoassay. A p24ag is first drawn and, if reactive, followed by a multispot Ab differentiation test as confirmation. The p24 can be reactive without the presence of HIV infectivity because of the presence of contamination by bacteria, infection (malaria, human African trypanosomiasis), or genetic differences. With discrepant results, HIV viral testing is performed. This allows diagnosis when the initial immunoassay is reactive with a second nonreactive immunoassay, but the presence of HIV RNA. It is a more sensitive test to detect acute and early HIV infection within 4–10 days of transmission (Fig. 5.2).

What provides the diagnosis for acquired immune deficiency syndrome (AIDS)?
The CDC considers people with HIV and CD4 counts of less than 200 cells/mm^3 to have AIDS, regardless of the presence of signs or symptoms of disease. Multiple opportunistic infections are

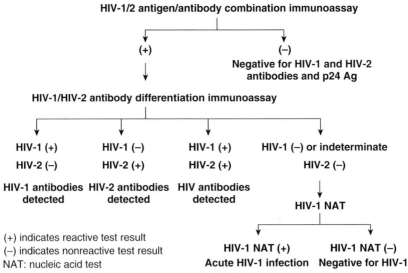

Fig. 5.2 HIV testing algorithm recommended in the United States. The recommended laboratory testing algorithm for HIV begins with a fourth-generation immunoassay, which detects HIV-1/HIV-2 antibodies and p24 antigen. If positive, the test proceeds to a confirmatory HIV-1/HIV-2 antibody differentiation immunoassay. If negative or indeterminate, the test proceeds to an HIV-1 nucleic acid test. Several potential combinations of test results are shown. *(From Smith C, McFarland E. Update on pediatric human immunodeficiency virus infection. Adv Pediatr. 2016;63:141–71. https://www.clinicalkey.com/#!/content/journal/1-s2.0-S006531011630007X?scrollTo=%231-s2.0-S006531011630007X-gr5)*

also AIDS-defining, including invasive cervical cancer, extrapulmonary coccidioidomycosis, cryptococcosis or histoplasmosis, HIV-related encephalopathy, Kaposi sarcoma, and others.

What laboratory, imaging studies, and management should be pursued?
Initial prenatal labs should be ordered for the patient including specific labs to assess her HIV status. Work-up should include routine prenatal labs (type and screen, rubella status, Pap smear, STI panel), a complete metabolic panel (CMP), complete blood count (CBC), CD4 count, HIV viral load (HIV RNA PCR), hepatitis panel, and urine drug screen (UDS).

Risk of HIV transmission increases with increasing viral loads; however, there is no clear threshold above which all women transmit the virus. Transmission usually does not occur with viral loads of less than 1000 copies/mL.

> The patient's lab evaluation reveals normal prenatal lab results; she has a negative UDS, negative hepatitis panel, and undetectable viral load. Her CD4 count is 1100 cells/mm^3. Ultrasound reveals presence of an intrauterine singleton gestation with a crown rump length of 18 mm and presence of cardiac activity. Bilateral adnexa appear normally.

What is the treatment for HIV during pregnancy?
ART is used during pregnancy to decrease perinatal transmission and optimize the health of the mother. The CDC recommends that ART should be initiated as early in pregnancy as possible and that antiretroviral drug-resistance studies should be performed to guide selection of regimens in women with HIV RNA levels above the threshold for resistance testing (>500–1,000 c/mL) unless previously performed. Therapy should not be delayed while awaiting these results. If ART was already initiated prior to such testing, the therapy should be modified based on the results. The preferred regimen for women who have not initiated ART includes a dual nucleoside reverse transcriptase inhibitor combination (abacavir/lamivudine or tenofovir disoproxil fumarate/emtricitabine or lamivudine) plus an integrase inhibitor (raltegravir) or a ritonavir-boosted protease inhibitor (atazanavir/ritonavir or darunavir/ritonavir). Once initiated, the HIV viral load usually becomes undetectable within 2 months.

CLINICAL PEARL   **STEPS 2/3**

The CDC recommends that women can be counseled that ART generally does not increase the risk of birth defects.

For decreasing CD4 counts, what is the appropriate prophylaxis?
Antimicrobial agents can be administered to decrease the risk of developing an opportunistic infection Table 5.1.

TABLE 5.1 ■ **Antimicrobial Prophylaxis**

Trimethoprim-sulfamethoxazole (TMP-SMX) for CD4 ≤200 cells/µL	Prophylaxis for *Pneumocystis jiroveci* pneumonia (PCP) and reactivation toxoplasmosis
Azithromycin for ≤75 cells/µL	Prophylaxis for disseminated infection with *Mycobacterium avium* complex (MAC).

Describe the management of labor, delivery and postpartum care for patients with HIV.

Women should continue ART during this time period. If the viral load is 400 copies/mL or higher or unknown near the time of delivery, then intravenous zidovudine (ZDV) should be administered. Common practice in many facilities, however, is administration of ZDV regardless of viral load due to patient discontinuation of ART prior to delivery and great benefit of ZDV in prevention of MTCT. Zidovudine 2 mg/kg bolus in 1 hour is administered followed by continuous infusion of 1 mg/kg every hour until delivery. If prior to cesarean delivery, ZDV should be administered 3 hours prior to surgery if possible. For a viral load of 1000 copies/mL or greater, cesarean delivery is recommended at 38 weeks' gestation (<1000 copies/mL may consider vaginal delivery).

CLINICAL PEARL   **STEPS 2/3**

For women without prior testing presenting at the time of labor, a rapid HIV test should be performed unless the patient opts out of screening. If positive, antiretroviral prophylaxis should be administered without waiting for confirmatory test results.

The patient undergoes an uncomplicated spontaneous vaginal delivery at term gestation.

How do you counsel the patient postpartum?

The patient should be counseled and encouraged to continue ART after delivery. Optimizing her health during this time and providing a network of support is critical. This includes contraceptive counseling, HIV specialty care, mental health services, and pediatric care for the neonate. In the United States, breastfeeding is not recommended for HIV-infected women due to possible breast milk transmission of HIV and the availability, affordability, and safety of replacement feeding. This recommendation, however, is different in resource-limited settings.

CLINICAL PEARL   **STEPS 2/3**

Neonates born to women with HIV receive combination ART for 6 weeks after birth to prevent HIV transmission. For full-term infants born to a mother who has received a standard combination ART regimen during pregnancy with sustained viral suppression, this may be decreased to a 4-week zidovudine regimen.

BEYOND THE PEARLS

- HIV testing during the first trimester of pregnancy is legally required in the United States; written informed consent for testing is not required in most states. Testing in the third trimester at less than 36 weeks is recommended by the CDC in order to allow medical treatment prior to delivery and decrease vertical transmission.
- Suppression of HIV RNA to undetectable levels should be achieved as rapidly as possible in pregnancy.
- Pregnant women with both HIV-1 and HIV-2 should be treated as per guidelines for HIV-1 with use of HIV-2–sensitive medications.

Case Summary

- A 27-year-old woman with HIV in pregnancy presents for initial prenatal care.
- The patient undergoes a detailed history and physical examination. Her laboratory assessment is significant for confirmation of HIV diagnosis.
- She delivers a healthy neonate at term gestation by spontaneous vaginal delivery.

References

Centers for Disease Control and Prevention (CDC). (2006). Achievements in public health: reduction in perinatal transmission of HIV infection- United States, 1985–2005. *MMWR Morbidity and Mortality Weekly Report*, *55*(21), 592–597.

Centers for Disease Control and Prevention (CDC). (2013). Detection of acute HIV infection in two evaluations of a new HIV diagnostic testing algorithm – United States, 2011–2013. *MMWR Morbidity and Mortality Weekly Report*, *62*(24), 489–494.

Centers for Disease Control and Prevention and Association of Public Health Laboratories. *Laboratory Testing for the Diagnosis of HIV Infection: Updated Recommendations*. http://stacks.cdc.gov/view/cdc/23447.

Connor, E. M., Sperling, R. S., Gelber, R., et al. (1994). Reduction of maternal-infant transmission of human immunodeficiency virus type 1 with zidovudine treatment. Pediatric AIDS Clinical Trials Group Protocol 076 Study Group. *The New England Journal of Medicine*, *331*(18), 1173–1180.

Garcia, P. M., Kalish, L. A., Pitt, J., et al. (1999). Maternal levels of plasma human immunodeficiency virus type 1 RNA and the risk of perinatal transmission. *The New England Journal of Medicine*, *341*(6), 392–402.

Klarkowski, D., O'Brien, D. P., Shanks, L., et al. (2014). Causes of false-positive HIV rapid diagnostic test results. *Expert Review of Anti-Infective Therapy*, *12*(1), 49–62.

Panel on Treatment of HIV-Infected Pregnant Women and Prevention of Perinatal Transmission. Recommendations for use of antiretroviral drugs in pregnant HIV-1–infected women for maternal health and interventions to reduce perinatal HIV transmission in the United States. http://aidsinfo.nih.gov/guidelines/html/3/perinatal-guidelines/0/.

Reitz, M., & Gallo, R. (2015). Human immunodeficiency viruses. In *Mandell, Douglas, and Bennett's Principles and Practice of Infectious Diseases, updated edition* (pp. 2054–2065.e3).

Townsend, C., Byrne, L., Cortina-Boria, M., et al. (2014). Earlier initiation of ART and further decline in mother-to-child HIV transmission rates, 2000–2011. *AIDS*, *28*(7), 1049–1057.

U.S. Department of Health and Human Services (2016). HIV medicines during pregnancy and childbirth. *AIDSinfo: HIV and Pregnancy*. https://aidsinfo.nih.gov/understanding-hiv-aids/fact-sheets/24/70/hiv-medicines-during-pregnancy-and-childbirth.

Joey England, MD

A 30-Year-Old Woman With Gestational Trophoblastic Disease

A 30-year-old G3P2 Asian-American woman at 16 weeks of gestation presents to the obstetric emergency department for headache and vaginal bleeding. Vital signs are taken and include a temperature of 36.6°C (98°F), blood pressure 180/105 mm Hg, a heart rate of 97/min, and oxygen saturation 100% on room air. On presentation, your patient is holding her head with her hands; she complains of nausea and the headache, which began overnight. She has tried Tylenol without relief of her headache. Her headache is not positional. She denies vision complaints. Her past medical history is significant for asthma, and she denies other medical problems. Her obstetric history includes two term spontaneous vaginal deliveries. She has not sought prenatal care at this point because of difficulty obtaining medical insurance.

On physical exam she is normocephalic, her cardiovascular exam is significant for a systolic ejection murmur with a normal pulmonary exam. Her neck palpates normally without lymphadenopathy. Her abdomen is mildly tender to palpation with normal bowel sounds, and her legs are mildly edematous with nonpitting edema. Pelvic exam reveals normal external female genitalia with dark purple blood in the vaginal vault. The uterus palpates approximately 18 weeks in size.

CLINICAL PEARL   **STEPS 2/3**

A systolic ejection murmur along the left sternal border is normal in pregnancy due to increased cardiac output (CO) through the aortic and pulmonary valves. Diastolic murmurs are never normal in pregnancy and must be investigated.

Cardiac output increases up to 50% in pregnancy, with the major increase by 20 weeks of gestational age. CO is the product of heart rate and stroke volume; both of these are increased during pregnancy.

What is the initial differential diagnosis for the patient?

Potential diagnoses to consider include preexisting hypertensive disease with exacerbation, chronic kidney disease, and preeclampsia. Preeclampsia is excluded due to the early gestational age (<20 weeks). Preexisting hypertensive disease and chronic kidney disease are less likely given patient's lack of prior medical problems. Secondary causes of hypertension can include pheochromocytoma, Cushing's syndrome, and hyperthyroidism. Illicit drug use can also cause severe hypertension, specifically cocaine use. Molar pregnancy should be considered given patient's hypertension prior to 20 weeks' gestation.

BASIC SCIENCE PEARL   **STEP 1**

Pheochromocytoma is a nonmalignant tumor of the adrenal medulla, the most common adrenal tumor in adults (vs. neuroblastoma, the most common in children). It is a catecholamine-secreting tumor and is associated with the classic triad of episodic headache, diaphoresis, and tachycardia.

What laboratory, imaging studies, and management should be pursued?

Initial work-up should include a complete metabolic panel (CMP), β-human chorionic gonadotropin (β-hCG), thyroid stimulating hormone (TSH), urine drug screen (UDS), and obstetric ultrasound. Blood type and antibody screen should be included due to presence of vaginal bleeding during pregnancy. Administration of antihypertensive medication and placement of intravenous (IV) access is performed.

> The patient's lab evaluation reveals a normal CMP and TSH, negative UDS, and a β-hCG of 180,000 mIU/mL. Her blood type is A positive with a negative antibody screen. Her repeat vital signs are improved, with exception to still elevated blood pressure of 140/90 mm Hg after administration of labetalol 20 mg slow IV push.
>
> A transvaginal ultrasound reveals absence of a fetus with numerous-well circumscribed hypoechoic lesions throughout the uterus. Bilateral adnexa are normal in appearance.

What is your diagnosis?

The elevated β-hCG and classic ultrasound findings provide the diagnosis of a complete molar pregnancy. The hypoechoic lesions within the uterus have been described as a "snowstorm" appearance. Additional ultrasound findings may demonstrate theca lutein cysts; these are associated with gestational trophoblastic disease and appear as a multiseptated cystic mass or multiple adjacent cysts within the adnexa (Figs. 6.1 and 6.2).

Gestational trophoblastic disease can include hydatidiform mole (complete and partial), invasive mole, and choriocarcinoma or placental site trophoblastic tumor. Hydatidiform mole is an abnormal pregnancy with varying degrees of trophoblastic proliferation and vesicular swelling of placental villi. Complete and partial moles are distinguished by differences in clinical presentation, pathology, genetics, and epidemiology (Table 6.1).

Gestational trophoblastic neoplasia (GTN) describes invasive mole, choriocarcinoma, or placental site trophoblastic tumor, which can progress, metastasize, and lead to maternal mortality if untreated.

CLINICAL PEARL   **STEPS 2/3**

GTN develops in approximately 15%–20% of patients with a complete mole and 1%–5% of patients with a partial mole. Management includes referral to a gynecologic oncologist for methotrexate administration alone; however, 30% of patients require additional, more intensive chemotherapy.

CLINICAL PEARL   **STEPS 2/3**

Choriocarcinoma is a malignant tumor arising from the trophoblast most commonly following noncomplete removal of hydatidiform mole. It can metastasize hematogenously, with the most common site of metastases as the lungs.

The patient is counseled regarding her diagnosis, and the recommendation is provided for surgery for removal of the molar pregnancy by dilation and curettage. In patients who desire permanent sterilization, a hysterectomy with the mole in situ can be considered.

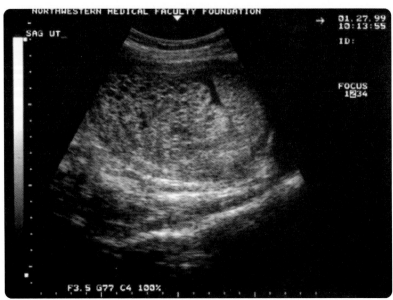

Fig. 6.1 Pelvic ultrasound of a complete hydatidiform mole with characteristic vesicular pattern of multiple echoes, holes within placental mass, and no fetus. *(From Lurain J. Gestational trophoblastic disease I: epidemiology, pathology, clinical presentation and diagnosis of gestational trophoblastic disease, and management of hydatidiform mole. Am J Obstet Gynecol. 2010:531–9. https://www.clinicalkey.com/#!/content/journal/1-s2.0-S0002937810008537?scrollTo=%231-s2.0-S0002937810008537-gr6)*

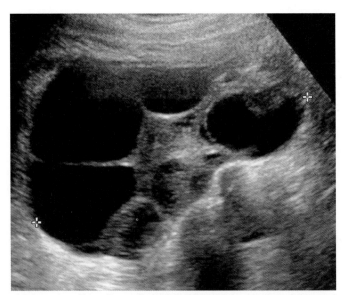

Fig. 6.2 Theca lutein cysts. *(From Brown D, Wall D. Ultrasound evaluation of the ovaries. In: Callen's ultrasonography in obstetrics and gynecology 2017:919–33. https://www.clinicalkey.com/#!/content/book/3-s2.0-B9780323328340000302?scrollTo=%233-s2.0-B9780323328340000302-f030-021-9780323328340)*

TABLE 6.1 ■ **Comparison of Complete Versus Partial Mole**

Complete Hydatidiform Mole	Partial Hydatidiform Mole
Diploid (46, XX -mainly; 46, XY); empty egg fertilized by two sperm	Triploid (69, XXY; 69, XYY; 69, XXX); 46 paternal chromosomes and 23 maternal chromosomes
Absent fetus/embryo	Abnormal fetus/embryo
Diffuse swelling of villi	Focal swelling of villi
Diffuse trophoblastic hyperplasia	Focal trophoblastic hyperplasia
hCG often >100,000 mIU/mL	hCG usually <100,000 mIU/mL
Medical complications	Rare medical complications

After signed, informed consent the patient opts for surgical treatment and undergoes dilation and curettage. The products of conception are sent to pathology. A baseline chest radiograph is obtained that reveals no abnormalities.

A karyotype of 46, XX and histopathology resulted, and these are consistent with complete molar gestation.

The patient is counseled that the risk of repeat molar pregnancy after one mole is approximately 1%. Additionally, due to the risk of development of invasive disease or gestational trophoblastic neoplasia, serial β-hCGs are drawn until there are three consecutive weekly assays of negative β-hCG followed by six monthly assays.

She is counseled and offered contraception during this time due to the increased risk of development of a second molar pregnancy. Her β-hCG levels are followed until undetectable serially.

BEYOND THE PEARLS

- Epidemiologic studies have reported wide regional variations in the incidence of hydatidiform mole. Specifically, estimates from North America, New Zealand, Australia, and Europe report incidence rates ranging from 0.57 to 1.1 per 1000 pregnancies. Studies in Japan and Southeast Asia report 2 per 1000 pregnancies.
- Contraception with oral contraceptive pills (OCPs) following molar pregnancy is preferable due to the advantage of suppressing endogenous luteinizing hormone, which may interfere with the measurement of β-hCG at low levels; studies have demonstrated no increased risk of postmolar trophoblastic neoplasia with OCPs.

Case Summary

- A 30-year-old Asian-American woman at 16 weeks of gestation presents to the obstetric emergency department for headache and vaginal bleeding.
- Her physical exam is significant for hypertension and dark purple vaginal bleeding. Lab evaluation is significant for elevated β-hCG with imaging significant for a complete molar pregnancy.
- The patient underwent treatment with dilation and curettage of the uterus and surveillance with serial measurements of β-hCG.

References

Atrash, H. K., Hogue, C. J. R., & Grimes, D. A. (1986). Epidemiology of hydatidiform mole during early gestation. *American Journal of Obstetrics and Gynecology, 154*, 906–909.

Bagshawe, K. D., Dent, J., & Webb, J. (1986). Hydatidiform mole in England and Wales 1973–1983. *Lancet, 2*, 673–677.

Berkowitz, R. S., & Goldstein, D. P. (1996). Chorionic tumours. *The New England Journal of Medicine, 335*, 1740–1748.

Berkowitz, R. S., Im, S. S., Bernstein, M. R., et al. (1998). Gestational trophoblastic disease: subsequent pregnancy outcome, including repeat molar pregnancy. *The Journal of Reproductive Medicine, 43*, 81–86.

Delcas, R. E., Miller, D. S., Rademaker, A. W., et al. (1991). The role of contraception in the development of postmolar gestational trophoblastic tumor. *Obstetrics and Gynecology, 78*, 221–226.

Feltmate, C. M., Batorfi, J., Fulop, V., et al. (2003). Human chorionic gonadotropin follow-up in patients with molar pregnancy: a time for reevalaution. *Obstetrics and Gynecology, 101*, 732–736.

Lurain, J. (2010). Gestational trophoblastic disease I: epidemiology, pathology, clinical presentation and diagnosis of gestational trophoblastic disease, and management of hydatidiform mole. *American Journal of Obstetrics and Gynecology*, 531–539.

Savage, P. (2013). Gestational trophoblastic disease. *First Consult.*

Jeff R. Temple, PhD

A 28-Year-Old Woman Presenting With Symptoms of Depression in the Postpartum Period

Emily, a 28-year-old woman, presents for her scheduled 6-week postpartum visit. Her physical examination is within normal limits. With the exception of sleep and appetite disturbances, she seems to be doing well. However, when you ask how she's been managing things at home with her new baby, Emily becomes teary-eyed and exclaims, "I just can't do it anymore."

Why is it important to ask about and discuss emotional health in postpartum women?
Postpartum depression is common and affects approximately 15% of mothers (30% of adolescent mothers). In addition to negatively affecting women's quality of life, postpartum depression may impact the child's development. Indeed, children of postpartum depressed women have been shown to have difficulty with attachment, be less responsive, and have more behavioral problems and cognitive deficits than children with nondepressed mothers. Thus, consistent with the stance of the American College of Obstetrics and Gynecology, you should routinely screen all postpartum women for depression.

An efficient and reliable screening tool is the Edinburgh Postnatal Depression Scale (EPDS) (Table 7.1),[6,9] in which women rate their current thoughts and feelings (past 7 days) on 10 items that assess symptoms consistent with depression (e.g., "I have felt sad or miserable"). The EPDS is a preferred screening tool because it (1) can be scored rapidly and provides the physician with a cutoff score indicative of depression and severe depression, (2) assesses suicidal ideation, and (3) distinguishes expected postpregnancy disturbances in quality of life from those that may be better attributed to depression (e.g., "I have been so unhappy that I have had difficulty sleeping").

Is it baby blues, depression, or psychosis?
It is important to distinguish postpartum depression from "baby blues," which are very common (50%–80% of postpartum women), transient, characterized by mild mood disturbances, and generally abate quickly with support and education. *Postpartum depression*, on the other hand, is characterized by more severe mood disturbances, of longer duration (persists for more than 2 weeks), and can present within weeks of delivery. Other symptoms include loss of interest or enjoyment in activities, frequent crying, fatigue, poor concentration, feelings of worthlessness (especially as it relates to motherhood), obsessing over the health and well-being of the baby, and unwanted and intrusive thoughts of harming baby. With respect to the latter, and unlike postpartum psychosis, there is little risk of depressed postpartum women harming the child. Indeed, women often hesitate to seek help and reveal these unsettling thoughts for fear that health care providers will remove the baby. While *postpartum psychosis* receives the abundance of media attention, it is extremely rare: about 1 or 2 per 1000 births. Characterized by psychotic

TABLE 7.1 ▓ Edinburgh Postnatal Depression Scale

In the past 7 days:
1. I have been able to laugh and see the funny side of things.
   __ As much as I always could
   __ Not quite so much now
   __ Definitely not so much now
   __ Not at all
2. I have looked forward with enjoyment to things.
   __ As much as I ever did
   __ Rather less than I used to
   __ Definitely less than I used to
   __ Hardly at all
3. I have blamed myself unnecessarily when things went wrong.
   __ Yes, most of the time
   __ Yes, some of the time
   __ Not very often
   __ No, never
4. I have been anxious or worried for no good reason.
   __ No, not at all
   __ Hardly ever
   __ Yes, sometimes
   __ Yes, very often
5. I have felt scared or panicky for no good reason.
   __ Yes, quite a lot
   __ Yes, sometimes
   __ No, not much
   __ No, not at all
6. Things have been getting on top of me.
   __ Yes, most of the time I haven't been able to cope at all.
   __ Yes, sometimes I haven't been coping as well as usual.
   __ No, most of the time I have coped quite well.
   __ No, I have been coping as well as ever.
7. I have been so unhappy that I have had difficulty sleeping.
   __ Yes, most of the time
   __ Yes, sometimes
   __ Not very often
   __ No, not at all
8. I have felt sad or miserable.
   __ Yes, most of the time
   __ Yes, quite often
   __ Not very often
   __ No, not at all
9. I have been so unhappy that I have been crying.
   __ Yes, most of the time
   __ Yes, quite often
   __ Only occasionally
   __ No, never
10. The thought of harming myself has occurred to me.
   __ Yes, quite often
   __ Sometimes
   __ Hardly ever
   __ Never

Response categories are scored 0, 1, 2, and 3 according to increased severity of the symptom. Items 3 and 5 through 10 are reverse scored (3, 2, 1, 0). The total score is calculated by adding together the scores for each of the 10 items.

From Cox JL, Holden JM, Sagovsky R. Detection of postnatal depression: development of the 10-item Edinburgh Postnatal Depression Scale. *Br J Psychiatry*. 1987;150:782. https://www.clinicalkey.com/#!/content/book/3-s2.0-B9780323321082000238?scrollTo=%23hl0000803

thoughts, delusions, and auditory and/or visual hallucinations (including, potentially, command hallucinations to cause harm to baby or self), postpartum psychosis is considered an emergent situation.

CLINICAL PEARL   **STEPS 2/3**

Postpartum mood disorders range from:
- "Blues" that affect approximately 50% of women, are self-limiting, and considered normal:
  - Occurs around day 3 postpartum with resolution after 1–2 weeks.
- Postpartum depression with incidence of 10%–15% of women;
  - Symptoms present for longer than 2 weeks and can persist for months.
- Psychosis has an occurrence of approximately 0.1%:
  - Onset is usually at the first 2 weeks after delivery.
  - Includes psychotic thoughts, elation, delusions, or unusual behavior.
  - May include thoughts of harming the baby or oneself.

Emily goes on to tell you that she cries every day, has difficulty sleeping, lacks energy, and has lost interest in things that she previously found enjoyable (e.g., exercising, reading, hanging out with friends). She reluctantly tells you that she resents her new baby, feelings of which she is incredibly ashamed, and feels guilty for wanting to return to work and for not being able to attend to her other two children (aged 2 and 6). She has not shared these feelings with anyone else, including her husband.

What are additional questions you need answered at this point?
While it appears that Emily's symptoms are more consistent with depression than with baby blues, additional information is needed, including (1) when did she first notice symptoms; (2) severity of symptoms; (3) personal and family history of depression, substance use, and other mental health problems; (4) presence of delusions or hallucinations (to rule out psychosis); and (5) thoughts of death or suicide. Physical causes of depression should also be ruled out, including hypothyroidism and anemia.

CLINICAL PEARL   **STEPS 2/3**

For diagnostic purposes, a woman presenting with symptoms of depression that began within 4 weeks of delivery,[a] is diagnosed with Major Depressive Disorder with peripartum onset. Five (or more) of the following criteria must have been present during the same 2-week period, represent a change from previous functioning, and at least one of the symptoms is either depressed mood or loss of interest or pleasure:
1. Depressed mood most of the day, nearly every day, as indicated by either subjective report (e.g., feels sad, empty, hopeless) or observation made by others (e.g., appears tearful).
2. Markedly diminished interest or pleasure in all, or almost all, activities most of the day, nearly every day (as indicated by either subjective account or observation).
3. Significant weight loss when not dieting or weight gain (e.g., a change of more than 5% of body weight in a month) or decrease or increase in appetite nearly every day.
4. Insomnia or hypersomnia nearly every day.
5. Psychomotor agitation or retardation nearly every day (observable by others, not merely subjective feelings of restlessness or being slowed down).
6. Fatigue or loss of energy nearly every day.
7. Feelings of worthlessness or excessive or inappropriate guilt (which may be delusional) nearly every day (not merely self-reproach or guilt about being sick).

Continued

CLINICAL PEARL—cont'd   **STEPS 2/3**

8. Diminished ability to think or concentrate, or indecisiveness, nearly every day (either by subjective account or as observed by others).
9. Recurrent thoughts of death (not just fear of dying), recurrent suicidal ideation without a specific plan, or a suicide attempt or a specific plan for committing suicide.

   Symptoms must cause clinically significant distress or impairment in social, occupational, or other important areas of functioning. Symptoms are not attributable to the physiological effects of a substance or to another medical condition, and there has never been a manic or hypomanic episode.

---

[a]Some researchers and clinicians have argued that postpartum onset should be extended to 6 months.

To assist with understanding patient needs, diagnosis, and treatment, clinicians should also be aware of risk factors and comorbidities associated with postpartum depression.

Emily meets the criteria for Major Depression. Moreover, you learn that Emily has little help at home. She recently moved her family across the state and away from her parents and friends to accommodate her husband's job. Her husband, while well-intentioned, is a medical resident and spends little time at home. While she receives some relief during the weekdays when her 6-year-old attends school, she is almost solely responsible for all three children, including her newborn, who has been especially "fussy" of late. She tells you that she did not have these symptoms after the birth of her first two children, but also reported that those were planned and prepared for and that those pregnancies "seemed easier." She found out that she was pregnant with her third child just as she was about to start graduate school. Emily has never taken psychiatric medication.

CLINICAL PEARL   **STEPS 2/3**

Risk factors and comorbidities for postpartum depression include:
- Age (higher with adolescents)
- Unplanned pregnancy
- Stressful life events/circumstances
- Interpersonal problems
- Difficult pregnancy or infant with health problems
- Prior history of depression, especially during a prior pregnancy/postpartum period
- Prior history of mental health problems, including posttraumatic stress disorder (PTSD) and substance use
- Family history of depression or other mood disorder
- Poor social support
- Chronic pain
- Obesity/inactive lifestyle

What immediate interaction and treatment should you undertake?

Perhaps most importantly, Emily's thoughts and feelings should be reflected and normalized. Acknowledge her recent stressors (newborn, moving, caring for three children with no time for herself, putting off graduate school) and let her know that her symptoms, while needing to be addressed, are somewhat expected. Normalize her feelings of guilt and resentment, and let her know that these are likely her depression "talking." Educate the patient on postpartum depression:

prevalence, course, common symptoms, and treatment. Reassure her that she does not have psychosis and that you are not worried about her developing this condition, nor are you worried about her harming the baby (provided this has been assessed and denied).

Next, help the patient shore up resources so that she can spend more time (1) alone or with friends, preferably doing something she enjoys (from her history, exercise for example), (2) with her husband in order to strengthen that partnership, (3) with her older children, and (4) resting/sleeping. While life circumstances (money, new to area, job) and the patient's guilt over leaving her child and obsessiveness with the child's welfare often make these changes difficult, they are essential for improvement. In Emily's case, it may mean her husband reducing his hours at work or flying in a family member/friend to assist.

BASIC SCIENCE PEARL   **STEP 1**

Patients with depression may show characteristic changes in sleep patterns including:
- Reduced slow-wave sleep
- Reduced rapid eye movement (REM) latency
- Increased REM early in sleep cycle
- Increased total REM sleep
- Early-morning awakening

What referral and long-term treatment is appropriate?

Referral will depend on the severity of symptoms and patient safety. If the patient is managing her symptoms, albeit with difficulty, a referral to a psychologist or other licensed mental health care professional is indicated. This is generally considered the treatment of choice, especially if the mother is breastfeeding (many psychiatric medications are contraindicated or have not been tested on breastfeeding mothers). Cognitive behavioral therapy may be used to manage and challenge a patient's negative thoughts (e.g., "I'm a horrible mother") and increase goal-oriented and pro-social behavior. A psychologist/therapist will also assist the patient in increasing resources and social support (e.g., mother's day out group).

If this approach does not reach the desired effect or if the patient's symptoms require more immediate attention, a referral should also be made to a psychiatrist with expertise in managing peripartum women. Selective serotonin reuptake inhibitors have been shown to be effective in treating symptoms of depression. Patients may need to discontinue breastfeeding and substitute with formula milk during their pharmacological treatment. You and the patient may need to discuss whether the benefits of treating depression with psychiatric medication outweigh any benefits of breastfeeding.

CLINICAL PEARL   **STEPS 2/3**

Lithium intake has been associated with Ebstein's anomaly. More recent data suggest that the risk of cardiovascular malformation following prenatal exposure to lithium is less than previously anticipated (1 per 2,000 versus 1 per 1,000) and may possibly not be a teratogen for Ebstein's anomaly.

Ebstein's anomaly refers to an abnormal tricuspid valve with apical displacement of the attachment of the septal leaflet, which may result in tricuspid regurgitation, tricuspid stenosis, and right heart dilation. Other associations may include atrial septal defect and pulmonary stenosis.

Case Summary

- A 28–year-old woman presents for her scheduled 6-week postpartum visit. The patient meets criteria for Major Depression and has little help at home.
- You recognize that it is important to acknowledge her recent stressors and normalize her feelings of guilt and resentment. Additionally, it is imperative to educate her regarding postpartum depression.
- You gather resources to assist the patient in spending more time doing something she enjoys, resting or spending time with her family.
- For patients with difficulty managing their symptoms, referral to a psychologist or other licensed mental health professional is indicated.

References

1. American Psychiatric Association (2013). *Diagnostic and statistical manual of mental disorders* (5th ed.). Washington, DC: Author.
2. Beck, C. T. (2001). Predictors of postpartum depression: an update. *Nursing Research, 5*, 275–285.
3. Bhat, A., Reed, S., & Unutzer, J. (2016). The obstetrician-gynecologist's role in detecting, preventing, and treating depression. *Obstetrics and Gynecology*, 129(1):157–163.
4. Cooper, P., & Murray, L. (1997). Prediction, detection, and treatment of postnatal depression. *Archives of Disease in Childhood*, 77(2), 97–99.
5. Cooper, P. J., & Murray, L. (1995). Course and recurrence of postnatal depression. Evidence for the specificity of the diagnostic concept. *The British Journal of Psychiatry, 166*(2), 191–195.
6. Cox, J. L., Holden, J. M., & Sagovsky, R. (1987). Detection of postnatal depression: development of the 10-item Edinburgh Postnatal Depression Scale. *The British Journal of Psychiatry, 150*, 782–786.
7. Melville, J. L., Reed, S. D., Russo, J., et al. (2014). Improving care for depression in obstetrics and gynecology: a randomized controlled trial. *Obstetrics and Gynecology, 123*, 1237–1246.
8. Robertson, E., Grace, S., Wallington, T., & Stewart, D. E. (2004). Antenatal risk factors for postpartum depression: a synthesis of recent literature. *General Hospital Psychiatry, 26*, 289–295.
9. Wisner, K. L., Parry, C. M., & Piontek, C. M. (2002). Postpartum depression. *The New England Journal of Medicine, 3*, 194–199.

Jean Cox, MS, RD

A 25-Year-Old Woman With Pica in Pregnancy

A 25-year-old woman is 27 weeks pregnant. She presents to her obstetrician's office for a routine prenatal visit. She has a past obstetric history significant for an intrauterine fetal demise at 30 weeks of gestation and recalls losing "a lot" of blood. Today she states that she feels very tired and short of breath. She starts to ask you something, but stops when her friend walks into the exam room. Later, in private, she asks if it is OK to eat "magnesia."

CLINICAL PEARL   **STEPS 2/3**

Pica is the craving and purposeful eating of items not culturally defined as foods or the consumption of foods in nonphysiological amounts. It has been reported worldwide and appears to be more common in warmer climates. It is difficult to estimate the prevalence of pica due to varying diagnostic criteria and likely underreporting. Prevalence among pregnant women in the United States has been documented as high as 77% but is more often estimated at 30%–40%. Cultural expectations affect the acceptability of disclosure of pica. The commonly reported substances also vary by cultures, but there can be considerable variability between individuals in both the substances reported and the willingness to disclose these cravings.

What are the critical questions to ask in anyone who reports eating or craving a nonfood substance?

The main issue is to identify the amount of risk that the patient is incurring. The local Poison Control Center (1-800-222-1222) can give valuable guidance in identifying which substances must be stopped immediately. For example, eating coffee grounds can cause caffeine toxicity, and eating cigarette filters may cause nicotine toxicity. While regular bleach usually causes nausea and vomiting, ultra bleach may cause erosion of the gastrointestinal (GI) tract. One case study reported consumption of large amounts of burnt matchsticks causing neonatal hemolysis and hyperbilirubinemia.

It is important to identify the substance and its source if possible. For example, what type of soil is being consumed? Sandy or clay? Where is it found? Is it imported from tropical areas, or is it found locally? Is it baked before consumption, or is it straight from the garden? However, even with that information, the actual risk of a particular substance may never be known.

Ask also about the quantity and duration of the consumption. Small tastes of baking soda are likely not of concern. However, eating a box a day of baking soda or large amounts of baking powder can cause symptoms mimicking preeclampsia. Large amounts of corn starch (1–2 boxes a day) have caused poor glucose control in women with diabetes.

It is helpful to distinguish between the normal cravings of pregnancy and pica. Ask the patient to describe her cravings, including whether or not she thinks she could resist them. Pica will be much more specific and also stronger. Pica cravings can be triggered by taste but also by smells and textures.

It is also important to identify the likely cause of the pica. When did the cravings start? Were they present before pregnancy? If not, did they appear early in pregnancy? If they have appeared later in gestation, are they associated with a decrease in iron? Is the craving improving or getting worse?

When identifying the modes for intervention, it is useful to understand the patient's beliefs about the pica. If she is craving something, is she actually eating it? If not, why not? Is she avoiding it? Does she feel she can resist eating it? Does she feel she should resist eating it? Has she tried any substitutions? Have they worked?

How does this information help you form a differential diagnosis?
There are some people who feel that their pica is just a normal sign of being pregnant or that it may have an emotional or religious benefit. However, many are often unwilling to discuss their pica because of embarrassment or fear that others will think they are "crazy." While pica may be a manifestation of a psychiatric disorder, including schizophrenia, obsessive-compulsive disorder, and anorexia nervosa, the fact that these cravings appear only during pregnancy makes that an unlikely diagnosis. Pica is also associated with celiac disease and renal dialysis. If it appears early in pregnancy, it may be associated with trying to control the nausea and vomiting of early pregnancy. Some behaviors (e.g., sniffing gasoline) may be associated with substance abuse.

CLINICAL PEARL   **STEPS 2/3**

While it is important to identify those behaviors that must be stopped immediately, the clinician is strongly advised to not overreact to what is being disclosed. When discussing the pica with the patient, it is helpful to treat this as a common part of pregnancy. This will enhance communication and compliance with your patient, which will lead to further discovery of the extent of disease and the best treatment approach.

When you ask if she is craving anything else, she reports that she craves dirt (geophagia). This craving is exacerbated for her if she smells wet dirt when it rains or notices small pieces of dirt mixed in with beans. While she eats the bean dirt a few times/week, she is afraid to eat the dirt outside her house because she knows the neighbor's dogs lie there. Eating "magnesia" helps her resist eating dirt.

What are the concerns that arise with the consumption of soils or "magnesia"?
Soil consumption may increase exposure to toxins and infectious agents. It may also reduce the effectiveness of medications and the absorption of micronutrients. Soil high in clay can cause GI obstruction, as can paper, cardboard, and foam rubber (Fig. 8.1). Clay can bind with micronutrients or form a matrix with the mucin layer of the gut, creating a barrier to absorption.

Sometimes called "magnesia de terrón" or "terrón de magnesia," the patient is referring to a block of magnesium carbonate. She reports eating small pieces from the block a few times a day, but recently she has wanted to eat it more often.

It is unknown whether consuming magnesium carbonate blocks is of concern. Magnesium carbonate has been used for the treatment of both constipation and heartburn, but there are also concerns about potential magnesium toxicity.

She reports that when she is not pregnant she rarely craves dirt and she doesn't want magnesia at all. In each of her other pregnancies, she has wanted dirt but it is getting worse now.

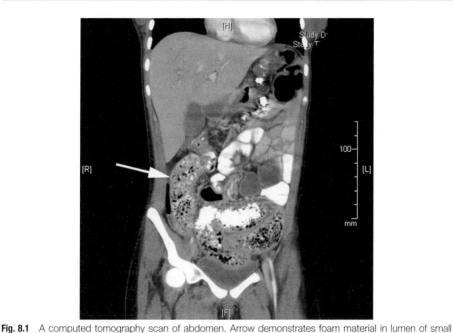

Fig. 8.1 A computed tomography scan of abdomen. Arrow demonstrates foam material in lumen of small intestine. Foam is also seen in distal large intestine. *(From Altepeter, T, Annes, J, Meller J. Foam bezoar: resection of perforated terminal ileum in a 17-year-old with sickle β+ thalassemia and pica. J Pediatr Surg. 2011:e31–2. https://www.clinicalkey.com/#!/content/journal/1-s2.0-S0022346811003174?scrollTo=%231-s2.0-S0022346811003174-gr1)*

CLINICAL PEARL **STEPS 2/3**

While the hematocrit or hemoglobin may be replaced within a few weeks or months after delivery, some women still have low serum ferritin (a measure of stored iron) 2 years after delivery.

For the last few weeks, she has also been eating many large glasses of ice (pagophagia) every day because she likes how it feels to chew it. She prefers the crushed ice from a local fast food restaurant and finds herself going out of her way to go there at least 2–3 times per day, getting the largest glass they serve and often dumping out the soda to get to the ice. While she also chews the ice cubes from home, they don't produce the same satisfying crunch. She has been told by her family that eating cold things, including ice, will worsen her pain during and after labor and delivery. However, even though she is afraid of it, she feels that the craving is so strong that she is unable to resist eating ice.

CLINICAL PEARL **STEPS 2/3**

While the evidence for iron, zinc, or other micronutrient deficiencies causing pica is limited, it is strongest between iron deficiency and the craving for ice.

Is consuming so much ice of concern?

While craving ice could be a response to dehydration or a way to treat mouth pain, there is no evidence that either is the cause in this case. The strength and the specificity of the craving described is often helpful in distinguishing pica from the food cravings common to pregnancy. Tooth breakage and jaw pain have been reported with ice consumption.

Although it is unknown why iron deficiency would cause someone to crave the crunch of ice, one hypothesis proposes that chewing ice may trigger the dive reflex, causing peripheral vasoconstriction and preferential perfusion of the vital organs, including the brain. There is evidence that chewing ice improves response times on neuropsychological tests in subjects with iron-deficiency anemia but not in healthy controls.

In her previous pregnancies in Latin America, she also ate the plaster and the adobe bricks from her wall, consuming 2–3 bricks (12 × 8 × 3-inch) over the course of her pregnancy. Her family wondered why her walls had holes in them, but she was afraid to tell them. The father of this baby knows nothing of that history, and she is embarrassed to tell him. Regarding her cravings now, she reports that she is afraid that eating dirt and magnesia might be dangerous for her baby, but she also can't seem to resist them.

CLINICAL PEARL   **STEPS 2/3**

The patient will often not mention her most concerning pica substance until she has seen your reaction to her previous disclosures. Discussing her pica as a way to help identify the iron-deficiency anemia common in pregnancy will help improve communication and therefore intervention. Reacting with shock or just telling her to stop the consumption of potentially dangerous things will likely only stop the disclosure and increase fear rather than stop the behavior.

Her prepregnancy body mass index is 21. Her weight gain at 27 weeks is 4.5 kg (10 lb), slightly low. Her most recent hematocrit was 28%, and her hemoglobin was 9 g/dL. No other iron studies were performed. However, iron studies and a peripheral smear can assist in the diagnosis of iron deficiency anemia (Fig. 8.2).

CLINICAL PEARL   **STEPS 2/3**

Iron studies are often done only after a patient fails to respond to intervention. The Dietary Reference Intakes (DRIs) for iron during pregnancy are nearly double that for nonpregnant women, making iron-deficiency anemia the most likely reason for the patient's low hematocrit and hemoglobin.

CLINICAL PEARL   **STEPS 2/3**

Liver is rich in preformed vitamin A, which has been associated with birth defects when consumed in large quantities. Therefore consumption of liver or liver products (paté, liverwurst, braunschweiger) in the first trimester should be limited. β-Carotene is not of concern.

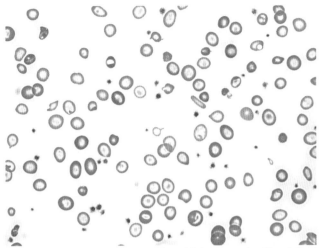

Fig. 8.2 A peripheral smear from a patient with severe iron-deficiency anemia with variation in size and shape of the red blood cells (anisopoikilocytosis). The cells are hypochromic with an enlarged area of central pallor. *(From Kroft, S, Monaghan S. Red blood cell/ hemoglobin disorders. In:* Hematopathology: a volume in foundations in diagnostic pathology series. *2012;3–54. https://www.clinicalkey.com/#!/content/book/3-s2.0-B9781437726060000019?scrollTo=%233-s2.0-B9781437726060000019-f001-010-9781437726060)*

> Her reported diet includes meat 1–2 times per week, mainly chicken. She drinks the liquid from cooked beans, but doesn't like to eat the beans. She seldom eats lentils. She has trouble taking pills and so is taking prenatal "gummy" multivitamins, two gummies per day. She takes no other supplements.

How do you approach treating the underlying iron deficiency?

Her reported diet is low in total iron and even lower in the better-absorbed heme iron. While there is a cultural belief that the liquid from cooked beans is high in iron, not all the iron moves to the cooking liquid and the beans should also be consumed. Lentils contain more iron than beans. However, all of the vegetable sources of iron are non-heme. Non-heme iron is poorly absorbed and is highly affected by the other dietary components.

Heme iron, found only in meats, is better absorbed and less affected by the rest of the diet. Foods highest in heme iron include red meats (beef, goat) and many wild meats (bear, deer, elk, buffalo, etc.). Those organ meats that include more iron than beef include liver (limit in the first trimester), kidneys, heart, and gizzards. Oysters, clams, mussels, and octopus are some of the higher heme iron seafood choices.

CLINICAL PEARL   **STEPS 2/3**

Enlisting the help of a registered dietitian can be critical in identifying foods that a patient is willing to eat and that are high enough in iron to treat her deficiency. Non-heme vegetable sources are not well enough absorbed to be useful, even if someone late in pregnancy were able to eat the large volume that would be required. Heme iron sources are a much better option.

Prenatal vitamins usually contain iron, but absorption is poor because they also contain the nonheme form. Some of the other minerals contained in those supplements may limit the bioavailability of iron. Of note, "gummies" rarely, if ever, contain iron or other minerals. Although there are iron supplements that contain heme iron, they are more expensive and have not been found to be superior to heme-rich foods.

While pica is often associated with iron-deficiency anemia, it is unclear whether iron is the only important variable. Zinc affects one's taste and smell perceptions. Zinc requirements increase during pregnancy, and good food sources of iron are also often high in zinc. There have been no studies examining the effectiveness of treatment with iron versus zinc. There have also been no studies directly looking at the effectiveness of supplements versus food sources. Iron supplements have not consistently been effective, but it is unknown whether that is because of the amount of iron prescribed, the poor bioavailability, or that iron may not be the only critical variable. Instituting a diet that features meats containing both iron and zinc addresses those concerns.

> The patient reports that she really doesn't want to eat the dirt and so eats the magnesia instead. However, when asked if she could stop, she replies that she "has to" eat it.

How do you approach addressing the actual pica substances?

In addition to the strength of the craving making resistance difficult, women are also often afraid not to eat the craved substance for fear that something will happen to the baby. Cultural beliefs vary but may include giving birth to a baby with something missing (cleft lip/palate or missing fingers) or with a birthmark or to an ill or stillborn infant. When she feels she shouldn't resist eating a craved substance, such as soil, which has potential for harmful consequences, have the patient try smelling wet dirt while she chews something that gives her the same mouth feel as the dirt she is craving. In this way, she is complying with the craving and lowering the perceived danger to the baby, but is consuming something that is less likely to be contaminated. In the meantime, treat her iron deficiency by prescribing a diet rich in red meats, and the cravings will disappear after just a few days or weeks.

> The patient chose to eat beef daily and liver 2–3 times per week for now. Although she will continue to eat beans, she will give priority to eating meats. She will also start taking ferrous sulfate supplements, taking 1–2 a day separately from each other, washing them down with water or juice, but she knows that she is getting more benefit from the meat than from the iron supplements. For the pica, she will eat a burned tortilla while she sniffs wet dirt. She will try to resist eating the magnesia but will continue to eat ice as long as her teeth don't hurt.

BASIC SCIENCE PEARL	**STEP 1**

Lab findings consistent with iron-deficiency anemia are as follows:
Elevated: Total iron binding capacity (TIBC), red cell distribution width (RDW)
Low: Serum iron, serum ferritin, reticulocyte count
Blood smear shows: Microcytic, hypochromatic red blood cells, doughnut cells with a large central area of pallor, or poikilocytosis.

> The patient returns to the clinic for her next obstetric visit at 30 weeks' gestation. She reports eating beef daily and eating liver a few times a week but that she is getting tired of it. She now reports that she feels less fatigued and denies shortness of breath. She says her head feels lighter and the cravings for dirt are less. Eating the burned tortilla helped, as did burned toast, but now she can resist eating dirt and doesn't need magnesia. While she still likes ice, she doesn't go out of her way to get it anymore. She reports no other cravings. Her follow-up hematocrit is now 34%.

How do you approach her long-term care?

If she had reported no improvement or a worsening of symptoms or cravings, further workup would have been done, including iron studies with zinc status. If she had not tried the substitutions, further interviewing regarding her decision-making choices should be pursued. Is her family counteracting our advice? Are there other beliefs and fears about the pica that have yet to be disclosed?

CLINICAL PEARL   **STEPS 2/3**

Zinc status is seldom monitored because of the low prevalence of zinc deficiency in the United States and the concern about the accuracy of lab assessment of zinc status, especially during pregnancy.

In this case, the patient should be reassured that she is on the right track and that both she and her baby are now safer. She will need to continue to eat red meats for the duration of the pregnancy and for a few weeks or months after delivery, but less frequently.

CLINICAL PEARL   **STEPS 2/3**

Replacement of serum ferritin, a measure of stored iron, takes at least 6 months after the hematocrit or hemoglobin have returned to normal.

BEYOND THE PEARLS

- Iron-deficiency anemia during pregnancy is associated with increased risk of preterm delivery, fetal growth restriction, and increased fetal and neonatal mortality.
- In addition, both increased fetal cortisol production and oxidative damage to fetal erythrocytes have been found.
- Maternal effects of iron-deficiency anemia include fatigue and dyspnea, but also increased risk of blood loss with uterine atony during delivery and impaired wound healing and immune function. There is also an increased risk of postpartum depression, poor maternal and infant interaction, and impaired lactation.
- Because of the decreased oxygen availability with long-term residency at high altitude (≥3000 ft), as well as with cigarette smoking, normal hemoglobin and hematocrit values should be adjusted to account for both. Standard cutoffs are available from the U.S. Centers for Disease Control (CDC).

Case Summary

- A 25-year-old pregnant woman presents with a craving for and consumption of dirt, ice, and blocks of magnesium carbonate.
- History reveals that the patient is fatigued and short of breath.
- Her laboratory evaluation is significant for a hematocrit of 28% and a hemoglobin of 9 g/dL.
- The diagnosis of pica (both geophagia and pagophagia) associated with iron-deficiency anemia is made. The patient was advised to eat beef daily and liver 2–3 times a week and will start taking ferrous sulfate. For the pica, she was advised to eat a burned tortilla while she smelled wet dirt.

References

Barraclough, K. A., Brown, F., Hawley, C. M., et al. (2012). A randomized controlled trial of oral heme iron polypeptide versus oral iron supplementation for the treatment of anaemia in peritoneal dialysis patients: HEMATOCRIT trial. *Nephrology, Dialysis, Transplantation, 27*(11), 4146–4153.

Bernardo, E. O., Matos, R. I., Dawood, T., et al. (2015). Maternal cautopyreiophagia as a rare cause of neonatal hemolysis: a case report. *Pediatrics, 135*(3), e726–e729.

Bodnar, L. M., Cogswell, M. E., & Scanlon, K. S. (2002). Low income postpartum women are at risk of iron deficiency. *The Journal of Nutrition, 132*(8), 2298–2302.

Centers for Disease Control and Prevention. (1998). Recommendations to prevent and control iron deficiency in the United States. Centers for Disease Control and Prevention. *MMWR. Recommendations and Reports, 47*(RR-3), 1–29. Available at: https://stacks.cdc.gov/view/cdc/7119/.

Fawcett, E. J., Fawcett, J. M., & Mazmanian, D. (2016). A meta-analysis of the worldwide prevalence of pica during pregnancy and the postpartum period. *International Journal of Gynaecology and Obstetrics, 133*(3), 277–283.

Hovdenak, N., & Haram, K. (2012). Influence of mineral and vitamin supplements on pregnancy outcome. *European Journal of Obstetrics, Gynecology, and Reproductive Biology, 164*(2), 127–132.

Hunt, M. G., Belfer, S., & Atuahene, B. (2014). Pagophagia improves neuropsychological processing speed in iron-deficiency anemia. *Medical Hypotheses, 83*(4), 473–476.

Lowe, N. M., Dykes, F. C., Skinner, A. L., et al. (2013). EURRECA: estimating zinc requirements for deriving dietary reference values. *Critical Reviews in Food Science and Nutrition, 53*(10), 1110–1123.

Rabel, A., Leitman, S. F., & Miller, J. L. (2016). Ask about ice, then consider iron. *Journal of the American Association of Nurse Practitioners, 28*(2), 116–120.

Young, S. L. (2010). Pica in pregnancy: new ideas about an old condition. *Annual Review of Nutrition, 30*, 403–422.

Kylie Fowler, MD

A 27-Year-Old Woman With Opiate Dependence in Pregnancy

A 27-year-old G2P1001 female at 25 weeks gestational age presents to obstetrical triage with symptoms of restlessness, tremors, nausea, and diarrhea for the past 36 hours. She has a history of opioid abuse, with last use approximately 24 hours ago.

Why is it important to screen for opioid abuse in pregnancy?

Substance use in pregnancy has a significant impact on the health of mothers and infants, as well as extensive implications for community public health. In the previous decade, maternal opiate use has increased dramatically from 1.19 per 1000 births in 2000 to 5.77 per 1000 births in 2009. Opioid abuse in pregnancy is associated with poor obstetrical outcomes including fetal demise, intrauterine growth restriction, preterm birth, and placental abruption as well as neonatal abstinence syndrome (NAS). Opioid abuse may take the form of illicit drug use or nonmedical use of opioid-containing pain medication. Use of other illicit substances in addition to opioid use can increase the severity of these adverse health outcomes.

What is a validated method to screen for substance abuse in pregnancy?

Pregnancy provides a unique opportunity to screen and treat for substance abuse. Women have more frequent contact with health care during pregnancy, with increased opportunity to maintain treatment for substance abuse. The *4 P's Plus(c)* is a validated substance abuse screening tool for use in pregnancy (Table 9.1).

Any question resulting in a positive answer should prompt a more formal and complete assessment of substance use. The last two questions regarding alcohol and tobacco use during the month prior to knowledge of pregnancy have the highest positive predictive validity for detecting illicit substance use in this population.

TABLE 9.1 ■ Screening With the Four P's Plus

Parents	Did either of your parents ever have a problem with alcohol or drugs?
Partner	Does your partner have a problem with alcohol or drugs?
Past	Have you ever drunk beer, wine, or liquor?
Pregnancy	In the month before you knew you were pregnant, how many cigarettes did you smoke? In the month before you knew you were pregnant, how many beers/how much wine/ how much liquor did you drink?

From Chasnoff IJ, Hung WC. *The 4P's plus*. Chicago: NTI Publishing; 1999. https://www.clinicalkey.com/#!/content/book/3-s2.0-B978032332108200055X?scrollTo=%23hl0001511

CLINICAL PEARL   **STEPS 2/3**

Tobacco abuse is common in opioid-dependent women. Tobacco use is an independent risk factor for intrauterine growth restriction, preterm birth, and fetal death. All pregnant women with tobacco use disorder should be assessed for their willingness to quit at each prenatal visit through use of motivational interviewing. If they express a desire to quit, smoking cessation resources should be provided with regular follow-up to track progress.

When a pregnant woman presents with concern for opiate withdrawal, what do you need to know about her history?

Because opioid abuse can take many forms with different implications for management and treatment, it is important to gain a complete drug use history. Heroin is a rapidly acting opioid and the most highly addictive. Patients who use heroin may have severe withdrawal symptoms within 4–6 hours of last use. Heroin may be injected, smoked, or nasally inhaled. Injection drug use is associated with high prevalence of blood-borne infectious diseases such as hepatitis B, hepatitis C, and human immunodeficiency virus (HIV). Intravenous (IV) injection can also result in severe infections such as bacterial endocarditis.

Use of narcotic pain medication, either obtained through prescription or illegal drug sale, will have different implications for withdrawal and treatment. For example, methadone is a long-acting opioid that is often sold as a street drug. It has a half-life of between 22 and 24 hours, with withdrawal occurring approximately 24–36 hours after last use. Therefore, specific opiate used, method of use, and timing of last use should be elicited.

Use of additional substances such as alcohol, tobacco, or other illicit drugs increases the risk of adverse neonatal and pregnancy outcomes, and therefore patients should be questioned about all substances used.

BASIC SCIENCE PEARL   **STEP 1**

The analgesic properties of opioids is primarily a result of their interaction with the mu opioid receptor. This receptor is in the G protein-coupled receptor family. Interaction with the mu opioid receptor induces cyclic AMP (cAMP) as a secondary messenger within the cell. Alterations in the levels of cAMP within cells after prolonged exposure to opioids can induce many cellular changes responsible for opioid tolerance and physical dependence.

You should also obtain a complete obstetric history for both the current and any previous pregnancies, as well as complete gynecologic history, past medical history, past surgical history, family and social history, medication list, allergies, and a complete review of systems. The social history may be of specific value as illicit drug use and addiction places the patient at significant risk for homelessness, high-risk activities such as prostitution or theft, and exposure to violence.

The patient reports a long history of heroin use starting at age 18. She primarily uses via IV injection. Her last heroin use was approximately 48 hours ago. In an attempt to self-alleviate her withdrawal symptoms she took 30 mg of methadone obtained from a friend approximately 24 hours ago. She denies use of any other illicit substances, although she does smoke 4–5 cigarettes a day.

She reports two previous prenatal visits in this pregnancy. Her estimated date of delivery is based on a 20-week ultrasound that demonstrated normal fetal anatomy and a posterior placenta. Her obstetrical history includes one previous pregnancy 3 years ago resulting in a term vaginal delivery of a female infant. This pregnancy was also complicated by opioid abuse, maintained on methadone therapy.

She reports irregular menses and an unknown last menstrual period. She denies a history of sexually transmitted infections (STIs) and is unsure of the date of her last Pap test.

Her past medical history is significant for posttraumatic stress disorder (PTSD) and depression. She has had no previous surgeries. She takes no medications and reports an allergy to penicillin resulting in a rash. Her family history is negative. Her social history reveals she is currently living with her grandmother and is unemployed. Her daughter is being raised by her daughter's father, and she has visitation rights on the weekends. She has previously engaged in prostitution to assist in heroin acquisition but states consistent condom use. Review of systems is positive for diffuse muscle and joint aches, mild rhinorrhea, nausea without emesis, diarrhea, and decreased sleep due to increased anxiety. She denies fevers, chills, chest pain or shortness of breath, loss of amniotic fluid, contractions, or vaginal bleeding.

What are important components of the physical exam for pregnant patients presenting with opioid withdrawal?

All pregnant patients presenting to obstetrical triage units should have a complete set of vital signs, and, for women at a gestational age over 24 weeks, a non–stress test (NST) should be performed. In addition to a complete physical exam, patients presenting for opiate withdrawal should have a Clinical Opiate Withdrawal Scale (COWS) performed to assess for severity of withdrawal (Table 9.2).

TABLE 9.2 ▓ Clinical Opiate Withdrawal Scale

Patient's Name:	Date and Time:

Reason for this assessment:

Resting Pulse Rate: _____ /minute *Measured after patient is sitting or lying for one minute* 0 pulse rate 80 or below 1 pulse rate 81–100 2 pulse rate 101–120 4 pulse rate greater than 120 Sweating: *over past ½ hour not accounted for by* *room temperature or patient activity.* 0 no report of chills or flushing 1 subjective report of chills or flushing 2 flushed or observable moistness on face 3 beads of sweat on brow or face 4 sweat streaming off face Restlessness *Observation during assessment* 0 able to sit still 1 reports difficulty sitting still, but is able to do so 3 frequent shifting or extraneous movements of legs/arms 5 unable to sit still for more than a few seconds Pupil size 0 pupils are pinned or normal size for room light 1 pupils possible larger than normal for room light 2 pupils moderately dilated 5 pupils so dilated that only the rim of the iris is visible Bone or Joint aches *If patient was having pain previously,* *only the additional component attributed to opiates* *withdrawal is scored* 0 not present 1 mild diffuse comfort 2 patient reports severe diffuse aching of joints/muscles 4 patient is rubbing joints or muscles and is unable to sit still because of discomfort Runny nose or tearing *Not accounted for by cold* *symptoms or allergies* 0 not present 1 nasal stuffiness or unusually moist eyes 2 nose running or tearing 4 nose constantly running or tears streaming down cheeks	GI Upset: *over last ½ hour* 0 no GI symptoms 1 stomach cramps 2 nausea or loose stool 3 vomiting or diarrhea 5 multiple episodes of diarrhea or vomiting Tremor *observation of outstretched hands* 0 no tremor 1 tremor can be felt, but not observed 2 slight tremor observable 4 gross tremor or muscle twitching Yawning *Observation during assessment* 0 no yawning 1 yawning once or twice during assessment 2 yawning three or more times during assessment 4 yawning several times/minute Anxiety or Irritability 0 none 1 patient reports increasing irritability or anxiousness 2 patient obviously irritable or anxious 4 patient so irritable or anxious that partici- pation in the assessment is difficult Gooseflesh skin 0 skin is smooth 3 piloerection of skin can be felt or hairs standing up on arms 5 prominent piloerection Total Score: _____ The total score is the sum of all 11 items Initials of person completing assessment: _____

Score 5–12 = mild; 13–24 = moderate; 25–36 = moderately severe; more than 36 = severe withdrawal

From Wesson DR, Ling W. The Clinical Opiate Withdrawal Scale (COWS). *J Psychoactive Drugs.* 2003;35(2):254–9.

Vital signs reveal a blood pressure of 132/78 mm Hg, a heart rate of 116/min, respiratory rate 22/min, and temperature 37.4°C (99.3°F). She is resting in bed, in no apparent distress. Her face appears flushed with moderately dilated pupils, no noticeable rhinorrhea, no yawning. Her heart has a regular rhythm with mild tachycardia and no murmurs. Lungs are clear to auscultation bilaterally; abdomen is soft, nontender, gravid with fundal height of 25 cm. Extremities are warm and well perfused; however, upper extremities show bilateral "track marks" from previous injection. When asked to extend her outstretched hands, you notice a mild bilateral tremor. Skin without rash or lesions, no notable piloerection.

Fetal NST reveals a baseline heart rate of 155/min, moderate variability, positive 10 × 10 accelerations and no decelerations. Tocometer without contractions.

Based on the history and physical exam for this patient, what is her COWS score?
Using the COWS, you calculate the following:
- Heart rate of 118: 2 points
- Notable flushing of patient's face: 2 points
- Reported restlessness but able to sit still: 1 point
- Pupils with moderate dilation: 2 points
- Nasal stuffiness: 1 point
- Reported nausea and loose stool: 2 points
- Slight observable tremor: 2 points
- No yawning during assessment: 0 points
- Patient reports increasing irritability or anxiety: 1 point
- No notable piloerection of skin: 0 points

Total score: 13 points, indicating moderate withdrawal.

What are the goals of treatment for opioid dependence in pregnancy?
Therapeutic goals in the treatment of opioid dependence are comprehensive and multidisciplinary. Initial treatment is focused on reducing acute symptoms of withdrawal, often through the use of opioid replacement with methadone or buprenorphine. Opioid replacement is also associated with improved compliance with regular prenatal care and decreased high-risk behaviors associated with illicit drug-seeking. Comprehensive treatment includes opioid maintenance therapy and behavior health treatment of addiction and co-occurring mental health disorders, as well as screening and treatment of other significant health concerns, such as infectious diseases, resulting in improved long-term health for both mother and infant.

What are the available options for opioid replacement therapy for pregnant women who are opioid dependent?
Methadone is the recommended first-line therapy for pregnant women with opioid dependence, with demonstrated efficacy since the 1970s. It is a full mu-opioid agonist distributed in federally approved substance abuse treatment clinics daily. There are many important pharmacokinetic aspects of methadone and its use in pregnancy.

CLINICAL PEARL   **STEPS 2/3**

The half-life of methadone decreases from 22–24 hours to approximately 8.1 hours in pregnancy. Therefore, close monitoring and dose adjustment, sometimes changing to twice-daily dosing, is necessary throughout pregnancy. Additionally, methadone is known to interact with several different medications including antiepileptics, antiretrovirals, and rifampin. Methadone doses are initiated at 10–30 mg per day, with dosage increases based on withdrawal assessment. NAS is a known complication of treatment; however, the dose of methadone does not appear to impact the severity of this syndrome.

Buprenorphine is a partial mu-opioid agonist used in the treatment of opioid dependence. It may be prescribed in the office setting by physicians who have been trained and obtained specific credentialing for its outpatient use. While there is less long-term data on its use in pregnancy, emerging evidence suggests some advantages to buprenorphine. In addition to the convenience of outpatient treatment without required daily visits to a licensed treatment program, buprenorphine has fewer drug interactions and a decreased risk of overdose. Additionally, it has been associated with less severe NAS when compared to methadone. Because it is a partial mu-agonist, buprenorphine may precipitate withdrawal. Disadvantages to buprenorphine include more difficult treatment initiation with potential for withdrawal, lack of long-term childhood outcomes data, and increased patient dropout rate, as well as potential increase in medication diversion.

A third option for treatment of opioid dependence in pregnancy is inpatient, supervised withdrawal. The American College of Obstetrics and Gynecologists does not recommend this as first-line treatment secondary to very high relapse rates. However, inpatient detoxification should be made available to women who express intent.

What is NAS?

NAS is characterized by hyperactivity of the central nervous system with accompanying dysfunction of the autonomic nervous system in infants born to opioid-dependent mothers. Infants with NAS may experience irritability, diarrhea, feeding difficulties, seizures, failure to thrive, and even death if left untreated. Treatment of infants with NAS often involves prolonged hospital stay with careful opioid-based pharmacologic treatment and weaning protocols.

How should you counsel a pregnant woman with opioid dependence who would like to begin opioid maintenance therapy?

Opioid-dependent pregnant women should be offered all options for opioid maintenance therapy as well as detoxification. The patient should be asked about her experiences and successes with previous opioid maintenance therapy. She should be counseled on methadone as current first-line therapy with the longest treatment history and most data available on its use in pregnancy. Distribution of methadone in licensed clinics on a daily basis should be reviewed and information on available clinics made available to the patient. While methadone is prescribed in specific outpatient licensed clinics by addiction specialists, the patient should know that her obstetrics providers will continue to provide comprehensive care for all facets of routine pregnancy in addition to coordinating any additional care she may need for her addiction. Providers should engage in an open discussion of NAS and its association with any form of opioid use during pregnancy. Patients should be offered the opportunity to meet with neonatal providers who may thoroughly counsel them on expectations for infant treatment following delivery.

With regards to buprenorphine, patients should be counseled on its distribution by licensed providers, and a list of the available providers should be given to the patient if you are not able to prescribe this medication. The limited long-term data regarding its use in pregnancy should be discussed. Providers should review the potential for induced withdrawal upon buprenorphine initiation. Providers should discuss emerging and consistent evidence that buprenorphine is associated with decreased severity of NAS. Patients should be advised that any opioid maintenance treatment will require very close follow-up as well as routine drug screening. Patients who would like to undergo supervised detoxification should be counseled that it is associated with high rates of relapse and will often require a prolonged hospital stay. However, this option is associated with the lowest rates of NAS.

Following comprehensive counseling, your patient decides that she would like to initiate methadone therapy as she was successfully maintained on this treatment in her previous pregnancy.

What additional testing should you perform prior to initiation of methadone therapy?
If not already performed as part of her prenatal care, testing should be performed for blood-borne infections including hepatitis B, hepatitis C, and HIV. Because she has engaged in high-risk sexual behavior, complete STI testing should also be performed. You should verify that all routine prenatal testing is up to date. Patients undergoing induction of opioid maintenance therapy should have a baseline urine drug screen performed to evaluate for poly-substance use that may impact treatment. Additionally, because methadone is associated with abnormalities of cardiac conduction, specifically prolongation of the QTc interval, a baseline electrocardiogram (ECG) should be obtained.

> The patient previously had routine prenatal care screening labs performed and records were obtained. You provide additional hepatitis C, hepatitis B, and HIV testing, which was negative. Complete STI testing was positive for chlamydia and single-dose azithromycin treatment was provided. Urine drug screen was positive for long- and short-acting opioids but no other substances. ECG revealed sinus tachycardia.

How should methadone opioid replacement therapy be initiated?
Methadone induction therapy may be initiated on an inpatient or outpatient basis. Maternal severity of withdrawal, gestational age, fetal monitoring, and availability of federally licensed outpatient methadone clinics are all factors in this decision. Initial doses are typically between 10 and 30 mg with titration based on withdrawal symptoms as objectively documented through use of the COWS assessment. Doses that do not adequately control withdrawal symptoms and cravings are associated with increased use of illicit opioid supplementation and associated high-risk behavior. ECG monitoring should be repeated with each dose increase and after steady-state has been reached on final maximal dosing. Additional monitoring, such as with routine repeated urine drug screens, will vary based on the protocol of individual clinics.

> After thorough counseling, your patient decides on outpatient methadone initiation. You provide her with an initial dose of 30 mg of methadone while in the obstetrical triage unit. She elects to continue methadone treatment at the clinic she attended previously. You give her a referral for this clinic and arrange an appointment the following morning.

What additional care will your patient need throughout her pregnancy?
While there is no specific data for antenatal monitoring in this patient population, consideration may be given for growth ultrasound evaluation every 4 weeks secondary to increased risk of intrauterine growth restriction and low-birth-weight infants. Additionally, twice weekly NST with weekly amniotic fluid index may be initiated at 32 weeks of gestational age due to increased risk of fetal death.

Additionally, patients presenting with opioid dependence should be screened for depression, anxiety, and suicidal ideation. Co-occuring mental illness occurs in up to 65% of opioid dependent women, with up to 12% reporting active suicidal thoughts. Regardless of co-occurring mental illness, patients should be referred to appropriate substance abuse and comprehensive psychiatric care.

> Your patient reports a history of depression and increased anxiety, as well as a history of PTSD. She is not currently experiencing active symptoms of major depressive disorder and denies active thoughts of self-harm. She feels safe with adequate support at her grandmother's home. You provide a follow-up appointment for your patient in your obstetrical outpatient clinic for the following week in addition to a referral to a psychiatrist. You provide her with emergency resources in case she experiences an increase in symptoms of withdrawal or worsening symptoms of depression.

BEYOND THE PEARLS

- Acute pain management for opioid dependent patients can be intimidating for even experienced providers. Multiple studies have shown, however, that appropriate treatment of acute pain does not increase risk for relapse, but untreated pain may result in illegal opioid-seeking behavior. Opioids with mixed agonist/antagonist properties (nalbuphine, butorphanol, pentazocine) should be avoided in patients on opioid replacement therapy as this can induce acute withdrawal. For acute pain, patients should receive scheduled nonsteroidal antiinflammatory medication (avoid use in the third trimester). Routinely given narcotics should be used to achieve adequate pain control, but studies have shown that patients receiving opioid replacement therapy may need as much as 50%–70% higher dosages· Patients should be monitored for respiratory depression while adequate pain control is obtained.
- As of 2016, 18 states consider substance use in pregnancy to be child abuse, and three consider it grounds for involuntary civil commitment to mental health or substance abuse treatment centers. Additionally, 18 states require reporting of suspected substance use in pregnancy. Despite these laws, the American College of Obstetricians and Gynecologist urges treatment of substance abuse as an illness and not as a moral failing. Every effort should be made to provide a safe and nonpunitive environment for obstetrical care and substance abuse treatment. Providers should be aware of mandatory reporting in their state, but every effort should be made to maintain and provide care outside of the legal system.

Case Summary

- A 27-year-old G2P1001 at 25 weeks of gestational age presents in acute opioid withdrawal.
- History and physical exam reveals a 9-year history of opioid dependence, with primary use of IV heroin. She received methadone opioid replacement therapy in her previous pregnancy with success. She has co-occuring depression, anxiety, and PTSD. Physical exam reveals reassuring fetal monitoring and moderate opioid withdrawal.
- She is thoroughly counseled regarding the risks and benefits of methadone and buprenorphine opioid maintenance as well as opioid detoxification, with specific emphasis on the severity of NAS associated with each treatment modality.
- Following counseling and appropriate screening, the patient decides to initiate opioid replacement therapy with methadone.
- Additional screening reveals a history of depression without active symptoms. In addition to obstetric and methadone therapy, appropriate referral is made for psychiatric care.

References

American College of Obstetricians and Gynecologists. (2011). Substance abuse reporting and pregnancy: the role of the obstetrician-gynecologists. Committee Opinion No. 473. *Obstetrics and Gynecology, 117*(1), 200–201.

American College of Obstetricians and Gynecologists. (2012). Opioid abuse, dependence, and addiction in pregnancy. Committee Opinion No. 524. *Obstetrics and Gynecology, 119*(5), 1070–1076.

Chasnoff, I. J., McGourty, R. F., Bailey, G. W., et al. (2005). The 4P's Plus© screen for substance use in pregnancy: clinical application and outcomes *Journal of Perinatology, 25*(6), 368–374.

Chasnoff, I. J., Wells, A. M., McGourty, R. F., et al. (2007). Validation of the 4P's Plus© screen for substance use in pregnancy. *Journal of Perinatology, 27*(12), 744–748.

Cleary, B. J., Donnelly, J., Strawbridge, J., et al. (2010). Methadone dose and neonatal abstinence syndrome-systemic review and meta-analysis. *Addiction, 105*(12), 2071–2084.

Guttmacher Institute. (2016). *Substance abuse during pregnancy. State Policies in Brief.* New York (NY): GI. https://www.guttmacher.org/state-policy/explore/substance-abuse-during-pregnancy.

Jone, H. E., Kaltenbach, K., Heil, S. H., et al. (2010). Neonatal abstinence syndrome after methadone or buprenorphine exposure. *The New England Journal of Medicine, 363*(24), 2320–2331.

Krans, E. E., Cochran, G., & Bogen, D. L. (2015). Caring for opioid dependent pregnant women: prenatal and postpartum care considerations. *Clinical Obstetrics and Gynecology, 58*(2), 370–379.

Stewart, R. D., Nelson, D. B., Adhikari, E. H., et al. (2013). The obstetrical and neonatal impact of maternal opioid detoxification in pregnancy. *American Journal of Obstetrics and Gynecology, 209*(3), 267 e1–e5.

Stover, M. W., & Davis, J. M. (2015). Opioids in pregnancy and neonatal abstinence syndrome. *Seminars in Perinatology, 39*(7), 561–565.

Vera von Bergen, MD

A 29-Year-Old G1P0 Woman With Hypothyroidism in Pregnancy

A 29-year-old G1P0 woman at 10 weeks gestational age is evaluated at the doctor's office with constipation and cold intolerance. Upon further questioning, her review of systems is positive for fatigue, muscle cramps, and weight gain. She has no past medical history. Her medications include prenatal vitamins, which she started taking 2 weeks ago.

What important questions should be asked to rule out other diagnoses?
A full medical history should be obtained including when her symptoms started. A list of medications she has taken in the past should also be obtained. A depression screening should be performed for this patient, given her symptoms. Further workup into her constipation is also warranted. Constipation can be common from prenatal vitamins (specifically associated with some forms of iron supplementation). Constipation is also common in pregnancy due to the hormonal effect of progesterone slowing down the intestines and intestinal compression in the last trimester. It is not common to have excessive weight gain in the first trimester of pregnancy, and this may serve as a red flag for other causes for weight gain. Cold intolerance is very unusual in a normal pregnancy.

On further questioning, the patient tells you that her symptoms started over a year ago. She states that she never made it to a physician for a checkup until she found out she was pregnant. She has never taken any prescription medications in the past. She denies any feelings of hopelessness or helplessness. She states that she is able to sleep well. She drinks eight glasses of water a day. Her constipation was present before she started taking her prenatal vitamins and before she found out she was pregnant. She has noticed a 15.9 kg (35-lb) weight gain over the past 6 months.

Findings: Her temperature is 36.7°C (98°F), blood pressure is 91/61 mm Hg, heart rate is 55/min, and respiration rate is 18/min; her body mass index is 37 kg/m². On physical examination she has edema, dry hair, and hair loss. Her thyroid exam in benign. Cardiac examination is normal except for slow heart rate. Respiratory examination is normal. Neurological examination demonstrates prolonged relaxation phase of her deep tendon reflexes.

What is your differential diagnosis at this point?
In a pregnant female with no past medical history and constipation, weight gain, cold intolerance, and fatigue, underactive thyroid disease should be at the top of the differential diagnosis. For many women, their first visit to a physician occurs when they find out they are pregnant. It is important to screen women for other medical conditions at their prenatal visits if their symptoms warrant further workup.

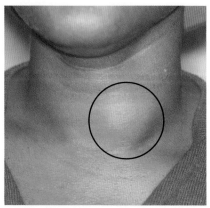

Fig. 10.1   A goiter caused by iodine deficiency in a pregnant woman (*circle*). *(From Castro L, Gambone J. Common medical and surgical conditions complicating pregnancy. In: Hacker & Moore's essentials of obstetrics and gynecology. 2016;201–23. https://www.clinicalkey.com/#!/content/book/3-s2.0-B97814557 75583000164?scrollTo=%233-s2.0-B9781455775583000164-f016-001-9781455775583)*

Does the thyroid exam have to be abnormal for thyroid disease?

On physical exam, a goiter is not always present for hypothyroidism. Goiters are more likely to be found in women with Hashimoto's thyroiditis (Fig. 10.1).

Hashimoto's thyroiditis is thought to be the most common cause of hypothyroidism in the United States. It is an autoimmune condition in which the thyroid gland does not produce enough thyroid hormone. Hashimoto's thyroiditis is diagnosed through serum testing for thyroid peroxidase antibodies.

What if a palpable nodule was noted on her thyroid exam?

Findings of a palpable solitary thyroid nodule during physical examination in pregnancy occurs in 1%–2% of patients. The risk of malignancy is 5%–43%, depending on whether or not there was prior radiation exposure, the patient's age, and the rate of growth. Solitary thyroid nodules are managed with a complete history and physical examination, serum TSH testing, and an ultrasound of the neck. Ultrasonographic characteristics associated with malignancy including hypoechoic pattern, irregular margins, and microcalcifications. If findings of ultrasound are suggestive of malignancy, fine-needle aspiration is warranted with testing for histologic tumor markers and immunostaining.

CLINICAL PEARL   **STEPS 2/3**

Radioactive iodine should not be administered in pregnancy or during breastfeeding because it crosses the placenta and can damage the fetal thyroid gland and is excreted in breast milk. If thyroid malignancy is diagnosed during the first or second trimester by fine-needle aspiration, thyroidectomy may be performed.

The ideal time for surgery during pregnancy is during the second trimester. Due to the possibility of accidental removal of parathyroid glands with thyroidectomy, many women and physicians delay surgery until after delivery. Surgical treatment is deferred to the immediate postpartum period for those diagnosed with thyroid cancer in the third trimester.

In addition to her prenatal labs and a dating ultrasound to confirm her due date, TSH level testing is indicated with a reflex free T4. Laboratory testing demonstrates a TSH level of 40 mIU/L and a reflex free T4 of 0.01 ng/dL.

CLINICAL PEARL   **STEPS 2/3**

Universal screening for thyroid disease in pregnancy is not recommended. Testing is only recommended for those at increased risk of overt hypothyroidism with a personal history of thyroid disease or symptoms of thyroid disease.

The first-line screening laboratory test is TSH. When the TSH is abnormally low or high (>0.1 mIU/L or >2.5 mIU/L in the first trimester), a follow-up free T4 level should be performed (Table 10.1). Measurement of antithyroid antibodies with overt thyroid disease is not generally recommended in pregnancy. Other lab abnormalities seen with overt hypothyroidism include hyponatremia, a macrocytic or normochromic normocytic anemia, hyperlipidemia, and elevated creatine phosphokinase. The anemia is generally due to decreased erythropoiesis but may reflect vitamin B_{12}, folic acid, or iron deficiency. If hyponatremia is noted, hypothyroidism should be in the differential diagnosis.

TABLE 10.1 ■ **Normal Values of Thyroid-Stimulating Hormone (TSH) by Trimester**

First trimester	0.1–2.5 mIU/L
Second trimester	0.2–3.0 mIU/L
Third trimester	0.3–3.0 mIU/L

CLINICAL PEARL   **STEPS 2/3**

Subclinical hypothyroidism is indicated by an elevated TSH level with a normal free T4 level. This occurs in 2%–5% of pregnancies. This is unlikely to progress to overt hypothyroidism during pregnancy, and treatment of subclinical hypothyroidism during pregnancy is not recommended.

Diagnosis: Overt hypothyroidism of pregnancy.

CLINICAL PEARL   **STEPS 2/3**

Worldwide, the most common cause for hypothyroidism is iodine deficiency. The most common cause for hypothyroidism in the United States is Hashimoto's thyroiditis.

What changes in the thyroid occur in pregnancy?

Physiologic thyroid changes occur during pregnancy and result in corresponding changes in thyroid laboratory tests (Table 10.2). Maternal thyroid volume grows 30% larger in the third trimester than in the first trimester. First, maternal thyroid-binding globulin increases in pregnancy, with an increase in maternal total or bound thyroid hormone. Second, TSH decreases in early pregnancy because of the weak stimulation of TSH receptors caused by elevated human chorionic

TABLE 10.2 ■ **Changes in Thyroid Function Test Results in Normal Pregnancy in Thyroid Disease**

Maternal Status	TSH	Free T4
Pregnancy	Varies by trimester	No change
Overt hyperthyroidism	Decrease	Increase
Subclinical hyperthyroidism	Decrease	No change
Overt hypothyroidism	Increase	Decrease
Subclinical hypothyroidism	Increase	No change

T4, Thyroxine; *TSH*, thyroid-stimulating hormone.

gonadotropin during the first 12 weeks of gestation. This leads to an increase in thyroid hormone secretion. The increased free thyroxine levels suppress the thyrotropin-releasing hormone (TRH) and limit further TSH secretion. After the first trimester, TSH returns to baseline and then increases in the third trimester due to placental growth and production of placental deiodinase. TSH does not cross the placenta and has no direct fetal effect.

How important is treatment for overt hypothyroidism in pregnancy?

During the first 12 weeks of gestation, maternal thyroxine is vitally important for normal fetal brain development. The fetal gland starts synthesizing thyroid hormone after 12 weeks' gestation.

Treatment of hypothyroidism is T4 replacement therapy, beginning with levothyroxine in dosages of 1–2 μg/kg per day or 100 μg daily.

What can happen if overt hypothyroidism is not treated in pregnancy?

Hypothyroidism warrants treatment in pregnancy, and adverse perinatal outcomes such as spontaneous abortion, preeclampsia, preterm birth, placental abruption, and intrauterine fetal demise may occur if the condition is left untreated. There is a significant increased rate of low birth weight and impaired neuropsychological development of the fetus without treatment.

How would you approach treatment?

With overt hypothyroidism, levothyroxine synthetic T4 replacement therapy, beginning in dosages of 1–2 μg/kg per or 100 μg daily is initiated. It takes 6–8 weeks of therapy for maximum effects. Liothyronine T3 replacement is three to four times more potent than levothyroxine; it has a shorter half-life of 24 hours and is not routinely used due to more frequent dosing requirements. Desiccated thyroid is obtained from animal sources and is less expensive than synthetic sources; however, due to protein antigenicity and product instability it is more difficult to monitor in the laboratory.

How do you adjust medication during pregnancy?

Treatment of hypothyroidism in pregnancy is initiated upon diagnosis. Therapy is then guided by measurement of TSH levels, with the dose of levothyroxine adjusted accordingly. TSH levels should be measured at 4- to 6-week intervals, with the dose adjusted by 25-μg to 50-μg increments. The goal is a normal TSH level. In women with a history of thyroidectomy or prior radioiodine ablation, it is recommended to anticipate at 25% increase in T4 replacement in pregnancy due to a pregnancy-related increase T4 requirement in one-third of supplemented women.

Due to medication interactions, is it recommended to administer thyroxine on an empty stomach, either 1 hour before meals, 4 hours after meals, or at bedtime. Also, thyroxine should be separated from prenatal vitamins and ferrous sulfate by at least 2–4 hours. Certain foods (e.g., bran, soy, coffee), calcium, vitamins, and certain drugs can interfere with intestinal absorption. The half-life of levothyroxine is 7 days, allowing for daily dosing.

> The patient is now in her third trimester and is experiencing nervousness, heat intolerance, episodes of palpitations, and tachycardia, with no weight gain over the past month.

What do you do if she experiencing symptoms of overtreatment?

These findings in our patient are concerning since they are symptom of excess thyroxine blood levels and overtreatment with T4. It will be important to monitor her serum TSH and free T4 levels for confirmation and to decrease her medication if warranted. Chronic overtreatment of hypothyroidism, especially in elderly patients, can increase the risk of atrial fibrillation and accelerated osteoporosis.

What nutritional requirements are there in pregnancy related to the thyroid?

Adequate maternal iodine intake is needed for maternal and fetal synthesis of T4. The recommended daily dietary intake of iodine is 150 μg outside of pregnancy. The recommended daily dietary intake of iodine increases to 220 μg for pregnant women and 290 μg for lactating women. Iodine is not found in all supplemental multivitamins, including prenatal vitamins, but it is found in many foods including seaweed, seafood, and plain yogurts. Iodine requirements increase in pregnancy due to increased thyroid hormone production, increased renal losses, and fetal iodine requirements. The World Health Organization has estimated that at least 50 million people worldwide have preventable brain damage due to iodine deficiency.

What is the patient's prognosis?

Complications from overt hypothyroidism of pregnancy are rare. The treatment dosage postpartum is reduced to the prepregnancy amount if applicable, and the TSH is measured 4–8 weeks postpartum.

Postpartum thyroiditis occurs in 5%–10% of women in the first year postpartum. Women with type 1 diabetes are three times more likely to develop this complication. Women with high thyroid autoimmune antibodies are affected. Symptoms include fatigue, palpitations, heat intolerance, and nervousness in the first phase. This phase lasts for 1–4 months and is destruction-induced thyrotoxicosis. Elevated free T4 and suppressed TSH are commonly seen on lab tests. Postpartum thyroiditis generally has an abrupt onset, with goiter sometimes present. Between 4 and 8 months, one-third of patients will have hypothyroidism. One-third of these patients will have permanent hypothyroidism. The course of postpartum thyroiditis varies, with some patients only experiencing a hyperthyroid phase and others only the hypothyroid phase.

Maternal thyroid inhibitory antibodies cross the placenta and cause fetal hypothyroidism in 1 out of 180,000 patients, a condition also known as *cretinism*. Newborn screening for congenital hypothyroidism has been implemented since 1974.

Myxedema coma is extremely rare in pregnancy and is an end state of untreated hypothyroidism. Patients present with altered mental status, weakness, hypothermia, hyperventilation, hypoglycemia, hyponatremia, shock, and death. It is a medical emergency requiring an intensive care unit stay and aggressive cardiopulmonary support. Patients with myxedema coma absorb

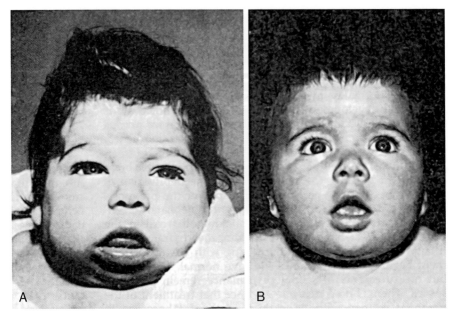

Fig. 10.2   Congenital hypothyroidism in an infant 6 months of age. The infant ate poorly in the neonatal period and was constipated. She had a persistent nasal discharge and a large tongue; she was very lethargic and had no social smile and no head control. A. Notice the puffy face, dull expression, and hirsute forehead. B. Four months after treatment, note the decreased puffiness of the face, the decreased hirsutism of the forehead, and alert appearance. *(From LaFranchi, S, Huang S. Hypothyrodism. Nelson textbook of pediatrics. 2016;2665–75. https://www.clinicalkey.com/#!/content/book/3-s2.0-B9781455775668005652?scroll To=%233-s2.0-B9781455775668005652-f565-001ab-9781455775668)*

drugs poorly from routes other than intravenous. Intravenous levothyroxine 300–400 μg initially followed by 50 to 100 μg daily is the recommended treatment. Intravenous opioids and sedatives should be used with extreme caution.

CLINICAL PEARL	STEPS 2/3

Outside of pregnancy, menstrual irregularities including anovulatory bleeding, heavy menstrual bleeding, and irregular menstrual bleeding can also be associated with hypothyroidism.

Case Summary

- A 29-year-old G1P0 woman presents at 10 weeks gestational age with constipation and cold intolerance. Upon further questioning, her review of systems is positive for fatigue, constipation, cold intolerance, muscle cramps, and weight gain. Her medications include prenatal vitamins, which she started taking 2 weeks ago.
- On physical exam she has edema, dry hair, hair loss, and a prolonged relaxation phase of her deep tendon reflexes. Her thyroid exam in benign.
- Laboratory testing demonstrates a TSH level of 40 mIU/L and a reflex free T4 of 0.01 ng/dL.
- The diagnosis is overt hypothyroidism of pregnancy.
- T4 replacement therapy, beginning with levothyroxine in dosages of 1–2 μg/kg per day or 100 μg daily is initiated.

References

American College of Obstetricians and Gynecologists (2015). Thyroid disease in pregnancy. Practice bulletin no. 148. *Obstetrics and Gynecology, 125*(4), 996–1005.

Bannerman, C. (2013). Thyroid and other endocrine disorders during pregnancy. In A. H. DeCherney, L. Nathan, N. Laufer, & A. S. Roman (Eds.), *CURRENT diagnosis and treatment: obstetrics and gynecology* (11th ed.). New York: McGraw-Hill. Available at: http://accessmedicine.mhmedical.com.ezproxyhost. library.tmc.edu/content.aspx?bookid=498&Sectionid=41008623.

Cunningham, F., Leveno, K. J., Bloom, S. L., et al. (Eds.). (2013). *Williams obstetrics* (24th ed.) New York: McGraw-Hill. Available at: http://accessmedicine.mhmedical.com.ezproxyhost.library.tmc.edu/content. aspx?bookid=1057&Sectionid=59789203.

Dong, B. J., & Greenspan, F. S. (2015). Thyroid and antithyroid drugs. In B. G. Katzung, & A. J. Trevor (Eds.), *Basic and clinical pharmacology* (13th ed.). New York: McGraw-Hill. Available at: http://accessmedic ine.mhmedical.com.ezproxyhost.library.tmc.edu/content.aspx?bookid=1193&Sectionid=69109748.

Nevena Krstic, MS, CGC ■ Aarti Ramdaney, MS, CGC

A 30-Year-Old Woman Undergoes Carrier Screening

A 30-year-old nulliparous Caucasian woman comes in for her routine gynecology appointment. She tells you that she would like to discontinue her birth control as she and her partner are planning to become pregnant in the next year. The patient says that one of her family members has cystic fibrosis (CF).

When is the optimal time to discuss the reported family history?
The ideal time to discuss potential genetic risk factors that may affect a pregnancy is actually before a pregnancy is achieved. During a preconception visit it is important to discuss routine screening options but also to obtain the patient's and her partner's personal, family, and pregnancy history to provide the couple with a personalized risk assessment and testing options. By having this conversation before a pregnancy, the patient or the couple can obtain information on their personal risk factors and be able to make the most informed decisions regarding their care and management.

What genetic testing is typically available in the preconception period?
Carrier screening for specific inherited genetic conditions, meant to identify couples at risk of passing on a genetic condition to their children, is available to all couples of reproductive age. Carrier screening for specific genetic conditions has traditionally been based on personal or family history or, in absence of family history, based on an individual's ancestry. However, with advances in screening technology and an increasingly multiethnic society, carrier screening is expanding to include multitudes of inherited genetic conditions. If carrier screening is done before pregnancy, couples have a broader range of options and more time for decision-making.

Upon review of the family history the patient tells you that the relative in question is her brother and that he was diagnosed at delivery with classic CF. The patient reports that no one in the family had previously had the condition and that the diagnosis had been very shocking. She tells you that she is very worried that her future children will also have the condition.

What is CF?
CF is an inherited disease characterized by the buildup of mucus that can damage many of the body's organs. The most common signs and symptoms of the disorder include progressive damage to the respiratory system and chronic digestive system problems, although the severity varies from classic CF to nonclassic CF. Intelligence is not affected. CF is inherited in an autosomal recessive manner and is caused by mutations in the CFTR gene. Severity is typically dependent on the type of mutations in the CFTR gene. CF is most common in the Caucasian population, with 1 in 25 individuals being a carrier, although it does occur in all ethnicity groups. As such, CF carrier screening is recommended by the American Congress of Obstetricians and Gynecologists

(ACOG) and the American College of Medical Geneticists (ACMG) for all individuals. CF is also screened for by state newborn screens.

BASIC SCIENCE PEARL	STEP 1

What is Autosomal Recessive Inheritance?

Autosomal recessive inheritance is one of several ways that a trait, disorder, or disease can be passed down through families. All individuals have two copies of every gene; we inherit one copy from our mother and one from our father. For conditions that follow autosomal recessive inheritance, both copies must have a mutation in order for the disease or trait to develop. This typically occurs when both parents of the affected individual are carriers of the condition—have one mutated gene and one normal gene—and both pass down the mutated gene. Carriers typically do not exhibit any symptoms. Autosomal recessive inheritance differs from autosomal dominant inheritance, in which only one copy of a gene must have a mutation in order for the disease or trait to develop. Autosomal recessive disorders are typically not seen in every generation of an affected family; instead, the mutation travels unobserved within a family and is expressed by one child or multiple siblings in a single generation. Examples of some diseases that follow autosomal recessive inheritance include CF, sickle-cell anemia, Tay-Sachs disease, and phenylketonuria.

CLINICAL PEARL	STEPS 2/3

What is Newborn Screening?

The purpose of newborn screening (NBS) is to evaluate newborns for serious, treatable inherited genetic disorders in order to facilitate and expedite diagnostic testing and interventions to prevent or minimize adverse outcomes. NBS is state mandated for every newborn and is composed of three parts: a "heel stick" to collect a small blood sample, pulse oximetry to look at the amount of oxygen in the baby's blood, and a hearing screen. All three parts are done within 48 hours of birth, and a few states may recommend a second sample several days later. While the U.S. Health Resources and Services Administration recommends uniform screening for at least 32 core genetic disorders and 26 secondary disorders, because NBS is state-mandated, the number of health conditions screened in each state varies. It is important to be aware of what conditions are screened for in your state. NBS does not replace carrier screening for parents. While in some states the carrier status of a newborn may be reported, NBS is designed to detect affected individuals, and, in an unaffected newborn, it may provide no information regarding the carrier status of the parents.

What is this patient's risk to be a carrier and have a child with CF?

Given that the patient's brother has CF, both of her parents are considered obligate carriers of CF. Using the Punnett Square (Table 11.1), carriers of the condition have a 1 in 4 (25%) chance of having a child with no mutations in the CFTR gene, a 1 in 2 (50%) chance of having a child who has one mutation and is a carrier of the condition, and a 1 in 4 (25%) chance of having a child with two mutations who would have CF. As the patient herself does not have CF, her risk of being a carrier is 2 in 3.

The risk for the patient's pregnancy to result in CF would depend on her partner's carrier status. Because CF is autosomal recessive, the only way the baby would be at risk of having CF is if both the patient and her partner are carriers of CF. If he has no previous family history of CF, his chance of being a carrier would depend on his ethnicity. (Table 11.2) He is reported to be of Hispanic ethnicity. The risk number can be obtained by multiplying the patient's chance of being a carrier (2/3) by the chance of the partner to be a carrier (1/58, based on his Hispanic ethnicity) by the chance of both passing on the genes with the mutation (1/4). Therefore, current risk for the patient to have a child with CF is 1/348.

TABLE 11.1 ■ Punnett Square Representing the Probability of a Specific Outcome for a Couple Who Are Both Carriers of Cystic Fibrosis (CF)

		Mother	
		A	A
Father	A	AA	Aa
	a	Aa	Aa

The uppercase A represents the nonmutated gene while the lowercase a is the mutated gene. Of note, the 1 in 4 (25%) risk in each pregnancy for CF applies regardless of previous pregnancy outcomes.

TABLE 11.2 ■ Cystic Fibrosis (CF) Carrier Frequencies Based on Ethnicity and Estimated Residual Risks Following 23-Mutation Panel Testing, as Reported by ACOG's Committee Opinion in 2011 (Reaffirmed in 2014)

Reported Ethnicity	Carrier Risk Before Testing	Estimated Detection Rate (%)	Residual Risk
Ashkenazi Jewish	1/24	94	1/380
Caucasian	1/25	88	1/200
Hispanic	1/58	72	1/200
African American	1/61	64	1/170
Asian American	1/94	49	1/180

Of note, the detection rate of various genotyping panels may vary between laboratories.

What testing should be offered to this patient?

Carrier screening for CF should be recommended. Given that the patient reported a family member diagnosed with the condition, it would be beneficial to ask if genetic testing was pursued to confirm the diagnosis. This would be beneficial in that there are more than 1700 different mutations that cause CF; if the mutations in her brother are known, it can be ensured that they would be detected by the testing offered to the patient.

Carrier screening is typically performed through "molecular" testing, and laboratories that offer carrier screening often use different molecular technologies, which can influence the detection rate and residual risk. The most common testing is *genotyping*, which determines a specific genetic variant or mutation an individual possesses. Most laboratories use genotyping to screen for a panel of the most common variants of a particular condition. ACOG recommends genotyping for 23 specific mutations in the CFTR gene. Because some mutations are more frequently found in specific ethnicities, the detection rate will vary by ethnicity. CF genotyping is most informative in the Caucasian and Ashkenazi Jewish population but has lower detection rates in individuals of other backgrounds. If her brother's genetic testing results are available and we know the specific mutations he has, we can also do *targeted genotyping* and only test the patient for those two specific mutations.

If her brother's genetic testing results are not available, carrier screening for CF can still be pursued, but the limitations and residual risk of being a carrier should be further discussed. In this case carrier screening via sequencing may be a better option. *Sequencing* is a method used to determine the exact sequence of a certain length of DNA and determines any genetic variant, common or rare, that an individual has. Sequencing is much more comprehensive than genotyping and provides a higher detection rate regardless of ethnicity, although it often comes at an increased cost. Sequencing may not always be appropriate for routine carrier screening because it may yield results that can be difficult to interpret, producing a situation referred to as a *variant of unknown significance*. Sequencing is generally offered for patients suspected of having CF, patients with a family history of CF, males with congenital bilateral absence of the vas deferens, and women carrying pregnancies with specific ultrasound findings concerning for CF.

Should you offer carrier screening for additional conditions?

As previously discussed, screening has traditionally been driven by family history and/or specific ethnicity. Various professional societies have recommendations or guidelines on carrier screening, but screening for additional conditions should be based on the couple's personal values and preferences in the presence of thorough counseling. Carrier screening should always remain voluntary, and patients have the right to decline screening at any time.

Currently, both ACOG and ACMG recommend CF screening to be offered for all women of reproductive age regardless of ethnicity. In addition to CF, carrier screening for Tay-Sachs' disease, Canavan's disease, and familial dysautonomia is recommended by ACOG and ACMG for individuals of Ashkenazi Jewish or Eastern European Jewish ancestry. ACMG recommends additional screening for the Ashkenazi Jewish population for mucolipidosis IV, Niemann-Pick disease type A, Fanconi anemia group C, Bloom's syndrome, and Gaucher's disease. ACMG also recommends routine carrier screening for spinal muscular atrophy (SMA) because the condition is present in all ethnic groups with a carrier frequency of approximately 1 in 40. ACOG recommends screening for hemoglobinopathies via electrophoresis for all individuals of African ancestry and individuals of Asian and Mediterranean ancestry who have had an abnormal complete blood count. This is often referred to as *ethnicity-based* or *traditional carrier screening,* and all of these conditions are inherited in an autosomal recessive manner.

What is important to keep in mind is that not all carrier screens that are commercially available are created equal. The majority of commercial laboratories offer "ACOG/ACMG" panels that test for some combination of the mentioned conditions. However, the conditions included on the ACOG/ACMG panel varies widely, as well as the methodology of testing (sequencing vs. genotyping vs. other biochemical testing). One example is the screen for an X-linked condition called fragile X syndrome. Fragile X carrier screening is not recommended by ACOG or ACMG for the general population and only recommended for those with a family history of unexplained intellectual disability, developmental delay, autism, and/or primary ovarian insufficiency. Women who do not meet that criteria may still request fragile X carrier screening, and genetic counseling is recommended to discuss the risks, benefits, and limitations of screening. However, fragile X is often included on ACOG/ACMG panels.

With advances in screening technology and an increasingly multiethnic society, carrier screening is expanding to include multitudes of inherited genetic conditions. This is often referred to as *expanded* or *universal carrier screening* and typically screens for hundreds of conditions regardless of ethnicity. There are advantages to offering carrier screening for the same set of diseases to all patients because it increases the information available to patients and does not solely rely on what may be inaccurate reporting of ethnicity and family history. However, it is also important to acknowledge that some of the conditions on these panels may not be fully understood in terms of population frequency, known detection rate, and natural history. Expanded carrier screens typically utilize a technology referred to as *next generation sequencing* (NGS) and thus there is also the potential of identifying variants of unknown clinical significance. Such variants may not have any clinical management recommendations but can lead to an unclear risk assessment for a pregnancy and increase parental anxiety. ACOG and ACMG, along with three other medical societies (National Society of Genetic Counselors, Society for Maternal-Fetal Medicine, and Perinatal Quality Foundation) published a joint statement in 2015 on the value and concerns of expanded carrier screening that health care providers should take into account as they consider offering such screening.

CLINICAL PEARL   **STEPS 2/3**

When is Molecular Testing Not Enough?
Genotyping or sequencing panels are not the most appropriate test for all types of genetic conditions and for all ethnicities. Screening for hemoglobinopathies is best performed using red cell indices on the complete blood count (CBC) and hemoglobin electrophoresis given that not every clinically significant mutation in the β-chain is found on a molecular-based test, and α-chain deletions are not screened for by every carrier panel. Screening for Tay-Sachs disease is performed most efficiently using hexosaminidase A enzyme analysis for ethnic groups with low carrier frequency (non-Ashkenazi Jewish). Therefore, it is not only important to keep in mind the conditions tested for on a panel, but also the methodology utilized for testing. It may be necessary to order two or three separate tests for an individual patient. While this may be inconvenient for the practitioner and patient, it will ensure that the patient is receiving the most appropriate and comprehensive screening.

The patient reports that she does not have any record of her brother's genetic testing results. She decides to pursue carrier screening via an ACOG/ACMG panel that assesses for CF by sequencing the CFTR gene as well as tests for SMA and fragile X syndrome. CF carrier screening identifies the patient as a carrier for the common δ-F508 mutation in CF.

Based on these results, what is this patient's risk of having an affected child with CF?
Given these results, the risk assessment has changed, and we would now assign a 1/1 (100%) chance for the patient to be a carrier of CF. However, the risk to the pregnancy is still dependent on the partner's carrier status, which is unknown. Therefore, current risk for the patient to have a child with CF is calculated at 1/232.

You inform the patient of these results, and the patient expresses to you that she is concerned about the 1/232 risk. She speaks to her partner, and the couple decides that they want to proceed with CF carrier screening for the partner.

What CF carrier screening, genotyping, or sequencing would you offer to the partner?
A referral to a genetics professional, such as a genetic counselor, should be considered in this situation to determine, in conference with the couple, the value of carrier screening via sequencing versus genotyping. Both of the screening options would be offered to the patient and the benefits and limitations of each methodology reviewed. Given that her partner is of Hispanic ethnicity, performing CF carrier screening via an ACOG-recommended genotyping panel will have a lower detection rate for CF, with a residual risk of approximately 1/200 if he screens negative compared to the current carrier risk of 1/58.

CF carrier screening via sequencing would produce a much higher detection rate and lower residual risk after a negative test, but it carries the risk of detecting variants of unknown significance which may be difficult to interpret. Additionally, sequencing often comes with a higher cost and lower insurance coverage.

| BASIC SCIENCE PEARL | STEP 1 |

What is Residual Risk?

Residual risk is the risk that remains after a negative test result. Given that carrier screening is not 100% accurate, it is possible for it to miss a mutation. Calculating residual risks is easy if the carrier frequency and detection rate is established for a particular disorder and can be done by using the following formula: (carrier frequency × [1 − detection rate]). Calculating the residual risk becomes more complicated, however, when conditions are rare and an exact carrier frequency or detection rate is not known. When counseling patients on negative carrier screening results it is important to emphasize that although a negative carrier screening result reduces the patient's chance to be a carrier, it is still possible to be a carrier and have an affected child.

In addition to being identified as a carrier of CF the patient is also revealed as an intermediate or "gray zone" carrier for fragile X syndrome with 52 and 30 CGG repeats (Table 11.3).

What is fragile X syndrome?

Fragile X syndrome is a genetic condition that causes a range of developmental problems including learning disabilities and cognitive impairment. Individuals with the condition can also develop seizures and have distinctive physical features that may become more apparent with age. Fragile X syndrome is the most common cause of inherited learning disabilities in males and occurs in approximately 1 in 4000 males and 1 in 8000 females. Nearly all cases of fragile X syndrome are caused by a mutation in which a DNA segment, known as the CGG triplet repeat, is expanded within the FMR1 gene on the X chromosome. Normally, this DNA segment is repeated from 5 to about 40 times. In individuals with fragile X syndrome, the CGG segment is repeated more than 200 times, and this leads to loss of certain protein functions. Loss or a shortage of this specific protein disrupts nervous system functions and leads to the signs and symptoms of fragile X syndrome.

Should you offer to test the patient's partner to see if he is a carrier for fragile X syndrome?

The vast majority of conditions on carrier screening are autosomal recessive, meaning that both parents must be carriers for a pregnancy to be at risk. Fragile X syndrome is an exception because it follows an X-linked inheritance pattern and only the mother has to be a carrier for a pregnancy to be at risk. There is a 50% chance that a mother will pass on the X chromosome with the abnormal number of CGG repeats. What is unique about triple repeat conditions, such as fragile X, is that the number of repeats can expand when passed on to the next generation. The risk for an expansion to more than 200 repeats depends on the number of maternal repeats.

TABLE 11.3 ■ **Risk of Expansion to Fragile X Syndrome Given Number of Maternal CGG Repeats, as Reported by ACOG's Committee Opinion in 2010 (Reaffirmed in 2014)**

Maternal Repeat Size (CGG)	Chance for Expansion to Full (200 CGG) Mutation (%)
55–59	4
60–69	5
70–79	31
80–89	58
90–99	80
100–200	98

BASIC SCIENCE PEARL   **STEP 1**

What is X-Linked Inheritance?

Disorders that follow X-linked inheritance are caused by mutations in genes on the X chromosome, which is one of the two sex chromosomes in each cell. Females have two X chromosomes while males have an X and Y chromosome. Males with an X-linked disorder typically have more severe symptoms given that they only have one X chromosome; however, females can manifest symptoms and be affected to the same degree as their male counterparts. Females with an X-linked disorder have a 1 in 2 (50%) risk of passing down the affected X chromosome to a male or female child. A distinct characteristic of X-linked inheritance is that fathers cannot pass the affected X chromosome to their sons (no male-to-male transmission), but all their daughters will be carriers. Some examples of X-linked disorders are fragile X syndrome, Duchenne muscular dystrophy, and hemophilia A and B.

What does it mean to be an intermediate carrier for fragile X?

Patients can either be intermediate or premutation carriers of fragile X. The key difference is the number of CGG repeats an individual possesses. Males and females with 55 to 200 repeats of the CGG segment are called *premutation carriers*. Most people with a premutation are intellectually normal and may not have any previous family history associated with fragile X syndrome. In some cases, however, individuals with a premutation can have mild versions of the physical features seen in fragile X syndrome and may experience emotional concerns, such as anxiety or depression. Some children with a premutation may also have learning disabilities or autistic-like behavior. The premutation is also associated with an increased risk of disorders called fragile X-associated primary ovarian insufficiency (FXPOI) and fragile X-associated tremor/ataxia syndrome (FXTAS). Female permutation carriers are at risk of having a child with fragile X syndrome, and preimplantation genetic diagnosis (PGD) and/or prenatal testing should be offered.

Individuals who have 45 to 54 repeats are considered to be *intermediate carriers* or in the "gray zone." These individuals typically do not have any signs or symptoms and are not at risk for other associated disorders. Women identified in the gray zone *are not* at risk of having a child with fragile X syndrome, but have up to a 50% risk of having children who are premutation carriers. PGD or prenatal diagnosis is not typically offered.

CLINICAL PEARL   **STEPS 2/3**

What is PGD?

Currently, PGD is the only way to predict whether an embryo is affected with a genetic condition prior to achieving pregnancy. PGD involves testing embryos prior to transfer to the woman's uterus. Embryos are obtained through in-vitro fertilization (IVF), and one cell is removed from each embryo and tested for the presence or absence of the specific mutations. Only embryos that do not carry mutation(s) tested for would be transferred to achieve pregnancy. PGD is expected to have a greater than 90% accuracy rate, but this may depend on the condition. PGD does not, however, replace prenatal diagnostic testing such as chorionic villus sampling (CVS)/amniocentesis, and diagnostic testing is recommended following PGD.

Is testing for fragile X syndrome recommended at delivery?

If a woman who is an intermediate carrier does not pursue preconception testing or prenatal diagnosis, fragile X carrier testing would only be necessary in childhood if a child shows signs or symptoms of fragile X syndrome. Otherwise, testing would be recommended once a child reaches reproductive age so that he or she can make informed decisions regarding fragile X carrier testing and available testing during pregnancy. Testing of asymptomatic children at delivery or in childhood is not recommended, to respect the autonomy and confidentiality of that child's health; as well, the medical implications of the result may not apply to the child until adulthood, and no interventions may be available until the onset of symptoms.

> The patient's partner elects to proceed with CF carrier screening via genotyping for 23 common mutations due to lack of insurance coverage and associated costs. He is identified as carrying a CF mutation (R334W).

What is the most appropriate next step?

Given that both the patient and her partner are confirmed to be carriers of CF, all of their pregnancies together will have a 1 in 4 (25%) chance of having CF. Remember, however, that symptoms of CF are variable and may depend on the type of mutations in the CFTR gene. Therefore, when a carrier screening result is positive it is important to double check that the reported mutation is known to be pathogenic and to check what the expected phenotype would be when a child inherits a δ-F508 and R334W mutation. While there may be various web-based resources as well as literature to help you determine this information, particularly for well-described conditions such as CF, these resources may be limited for other conditions. Therefore, a referral to a genetics specialist, such as a genetic counselor, is appropriate in this situation.

> Upon review of literature, you find that, in combination, the δ-F508 and R334W mutation cause classic CF symptoms, expected to be similar in severity to the patient's brother's symptoms. The patient and her partner express that they do not wish to have a child with CF.

Should you recommend that they do not attempt a pregnancy?

Couples who are carriers of a recessive condition have several options. While one option is not to pursue a pregnancy, a carrier couple may choose to become pregnant and test the fetus in pregnancy via a diagnostic procedure such as CVS or amniocentesis, electing not to continue the pregnancy if the fetus is affected. Prenatal diagnosis is still recommended and should be offered to couples who choose not to change pregnancy management because the information can be beneficial for preparation purposes. A carrier couple may also choose to pursue IVF with PGD for CF, they may choose to use donor egg or sperm, or to adopt. Because pregnancy and potential termination can be sensitive topics, remember to offer the couple empathy and support on whatever decision they make.

> Although the couple expresses interest in the option for PGD, they are concerned with the financial cost of pursuing IVF. They will try and conceive naturally and make a plan to pursue prenatal diagnosis in the first trimester of pregnancy. You provide them with contact information for a local genetic counselor.

Case Summary
- A 30-year-old nulliparous Caucasian woman expresses plans to become pregnant in the future and reports a family history of CF that should be addressed in the preconception period. Some points to consider are the number and type of conditions the patient should be screened for and the type of technologies utilized by a laboratory that would be most informative and appropriate.

- Carrier screening reveals that the patient is a carrier for CF. The patient's partner also elects to pursue screening for CF to clarify the risk assessment and is revealed to be a carrier. Any pregnancies pursued by the couple will have 1 in 4 (25%) risk of having CF. Testing options would include PGD via IVF and prenatal diagnosis.
- The patient is also revealed to be an intermediate carrier for fragile X syndrome. Given this result, the patient is not at risk of having a child with the disorder, and no further testing is recommended.

References

American Congress of Obstetricians and Gynecologists (ACOG) (2010). Carrier screening for fragile X syndrome. ACOG committee opinion no. 469. *Obstetrics and gynecology, 116*(4), 1008–1010.

American Congress of Obstetricians and Gynecologists (ACOG) (2009). Preconception and prenatal carrier screening for genetic diseases in individuals of Eastern European Jewish descent. ACOG committee opinion no. 442. *Obstetrics and gynecology, 114*(4), 950–953.

American Congress of Obstetricians and Gynecologists (ACOG) (2009). Spinal muscular atrophy. ACOG committee opinion no. 432. *Obstetrics and gynecology, 113*(5), 1194–1196.

American Congress of Obstetricians and Gynecologists (ACOG) (2011). Update on carrier screening for cystic fibrosis. ACOG committee opinion no. 486. *Obstetrics and gynecology, 117*(4), 1028–1031.

Braude, P., Pickering, S., Flinter, F., et al. (2002). Preimplantation genetic diagnosis. *Nature Reviews. Genetics, 3*(12), 941–955.

Edwards, J. G., Feldman, G., Goldberg, J., et al. (2015). Expanded carrier screening in reproductive medicine—points to consider: a joint statement of the American College of Medical Genetics and Genomics, American College of Obstetricians and Gynecologists, National Society of Genetic Counselors, Perinatal Quality Foundation, and Society for Maternal-Fetal Medicine. *Obstetrics and gynecology, 125*(3), 653–662.

Ethics Committee of the American Society for Reproductive Medicine. (2013). Use of preimplantation genetic diagnosis for serious adult onset conditions: a committee opinion. *Fertility and Sterility, 100*(1), 54–57.

Grody, W. W., Cutting, G. R., Klinger, K. W., et al. (2001). Laboratory standards and guidelines for population-based cystic fibrosis carrier screening. *Genetics in Medicine, 3*(2), 149–154.

Grody, W. W., Thompson, B. H., Gregg, A. R., et al. (2013). ACMG position statement on prenatal/preconception expanded carrier screening. *Genetics in Medicine, 15*(6), 482–483.

Gross, S. J., Pletcher, B. A., & Monaghan, K. G. (2008). Carrier screening in individuals of Ashkenazi Jewish descent. *Genetics in Medicine, 10*(1), 54–56.

Grosse, S. D., Boyle, C. A., Botkin, J. R., et al. (2004). Newborn screening for cystic fibrosis: evaluation of benefits and risks and recommendations for state newborn screening programs. *MMWR. Recommendations and Reports, 53*(RR-13), 1–36.

McConkie-Rosell, A., Finucane, B., Cronister, A., et al. (2005). Genetic counseling for fragile X syndrome: updated recommendations of the national society of genetic counselors. *Journal of Genetic Counseling, 14*(4), 249–270.

Pletcher, B. A., & Bocian, M. (2006). Preconception and prenatal testing of biologic fathers for carrier status. *Genetics in medicine, 8*(2), 134–135.

Prior, T. W. (2008). Carrier screening for spinal muscular atrophy. *Genetics in Medicine, 10*(11), 840–842.

Rose, N. C., & Dolan, S. M. (2012). Newborn screening and the obstetrician. *Obstetrics and Gynecology, 120*(4), 908.

Sherman, S., Pletcher, B. A., & Driscoll, D. A. (2005). Fragile X syndrome: diagnostic and carrier testing. *Genetics in medicine, 7*(8), 584–587.

U.S. Department of Health and Human Services. Advisory Committee on Heritable Disorders in Newborns and Children. Available at: http://www. hrsa. gov/advisorycommittees/mchbadvisory/heritabledisorders/index. html.

Watson, M. S., Cutting, G. R., Desnick, R. J., et al. (2004). Cystic fibrosis population carrier screening: 2004 revision of American College of Medical Genetics mutation panel. *Genetics in Medicine, 6*(5), 387–391.

Hind N. Moussa, MD

CASE 12

A 36-Year-Old Woman With Headache in Pregnancy

A 36-year-old African-American G1P0 woman at 33 weeks 2 days gestation presents with worsening headache of 2 days duration. The pain is not severe, but is persistent and is currently affecting her vision. She had migraines in the past and thought she might be having one, but this headache is different and she is having blurry vision rather than her usual photophobia. Her medications include prenatal vitamins and ferrous sulfate.

Why is it important to ask about headache in pregnancy?

Neurologic symptoms in pregnancy and the postpartum period may be caused by exacerbation of a preexisting neurologic condition, the initial presentation of a non–pregnancy-related problem, or the development of a new neurologic problem.

The most common pregnancy-related diagnosis remains preeclampsia. It is estimated that hypertensive disorders of pregnancy complicate about 10% of pregnancies, and preeclampsia complicates about 3% of pregnancies in the United States.

When a woman has headache in pregnancy, what do you need to know about her history? What clues in the history might point toward preeclampsia?

Headache is a symptom. A detailed evaluation should include prior history of headaches, because those may continue during pregnancy. Asking about characteristic symptoms of the headache as well as other associated symptoms is important. Neurologic emergencies should be suspected early, and indications for neuroimaging and lumbar puncture are similar to those in nonpregnant adults.

Careful and detailed history should include prepregnancy hypertension because it is the second most common cause of maternal death in the United States, and African-American women have a fourfold increased mortality rate. The mortality rate is also increased in women over the age of 35.

Preeclampsia must be considered in every pregnant woman over 20 weeks of gestation who presents with headache. This patient, despite a long-standing history of migraine headaches, reports that her headache is different from her typical migraine headache. It is different in nature as well as worsening. Preeclampsia-related headache is typically diffuse, constant, and mild to severe in intensity. Also, the associated visual changes are typical of preeclampsia, with blurry vision or scotomata, and thus support the diagnosis of preeclampsia.

In addition to her headache, what other information should be gathered from this patient?

Symptoms of preeclampsia include cerebral/visual symptoms, severe persistent right upper quadrant/epigastric pain unresponsive to treatment, and pulmonary edema. She should be asked about any recent pain medication intake. In addition, if she complains of any chest pain

---

CLASSIFICATION OF HYPERTENSIVE DISORDERS IN PREGNANCY   BOX 12.1

I. **Gestational hypertension**
   - Systolic <160 mm Hg or
   - Diastolic <110 mm Hg
   No proteinuria *and* no symptoms.
II. Preeclampsia (hypertension ≥20 weeks+ proteinuria)
   Proteinuria Definition:
   ≥300 mg/24 hour
   or
   Protein/creatinine ratio ≥0.30
   or
   ≥1+ on dipstick
III. Preeclampsia with severe features: New-onset hypertension with any of the following
   Severe hypertension:
   - Systolic ≥160 mm Hg *or*
   - Diastolic ≥110 mm Hg
   - Persistently severe cerebral symptoms
   - Thrombocytopenia 100,000/µL
   - Elevated liver enzymes >2× upper limit normal
   - Pulmonary edema
   - Serum creatinine 1.1 mg/dL
IV. Chronic hypertension
   Hypertension before pregnancy
   Hypertension before 20 weeks' gestation
V. Superimposed preeclampsia
   Exacerbation of hypertension
   and/or
   New-onset proteinuria
   and/or
   Sudden increase in proteinuria
VI. Superimposed preeclampsia with severe features: CHTN with any of criteria from III.

**Changes have to be substantial and sustained.

---

or shortness of breath she should be evaluated for pulmonary edema. Edema in dependent and nondependent regions is common in pregnancy and is not an essential diagnostic criterion, although it is commonly present in the setting of preeclampsia. Preeclampsia syndrome can be subdivided into preeclampsia with and without severe features. The distinction between the two is based on the severity of hypertension as well as the involvement of other organ systems. The Task Force on Hypertension in Pregnancy no longer classifies preeclampsia as mild versus severe, but rather by having evidence of hypertensive pathology; its severe form is defined by having severe features (Box 12.1).

Are there any fetal considerations that need to be evaluated?
In regards to fetal outcomes, perinatal mortality and perinatal death are higher in pregnancies complicated by preeclampsia (Box 12.2). Fetal growth restriction is more common with chronic hypertension and is usually associated with superimposed preeclampsia. Fetal assessment should be done through ultrasonographic evaluation of estimated fetal weight and amniotic fluid index, nonstress test (NST), and biophysical profile (BPP). Sonographic evaluation of fetal growth as well as well-being is needed in our patient. In addition, fetal heart tones must be monitored because she is at increased risk for poor uteroplacental perfusion as well as placental abruption.

FETAL-NEONATAL COMPLICATIONS	**BOX 12.2**

- Severe intrauterine growth restriction
- Oligohydramnios
- Preterm delivery
- Hypoxia-acidosis
- Neurologic injury
- Death

On physical exam, the patient has a temperature of 36.5°C (97.8°F), a heart rate of 95/min, an oxygen saturation of 99% on room air, and a blood pressure (BP) of 165/100 mm Hg. She looks uncomfortable, but not in acute distress. Her abdomen is gravid, soft, and nontender to palpation. She has a normal neurologic exam except for brisk deep tendon reflexes. Ultrasound reveals a normally grown fetus, with a BPP of 8/8. Continuous fetal heart rate monitoring is consistent with category I tracing. What would be the next step in the management of this patient?

In the presence of severe hypertension, defined as a systolic BP of 160 mm Hg or higher and/or a diastolic BP of 110 mm Hg or higher, stabilization of maternal status through antihypertensive therapy is recommended. Our patient meets the criteria for medical management of her BP as her systolic BP was persistently elevated above the threshold of 160 mm Hg. The choice of antihypertensive medication should be based on potential adverse effects as well as the clinician's individual experience and familiarity with a particular medication. Intravenous (IV) labetalol, IV hydralazine, and oral nifedipine are first line-agents for lowering BP in the acute hospital settings. Magnesium sulfate should also be administered for the prevention of an eclamptic seizure.

In women with severe preeclampsia and a viable fetus at 33 6/7 weeks or less, it is suggested that glucocorticoids for promotion of fetal lung maturity be used and delivery deferred for 48 hours, without the presence of any contraindications to expectant management or any associated complications. These include pregnancy complications such as preterm premature rupture of membranes, labor, and oligohydramnios. In the same group of patients, it is recommended that delivery not be delayed regardless of gestational age if maternal condition is complicated by uncontrollable severe hypertension, eclampsia, pulmonary edema, abruptio placentae, disseminated intravascular coagulation, evidence of nonreassuring fetal status, or fetal demise.

Directly after her IV access line was inserted and blood drawn for labs the patient becomes unresponsive and starts having tonic-clonic movements.

What is your diagnosis at this time, and how would you manage her?
Eclampsia is defined as preeclampsia accompanied by development of new-onset grand mal seizures or coma during pregnancy or the postpartum period not attributable to other causes. With her new-onset seizure, the patient now meets criteria for eclampsia. Usually eclamptic seizures are short in duration. Prevention of maternal trauma is important. At the bedside, it is important to protect the patient's airway and secure a padded area to protect the patient from trauma. Padded bedrails can be created for the patient. Also, she should be placed in a lateral position, if possible.

Recurrent seizures are prevented through the administration of magnesium sulfate. Since she has an IV access, IV magnesium sulfate is given in a loading as well as a maintenance dose, with

TABLE 12.1 ■ Magnesium Sulfate: Dosages, Serum Levels, and Associated Findings

Magnesium Doses	
Loading dose:	6 g IV over 20–30 min (6 g of 50% solution diluted in 150 mL D$_5$W)
Maintenance dose:	2–3 g IV per hour (40 g in 1 L D$_5$LR at 50 mL/h)
Recurrent seizures:	Reload with 2 g over 5–10 min, 1–2 times and/or 250 mg sodium amobarbital IV

Magnesium Levels and Associated Findings	
Loss of patellar reflexes	8–12 mg/dL
Feeling of warmth, flushing, double vision	9–12 mg/dL
Somnolence	10–12 mg/dL
Slurred speech	10–12 mg/dL
Muscular paralysis	15–17 mg/dL
Respiratory difficulty	15–17 mg/dL
Cardiac arrest	20–35 mg/dL

the plan now to proceed with delivery once stabilized (Table 12.1). Studies on magnesium sulfate for the management and prevention of eclampsia have shown it superior to other anticonvulsants such as phenytoin and diazepam. Patients being treated for eclamptic seizures should receive an IV loading dose of 4–6 g of magnesium sulfate followed by a maintenance dose of 1–2 g/h for at least 24 hours. It is recommended that women with eclampsia should undergo delivery after initial stabilization. If undergoing cesarean delivery, the Task Force recommends intraoperative administration of parenteral magnesium sulfate.

An emergent cesarean delivery was performed once the patient was stabilized. After her delivery, the patient recovers and does not remember much about her antepartum course.

Are there any special considerations for her postpartum care?

Postpartum follow-up is essential for monitoring and management of hypertensive disorders affecting pregnancy. For women in whom gestational hypertension, preeclampsia, or superimposed preeclampsia is diagnosed, it is suggested that BP be monitored in the hospital or that equivalent surveillance be performed at least 72 hours postpartum and again 7–10 days after delivery. For all women in the postpartum period (not just women with preeclampsia), it is suggested that discharge instructions include information about the signs and symptoms of preeclampsia as well as the importance of prompt reporting of this information to their health care providers. For women with persistent postpartum hypertension (BP of 150 mm Hg systolic or higher or 100 mm Hg diastolic or higher on two or more occasions, 4–6 hours or longer apart), antihypertensive therapy is recommended. Persistent BP of 160 mm Hg systolic or 100 mm Hg diastolic or higher should be treated within 1 hour.

What does the patient need to do at home, and can this happen again in a future pregnancy?

It is thought that preeclampsia can develop secondary to alterations in systemic prostacyclin-thromboxane balance. There is also increased inflammation. Therefore, low dose-aspirin (81 mg or less), an antiinflammatory agent blocking thromboxane synthesis, has been shown to be effective for prevention of preeclampsia. For women with a history of early-onset preeclampsia and preterm delivery at less than 34 weeks of gestation or preeclampsia in more than one prior pregnancy, it is recommended to initiate daily low-dose aspirin beginning in the late first trimester. Our patient meets criteria for using baby aspirin for preeclampsia prevention in a future pregnancy.

The administration of vitamin C or vitamin E has not been proved to be of any effect in prevention of preeclampsia. It is recommended that dietary salt not be restricted during pregnancy for the prevention of preeclampsia. Bed rest or physical activity restriction is not recommended for the prevention of preeclampsia and its complications.

Case Summary
- A 36-year-old woman G1P0 at 33 weeks 2 days of gestation presents with worsening headache of 2 days duration. She is also having blurred vision.
- History and physical reveals that the patient has preeclampsia, which is a common yet serious etiology of headache in pregnancy. She is also at less than 34 weeks' gestation and thus requires consideration for expectant management.
- The patient has an eclamptic seizure requiring delivery and further management.
- After her delivery, the patient recovers and has appropriate postpartum follow-up as well as preconceptional counseling for future pregnancy.

BEYOND THE PEARLS

- Preeclampsia must be considered in every pregnant woman of over 20 weeks of gestation with headache.
- Symptoms of preeclampsia include cerebral/visual symptoms, severe persistent right upper quadrant/epigastric pain unresponsive to treatment, and pulmonary edema.
- Preeclampsia syndrome can be subdivided into preeclampsia with and without severe features. The distinction between the two is based on the severity of hypertension as well as the involvement of other organ systems. The Task Force on Hypertension in Pregnancy no longer classifies preeclampsia as mild versus severe, but rather by having evidence of hypertensive pathology; its severe form is defined by having severe features.
- In the presence of severe hypertension, as defined as systolic BP of 160 mm Hg or higher and/or diastolic BP of 110 mm Hg or higher, stabilization of maternal status through antihypertensive therapy is recommended.
- Contraindications to expectant management or any associated complications include pregnancy complications such as preterm premature rupture of membranes, labor, and oligohydramnios. In the same group of patients, it is recommended that delivery not be delayed, regardless of gestational age, if maternal condition is complicated by uncontrollable severe hypertension, eclampsia, pulmonary edema, abruptio placentae, disseminated intravascular coagulation, evidence of nonreassuring fetal status, or fetal demise.

BEYOND THE PEARLS

- Eclampsia is defined as preeclampsia accompanied by development of new-onset grand mal seizures or coma during pregnancy or the postpartum period not attributable to other causes.
- The prevention of recurrent seizure is through the administration of magnesium sulfate.
- Postpartum follow-up is essential for monitoring and management of hypertensive disorders affecting pregnancy.
- For women with a history of early-onset preeclampsia and preterm delivery at less than 34 weeks of gestation or preeclampsia in more than one prior pregnancy, it is recommended to initiate daily low-dose aspirin beginning in the late first trimester.

References

Amro, F. H., Moussa, H. N., Ashimi, O. A., & Sibai, B. M. (2016). Treatment options for hypertension in pregnancy and puerperium. *Expert Opinion on Drug Safety*, *15*(12), 1635–1642.

Gillon, T. E. R., Pels, A., von Dadelszen, P., MacDonell, K., & Magee, L. A. (2014). Hypertensive disorders of pregnancy: a systematic review of international clinical practice guidelines. *PLoS ONE*, *9*(12), e113715.

Moussa, H. N., Ontiveros, A. E., Haidar, Z. A., & Sibai, B. M. (2015). Safety of anticonvulsant agents in pregnancy. *Expert Opinion on Drug Safety*, *14*(10), 1609–1620.

Roberts, J. M., August, P. A., Bakris, G., et al. (2013). Hypertension in pregnancy report of the American College of Obstetricians and Gynecologists' Task Force on hypertension in pregnancy. *Obstetrics and Gynecology*, *122*(5), 1122–1131.

CASE 13

Joey England, MD

A 20-Year-Old Woman With Preterm Premature Rupture of Membranes

A 20-year-old G1P0 woman at 28 weeks' gestation presents to the obstetrical emergency department after experiencing a vaginal gush of fluid.

What is the differential diagnosis during pregnancy for suspected vaginal loss of fluid?
The differential diagnosis includes vaginal infection, preterm premature rupture of membranes (PPROM), recent intercourse, and urinary incontinence.

What is the next step in evaluating this patient?
A thorough history and physical exam should be performed and includes obtaining her vital signs, history of genitourinary infections, history of urinary incontinence, time of last intercourse, and other associated symptoms including fevers or chills, abdominal or pelvic pain, or costovertebral angle tenderness (CVAT, or back pain). Physical exam includes a complete physical with focus on signs of labor (abdominal tenderness, uterine tenderness), back pain or CVAT, and vaginal discharge. A sterile speculum examination should be performed and include collection of vaginal fluid to evaluate for rupture of membranes. Digital cervical exam is avoided if possible due to introduction of vaginal organisms into the cervical canal and increased risk for infection.

CLINICAL PEARL	**STEPS 2/3**

To evaluate for rupture of membranes, vaginal fluid can be tested by:
- Application of Nitrazine paper (turns blue at pH >6); amniotic fluid is basic and usually has a pH of 7.1–7.3 as compared to the vagina's pH of 4.5–6
- Pooling of the amniotic fluid in the vaginal vault
- Expulsion of fluid from the cervix with maternal Valsalva maneuver
- Visualization of ferning (arborized crystals) characteristic of amniotic fluid under microscopy (Fig. 13.1)

Also useful are commercially available point-of-care tests. For example, the rapid slide test for placental α-macroglobulin-1 protein assay (AmniSure) or insulin-like growth factor binding protein 1 (Actim PROM) may be utilized to assess for PPROM; however, in the United States, these are not widely used due to cost and availability.

Vaginal cultures should be obtained to evaluate for the presence of infection including group B streptococci (GBS), trichomonas, yeast, bacterial vaginosis, *Neisseria gonorrhoeae*, or *Chlamydia trachomatis*.

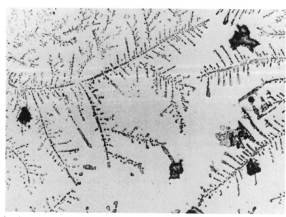

Fig. 13.1 A typical ferning appearance is seen with a vaginal swab and the specimen was smeared on a glass slide and allowed to air dry. The sample was obtained from a patient with premature rupture of the membranes. *(From Mercer B. Premature rupture of the membranes. In: Creasy and Resnik's maternal-fetal medicine: principles and practice. 2014;663–72. https://www.clinicalkey.com/#!/content/book/3-s2.0-B9781455711376000428?scrollTo=%233-s2.0-B9781455711376000428-f042-001-9781455711376)*

You perform a physical exam. Her temperature is 37.1°C (98.8°F), blood pressure is 110/70 mm Hg, pulse is 80/min, respiration rate is 16/min, and oxygen saturation is 99% on room air. She has a normal cardiopulmonary and abdominal exam. Her sterile speculum exam reveals clear pooling fluid in the vaginal vault, with positive fluid extrusion from the cervix upon maternal Valsalva maneuver and absence of bleeding. The cervix appears visually 1 cm dilated. Nitrazine paper turns blue on contact with vaginal fluid, and under microscopy the vaginal fluid is positive for ferning.

CLINICAL PEARL   **STEPS 2/3**

False-positive test results can occur in the presence of blood or semen, alkaline antiseptics, or bacterial vaginosis. False-negative test results can occur with prolonged membrane rupture and minimal vaginal fluid present for testing.

What is the appropriate laboratory and imaging evaluation?

A complete blood count (CBC), urine culture, and cultures as listed previously should be collected with review of the patient's prenatal lab results. Ultrasound imaging should assess fetal presentation, amniotic fluid volume, gestational age, location of the placenta, and an anatomic survey (if not already performed).

The patient's lab evaluation reveals normal prenatal results. CBC is normal, and vaginal cultures are negative after allowing for growth in the laboratory. Ultrasound reveals presence of an intrauterine singleton gestation in cephalic presentation with an estimated fetal weight of 1250 grams (60th percentile for weight) and normal anatomy. The amniotic fluid volume measures 1 cm, consistent with oligohydramnios. Bilateral adnexa appear normally.

What is your diagnosis?

The diagnosis is PPROM, which accounts for 30%–40% of preterm deliveries and is a leading cause of perinatal morbidity and mortality.

What are the etiology and risk factors for PPROM?

Shearing forces created by uterine contractions and intra-amniotic infection can cause PPROM. Risk factors associated with PPROM include prior pregnancy affected by PPROM, short cervical length, low body mass index, tobacco or illicit drug use, low socioeconomic status, and second- or third-trimester bleeding.

How do you counsel the patient regarding this diagnosis?

The primary factor for prognosis of the neonate is preterm delivery and relies upon gestational age at delivery. Preterm delivery occurs in approximately 12% of all births in the United States. About 3% of all pregnancies in the United States are complicated by PPROM. Potential complications with PPROM and preterm delivery include respiratory distress syndrome (RDS), necrotizing enterocolitis (NEC), intraventricular hemorrhage (IVH), and sepsis. Pulmonary hypoplasia occurs in 0%–26.5% of infants delivering after PPROM between 16 and 26 weeks' gestation. Early PPROM (<20 weeks) carries the highest risk for lethal pulmonary hypoplasia. This is uncommon (0%–1.4%) with PPROM after 24–26 weeks' gestation due to adequate alveolar development. Long-term complications can occur, such as mental delay, visual or hearing difficulties, chronic lung disease, and cerebral palsy. These are much less common after 32 weeks gestational age.

Maternal risks can include chorioamnionitis, endometritis, placental abruption, and retained placenta. Although rare, maternal sepsis is a complication occurring in approximately 1% of women with PPROM. Maternal death has been reported in this setting.

What is the next step in management?

Because delivery prior to 32 weeks' gestation is associated with a high risk for perinatal morbidity and mortality with long-term sequelae, women should usually be managed expectantly to prolong pregnancy unless there is evidence of chorioamnionitis, placental abruption, or umbilical cord accident with non-reassuring fetal heart rate. Antenatal well-being is assessed as the mother is hospitalized until delivery; daily surveillance can include daily fetal heart rate monitoring by nonstress test or biophysical profile.

CLINICAL PEARL   STEPS 2/3

A composite biophysical score is derived from assigning two points for each of five parameters if present:
- Heart rate accelerations (noted on the nonstress test)
- Breathing movement
- Body and limb movement
- Tone
- Amniotic fluid volume (oligohydramnios may be present due to PPROM)

CLINICAL PEARL   STEPS 2/3

Chorioamnionitis increases the risk for perinatal mortality and intraventricular hemorrhage. The diagnosis is clinical with the presence of maternal fever (38°C [100.4°F]) with uterine tenderness or with maternal or fetal tachycardia in the absence of another source of infection.

The most common acute morbidity with conservatively managed neonates with maternal PPROM is RDS. Antenatal corticosteroid administration has been extensively studied demonstrating significantly reduced risks for RDS (20% vs. 35.4%), IVH (7.5% vs. 5.1%), and NEC (0.8% vs. 4.6%) without increasing maternal or neonatal risk.

You counsel the patient regarding her diagnosis, prognosis, and recommendation for hospitalization and antenatal corticosteroid administration to decrease the risk of prematurity of her baby. Additionally, you discuss with her the recommendation to administer antibiotics (ampicillin/amoxicillin plus erythromycin) for 7 days to treat or prevent ascending infection, to prolong the pregnancy and reduce morbidity while limiting the risk for neonatal infection. After counseling, the patient opts for antibiotic and corticosteroid administration with expectant management. As cerebral palsy risk is reduced with administration of intravenous magnesium sulfate prior to 32 0/7 weeks' gestation with preterm delivery, the patient opts to receive this medication.

Describe the management of labor, delivery, and postpartum care for patients with PPROM
The optimal gestational age for delivery is controversial; however, the American College of Obstetricians and Gynecologists (ACOG) recommends delivery for all women with PPROM at 34 0/7 weeks' gestation. Additionally, if desired, delivery may be considered up to 37 0/7 weeks' gestation, although the risks and benefits must be extensively counseled with the patient, including chorioamnionitis, neonatal sepsis, and possible stillbirth.

The patient remains hospitalized with antenatal surveillance with daily nonstress tests, and she undergoes an uncomplicated spontaneous vaginal delivery with induction of labor at 34 weeks' gestation.

How do you counsel the patient regarding future pregnancy?
Women should be offered weekly progesterone therapy starting at 16–24 weeks' gestation due to the potential benefit to decrease recurrent PPROM and preterm delivery. Similar to women with a prior history of preterm delivery, transvaginal cervical length screening by ultrasound can be performed. With a cervical length of less than 25 mm prior to 24 weeks' gestation in the subsequent pregnancy, cerclage placement may be considered.

CLINICAL PEARL   **STEPS 2/3**

Cervical cerclage is the placement of a suture or tape circumferentially to occlude the uterine cervix to reduce the risk of preterm delivery (Fig. 13.2). Several methods are the McDonald cerclage (simple purse-string closure), the Shirodkar cerclage (submucosal closure), and the abdominal cerclage. The abdominal cerclage is considered for patients with an extremely shortened cervix (possibly as a result of prior cervical excisional procedure) or failed vaginally placed cerclage. The abdominal cerclage is placed by a laparotomy with elevation of the uterus to allow access to the isthmus and cervix, identification of the ureters and uterine vessels, and placement of the cerclage in an avascular plane between the uterine vessels and isthmus. This method precludes a vaginal delivery and the suture remains in place permanently. On the other hand, a vaginally placed cerclage is usually removed at approximately 36 weeks' gestation and the patient is allowed to labor.

BEYOND THE PEARLS

- Previously with a challenging diagnosis of rupture of membranes, an amniodye test was performed. Intra-amniotic dye instillation can be performed by ultrasound-guided amniocentesis. Indigo carmine is injected into the amniotic cavity under sterile conditions with a tampon placed vaginally. A positive test occurs with blue coloration of the tampon in 30 minutes. Indigo carmine dye, however, is no longer available in the United States.

Surgical Management of Cervical Incompetence (Cerclage)

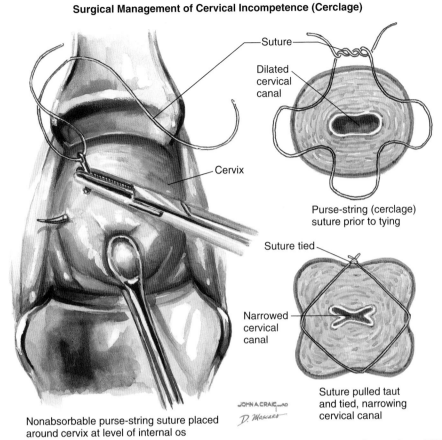

Fig. 13.2 Cervical cerclage. *(From Smith, R. Cervical cerclage. Netter's obstetrics and gynecology. 2008; 585–86. Kansas City: Elsevier https://www.clinicalkey.com/#!/content/book/3-s2.0-B9781416056829502389? scrollTo=%233-s2.0-B9781416056829502389-fx1)*

- Prolonged oligohydramnios can cause fetal deformations, including Potter-like facies (low set ears and epicanthal folds) and limb contractures or other positioning abnormalities.
- Historically, infection of the chorion, amnion, or both was termed "chorioamnionitis." In 2015, a National Institute of Child Health and Human Development Workshop expert panel recommended use of the term "triple I," describing intrauterine inflammation or infection or both. A presumptive diagnosis relies on criteria including maternal fever without another clear source and either fetal tachycardia, maternal white cell count of greater than 15,000/mm^3, or purulent-appearing fluid from the cervical os. Confirmatory diagnosis includes the preceding criteria and either a positive amniotic fluid Gram stain or histopathological evidence of inflammation or infection in the placenta, fetal membranes, or umbilical cord vessels.

Case Summary

- A 20-year-old woman at 28 weeks' gestation presents to the obstetrical emergency department after experiencing a vaginal gush of fluid.
- The patient undergoes a detailed history and physical examination. Her laboratory assessment is within normal limits, including vaginal and urine cultures and CBC.

- Her diagnosis of PPROM is made by sterile speculum exam positive for ferning under microscopy, blue-turning Nitrazine paper, and pooling of amniotic fluid, which is seen with extrusion of fluid from the cervical os. After counseling, she decides to receive corticosteroids, magnesium sulfate, and antibiotics with expectant management until 34 weeks' gestation.
- She delivers a preterm neonate at 34 weeks' gestation after induction of labor.

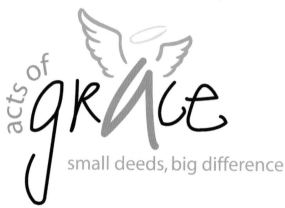

(http://www.actsofgracefoundation.org/)

Acts of Grace Foundation

Dedicated to pregnant women who experience hospital bed rest. These women may have nothing in common, but they have a common goal of bringing healthy babies into this world. Acts of Grace Foundation's mission is to transform a small deed into a big difference for pregnant women on hospital bedrest.

References

Alexander, J. M., Mercer, B. M., Miodovnik, M., et al. (2000). The impact of digital cervical examination on expectantly managed preterm rupture of membranes. *American Journal of Obstetrics and Gynecology, 183*(4), 1003–1007.

Berghella, V., Rafael, T. J., Szychowski, J. M., et al. (2011). Cerclage for short cervix on ultrasonography in women with singleton gestations and previous preterm birth: a meta-analysis. *Obstetrics and Gynecology, 117*(3), 663–671.

Harding, J. E., Pang, J., Knight, D. B., et al. (2001). Do antenatal corticosteroids help in the setting of preterm premature rupture of membranes? *American Journal of Obstetrics and Gynecology, 184*(2), 131–139.

Marcellin, L., Anselem, O., Guibourdenche, J., et al. (2011). Comparison of two bedside tests performed on cervicovaginal fluid to diagnose premature rupture of membranes. *Journal de Gynecologie, Obstetrique et Biologie de la Reproduction, 40*(7), 651–656.

Mercer, B. M., Goldenberg, R. L., Meis, P. J., et al. (2000). The Preterm Prediction Study: prediction of preterm premature rupture of membranes through clinical findings and ancillary testing. The National Institute of Child Health and Human Development Maternal-Fetal Medicine Units Network. *American Journal of Obstetrics and Gynecology, 183*(3), 738–745.

Mercer, B. M. (2003). Preterm premature rupture of the membranes. *Obstetrics and gynecology, 101*(1), 178–193.

Rotschild, A., Ling, E. W., Puteman, M. L., et al. (1990). Neonatal outcome after prolonged preterm rupture of the membranes. *American journal of obstetrics and gynecology, 162*(1), 46–52.

Waters, T. P., Mercer, B. (2011). Preterm PROM: prediction, prevention, principles. *Clinical obstetrics and gynecology, 54*(2), 307–312.

Sandra Herrera, MD

A 36-Year-Old Woman at 33 Weeks' Gestation With Bleeding

A 36-year-old G4P3 woman at 33 weeks' gestation presents to labor and delivery for vaginal bleeding. She reports a gush of bright red blood vaginally that first happened about 1 hour ago while she was enjoying dinner with her family. She noticed the blood soaked her clothes and dripped to the floor. She has had limited prenatal care but denies any complications with this pregnancy.

What are critical questions to ask anyone who presents with vaginal bleeding in the third trimester?

Any pregnant patient who presents with vaginal bleeding in the third trimester should be evaluated immediately to rule out potentially life-threatening causes. Third-trimester vaginal bleeding can range from spotting to massive hemorrhage, so asking the patient about the quantity of blood, presence of blood clots, and even the color of the blood is important. Another important question to ask is whether the patient is experiencing any type of pain. In most cases, painless third-trimester bleeding can be associated with placenta previa and less likely to be placental abruption.

Other important questions to ask include whether the patient has had an ultrasound during this pregnancy to evaluate the placenta location, the last time of intercourse, if she has she experienced any type of trauma, and any drug use.

These questions can help develop your differential diagnosis that includes bloody show from cervical changes in labor, abruptio placentae, placenta previa, vasa previa, trauma/genital lacerations, uterine rupture, cervicitis, foreign body, postcoital bleeding, and carcinoma.

The patient denies contractions, cramping, or abdominal pain. She says last sexual intercourse was more than 2 weeks ago. She denies any recent trauma. She denies drug use but does smoke cigarettes. Her three previous babies were delivered by cesarean section. She otherwise has a negative medical or surgical history.

How does this information help you narrow your differential diagnosis?

The patient is experiencing what appears to be a significant amount of vaginal bleeding and denies any associated pain. She has had three previous cesarean deliveries, making her risk of abnormal placentation greater since the most important risk factor is a previous cesarean delivery. She smokes cigarettes and is of advanced maternal age (>35 years), both of which have been associated with a greater incidence of placenta previa. She denies recent sexual activity, which can be a cause of light vaginal bleeding in pregnancy. She denies drug use, specifically cocaine abuse, which has been associated with placenta abruption. She also denies trauma, which can rule out any type of vaginal or perineal laceration. The patient has several risk factors for placenta previa. Placenta previa accounts for about 20% of cases of third-trimester bleeding. Other risk factors specific to placenta previa include multifetal gestation and prior cesarean delivery.

> On physical examination, you notice she is responsive, cooperative, but pale. Her blood pressure is 95/68 mm Hg, heart rate is 135/min, respiration rate is 28/min, and temperature 37.2°C (98.9°F). Her abdomen is soft, nondistended; no guarding or rebound is present. The uterus is nontender, firm but not rigid. Fundal height is 34 cm. Fetal heart tones are in the 130s with good variability. The external monitor reveals uterine irritability only. On pelvic exam, there is a steady stream of blood coming from her vagina.

How do you assess a patient like this in triage?

As with any patient who may be experiencing a life-threatening bleed, you should remember your ABCs: Airway, Breathing, and Circulation. She is tachycardic, pale, and hypotensive. She is responsive but pale. She is breathing on her own, unlabored it appears, but preparations should be made to move toward delivery. The patient should have two large-bore IVs placed, and the anesthesia team should be notified. Fluid resuscitation should be initiated and a Foley catheter placed to monitor urine output. Her abdomen is soft, and no contractions are palpated, which make placenta abruption less likely. Her fetus has an appropriate fetal heart rate with good variability, making vasa previa and uterine rupture less likely. Given your strong suspicion of placenta previa, avoid a cervical exam. This would only exacerbate the bleeding.

What laboratory values or imaging should you obtain?

In the acute setting of hemorrhage with placenta previa, obtain a type and cross, complete blood cell count to evaluate severity of anemia, and coagulation studies to evaluate for disseminated intravascular coagulopathy (DIC). The patient's Rhesus (Rh) blood group should be determined and a Kleihauer-Betke test may be considered. Imaging studies in the acute study are not necessary, but previous examination of the placenta location should be investigated. If the patient is stable and ultrasound equipment is readily available, a complete placenta previa (Fig. 14.1) may be seen on a transabdominal ultrasound.

Maternal body habitus and advanced gestational age may make imaging more challenging in an acute setting.

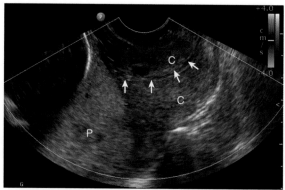

Fig. 14.1   Posterior complete placenta previa. Transvaginal ultrasound reveals the placenta completely covering the internal os. *Arrows* indicate cervical canal. *C*, Cervix; *P*, placenta. *(From Pri-Paz S, D'Alton M. Placenta previa. Obstetric imaging, Philadelphia, 2012, Elsevier, pp 499–502. https://www.clinicalkey.com/#!/content /book/3-s2.0-B9781437725568001088?scrollTo=%233-s2.0-B9781437725568001088-f108-001- 9781437725568)*

CLINICAL PEARL   **STEPS 2/3**

Kleihauer-Betke testing is an acid elution test. Adult hemoglobin is separated from fetal hemo-globin by exposing maternal blood to an acid bath. Adult hemoglobin is eliminated while fetal hemoglobin is resistant, and subsequent staining makes fetal cells appear pink. This is used to determine the fetal-to-maternal hemorrhage in excess of that which can be treated with a standard dose of 300 µg Rho(D) immune globulin (RhoGAM). Administration of RhoGAM is utilized to prevent rhesus (Rh) isoimmunization.

What other complications can arise from a placenta previa?

Placenta previa increases the risk of abnormal placentation: placenta accreta, increta, and percreta (Fig. 14.2).

Placenta accreta occurs when the placenta adheres directly to the uterus without the usual intervening decidua basalis. The risk of a placenta accreta in the setting of a previa increases with number of previous cesarean deliveries. Placenta increta occurs when the placenta invades the myometrium but does not cross the serosa. Placenta percreta penetrates the entire uterine wall, potentially growing into bladder or bowel. Any form of abnormal placentation would necessitate delivery via a cesarean hysterectomy and increased risk of hemorrhage and need for blood transfusion. Placenta previa is also associated with fetal malpresentation, preterm premature rupture of membranes, intrauterine growth restriction, velamentous cord insertion, and vasa previa.

What are the classifications of placenta previa?

A recent Fetal Imaging Workshop sponsored by the National Institutes of Health recommended the following classification in an attempt to simplify the nomenclature:

Placenta previa and low-lying placenta. A low-lying placenta is defined as implantation in the lower uterine segment in which the placental edge does not reach the internal os and remains outside a 2-cm wide perimeter around the os. Placenta previa now specifically describes a pregnancy in which the internal os is covered partially or completely by the placenta.

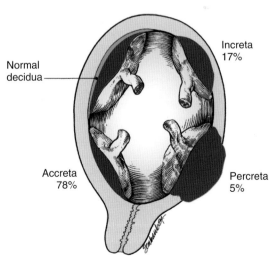

Fig. 14.2 Uteroplacental relationships found with invasive placentation. *(From Jauniaux E, Bhide A, Wright J. Placenta accreta. In: Obstetrics: normal and problem pregnancies, Philadelphia, 2017, Elsevier, pp 456–66. https://www.clinicalkey.com/#!/content/book/3-s2.0-B9780323321082000214?scrollTo=%233-s2.0-B9780323321082000214-f021-001-9780323321082)*

The patient is taken to the operating room and undergoes a repeat cesarean section. While performing the low transverse hysterotomy, the physicians note a posterior placenta previa. The fetus is delivered without complications and is crying immediately after birth. The placenta is removed manually without hemorrhage or evidence of invasion into the myometrium. The surgery concludes without complications, and the patient recovers well.

What other life-threatening causes must be considered?

Placental abruption should always be considered in a patient with third-trimester bleeding. It accounts for up to one-third of all antepartum bleeding. Placental abruption is caused by the premature separation of the placenta from the uterine wall due to maternal/uterine bleeding into the decidua basalis. Placental abruption can be chronic or traumatic. Traumatic abruptions usually occur from external trauma, usually from motor vehicle accidents or aggravated assault. This type of abruption is more commonly associated with fetal-to-maternal hemorrhage, and nonreassuring fetal heart tracing may be seen on evaluation (sinusoidal heart rate is one example) Fig. 14.3.

On the other hand, chronic abruptions may begin early in pregnancy with no evidence of fetal compromise. These patients may have chronic minimal vaginal bleeding. These pregnancies may have abnormally elevated serum levels of α-fetoprotein.

Patients with acute placental abruption usually present with painful, tetanic contractions.

CLINICAL PEARL	STEPS 2/3

If the patient experiences rupture of membranes, either artificial or spontaneous, the vessels could rupture and result in fetal hemorrhage, exsanguination, or even death. Fortunately, fetal mortality for pregnancies complicated by vasa previa is less than 10% due to improved prenatal diagnosis with ultrasound. The incidence of vasa previa is 1 in 2500.

Another potential life-threatening cause of vaginal bleeding is vasa previa. Vasa previa occurs when the fetal blood vessels are unprotected by the umbilical cord or placenta, traverse through the amniotic membranes, and cross the cervix (Fig. 14.4).

CLINICAL PEARL	STEPS 2/3

Risk factors for placental abruption include maternal hypertension, advanced maternal age, multiparity, tobacco use, cocaine use, chorioamnionitis, and trauma. Placenta abruption may have serious maternal complications such as hemorrhagic shock and DIC.

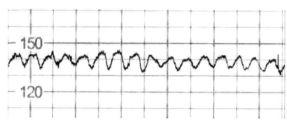

Fig. 14.3 Sinusoidal pattern of fetal heartbeat. *(From Peng Hsiu-Heui, Ng Zooi-Ping. Term pregnancy with choriocarcinoma presenting as severe fetal anemia and postpartum hemorrhage.* Taiwan J Obstet Gynecol. *2016;430–3. https://www.clinicalkey.com/#!/content/journal/1-s2.0-S1028455916300432?scrollTo=%231-s2.0-S1028455916300432-gr1)*

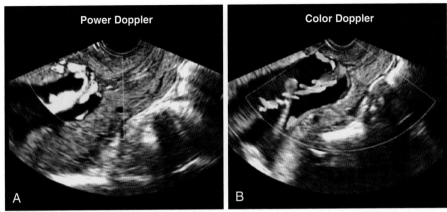

Fig. 14.4 Vasa previa diagnosed antenatally by ultrasound with color (B) and pulsed Doppler (A) mapping. Transvaginal ultrasound images show vasa previa and velamentous cord. The placenta is posterior with an anterior succenturiate lobe. *(From Francois K, Foley M. Antepartum and postpartum hemorrhage. In: Obstetrics: normal and problem pregnancies, Philadelphia, 2017, Elsevier, pp 395–424. https://www.clinicalkey.com/#!/content/book/3-s2.0-B9780323321082000184?scrollTo=%233-s2.0-B9780323321082000184-f018-007ab-9780323321082)*

In addition to placenta previa other risk factors of vasa previa are velamentous cord insertion, succenturiate placental lobe, low-lying placenta, and in vitro fertilization. Pregnancies with vasa previa can be managed as outpatient or inpatient. The decision should be individualized and depends on the patient's history of spontaneous preterm birth, presence or absence of symptoms, and logistics (transportation, distance from the hospital, etc.). The goal is to deliver the patient before rupture of membranes while minimizing the risks of prematurity. Current recommendations are for delivery via cesarean section at 34–37 weeks of gestation.

How do you counsel patients who experienced third-trimester bleeding in future pregnancies?

Of all the causes of third-trimester bleeding, placental abruption is the one associated with a high recurrence risk. Some studies have estimated a recurrence risk of between 12% and 22% in subsequent pregnancies. It is important to individualize counseling for each patient given her risk factors and encourage lifestyle modifications if appropriate. This patient should be counseled regarding her increased risk of placenta previa and subsequent increased risk for placenta accreta at next pregnancy.

BEYOND THE PEARLS

- The pathogenesis of placenta previa is unknown. One hypothesis is that the presence of areas of suboptimal vascularized endometrium in the upper uterine cavity due to prior surgery or pregnancies promotes implantation of trophoblasts toward the lower uterine cavity.
- Two types of vasa previa have been described:
  - Type I occurs in the setting of a velamentous cord insertion between the umbilical cord and placenta, and the fetal vessels run freely within the amniotic membranes and overlie the cervix or are in close proximity to it (<2 cm). Patients who have a resolved placenta previa or low-lying placenta are at risk for type I.
  - Type II occurs when the placenta contains a succenturiate lobe or is multilobed (typically bilobed) and fetal vessels that connect the two placental lobes course over or near the cervix (<2 cm).

Case Summary

- A 36-year-old G4P3 woman at 33 weeks' gestation presents with painless, bright red vaginal bleeding.
- History and physical exam reveal that she has had three previous cesarean sections and she smokes cigarettes. She has had limited prenatal care. She is tachycardic and pale on exam but responsive, with good fetal heart tones.
- The patient underwent a repeat cesarean delivery in which the placenta is noted to be a posterior previa without evidence of accreta.

References

Cunningham, F., Leveno, K. J., Bloom, S.L., et al. Obstetrical hemorrhage. In F. Cunningham, K. J. Leveno, S. L. Bloom, C. Y. Spong, J. S. Dashe, B. L. Hoffman, B. M. Casey, & J. S. Sheffield, (Eds.), *Williams obstetrics* (24th ed.). Retrieved October 13, 2016 from http://accessmedicine.mhmedical.com/content.aspx?bookid=1057&Sectionid=59789185.

Dashe, J. S., McIntire, D. D., Ramus, R. M., et al. (2002). Persistence of placenta previa according to gestational age at ultrasound detection. *Obstetrics and Gynecology, 99*(5), 692–697.

Oppenheimer, L. W., & Farine, D. (2009). A new classification of placenta previa: measuring progress in obstetrics. *American Journal of Obstetrics and Gynecology, 201*(3), 227–229.

The Society of Maternal Fetal Medicine. (2015). Publications Committee. diagnosis and management of vasa previa. *American Journal of Obstetrics and Gynecology, 213*(5), 615–619.

The Society of Maternal Fetal Medicine. (2010 Nov). Publications Committee. Placenta accreta. *American Journal of Obstetrics and Gynecology, 203*(5), 430–439.

Alexandria J. Hill, MD

CASE 15

A 36-Year-Old Woman With Placental Abruption

A 36-year-old G1P0 woman at 33 weeks; gestation presents to triage with acute onset of abdominal pain. She reports this began at home earlier in the day and continually worsened. Her vital signs are stable and she describes the pain as sharp and intermittent.

What are the critical questions to ask a pregnant woman with abdominal pain in the third trimester?

It is important to inquire if the patient is experiencing any vaginal bleeding or contractions given the acute onset of new abdominal pain in the third trimester. The location, duration, and intensity of the pain should be described. Is the pain associated with dysuria, diarrhea, constipation, fevers, chills, difficulty breathing, cough, or ingestion of food? A complete review of systems must be performed. Abdominal pain in this setting can be obstetric or non-obstetric (Table 15.1).

In women with acute abdominal pain that is new and sharp in nature, placental abruption is at the top of the differential. Obtaining a detailed history is important; it is imperative to inquire about any history of drug use. Cocaine and tobacco use increases the risk of placental abruption. Additional risk factors for abruption include advanced parity, hypertension, advanced maternal age, higher order multiples, preterm premature rupture of membranes, and a history of prior placental abruption. Inquiring about trauma to the abdomen or any recent fall is prudent, as even minor shearing forces between the placenta and the uterine wall can cause tearing of the interface and lead to placental abruption.

The patient states that she has not experienced vaginal bleeding or loss of amniotic fluid. She reports that the pain is sharp in nature and worsens (to a 6/10) when she feels contractions. She denies any trauma to the abdomen. Her medical history is negative for any drug or tobacco use, and she has no history of hypertensive disorders. Her body mass index is 38 and she has normal vital signs (blood pressure (BP) 124/83 mm Hg, heart rate (HR) 88/min, oxygen saturation of 98% on room air, respiratory rate 18/min). She denies fevers, chills, nausea, vomiting, diarrhea, constipation, or association of pain with food intake.

What lab evaluation is necessary?

There is concern for a placental abruption given her medical history and her complaint of contractions. The next step is to obtain intravenous (IV) access and draw a complete blood count (CBC) and type and cross. Further lab evaluation directed at eliciting the etiology of the abdominal pain may include liver function tests, amylase, lipase, and urine analysis and culture. A coagulation panel (consisting of PT, PTT, INR, and fibrinogen) and a Kleihauer-Betke (KB) test would be recommended given the concern for placental abruption. The type and cross is imperative because if the patient requires emergent delivery, and she indeed has a placental abruption, she would carry a high risk of hemorrhage. Knowing the patient's coagulation status prior to delivery will help you to assess

TABLE 15.1 ■ **Differential Diagnosis for Abdominal Pain During Pregnancy**

Pregnancy-Related Causes	Nonpregnancy-Related Causes
Miscarriage	Gastroesophageal reflux
Ectopic pregnancy	Cholecystitis
Labor	Pneumonia
Placental abruption	Appendicitis
Uterine rupture	Nephrolithiasis
Preeclampsia with severe features	Inflammatory bowel disease
Chorioamnionitis	Bowel obstruction
Acute fatty liver	Sickle-cell crisis
	Pubic symphysis separation
	Ovarian torsion

future coagulation studies if needed. The type and screen is important to verify the patient's rhesus (Rh) status. The KB test will be helpful to calculate the amount of RhoGAM that needs to be administered to a patient who is Rh negative that is antibody (indirect Coombs) negative.

What imaging would you like to perform for this patient?
Performing a targeted obstetric ultrasound will allow imaging of the placental location (particularly to assess for presence of a placenta previa). Fetal presentation and weight can also be quickly assessed. Ultrasound carries a low sensitivity of 25%–50% in detecting placental abruption; however, if ultrasound findings are concerning for abruption, the positive predictive value is 88%.

Likewise, physical examination does not always diagnose placental abruption. If a patient does not have vaginal bleeding, you cannot completely rule out placental abruption because the region of abruption could be concealed. It is important to recall that about 10%–20% of the time patients with a placental abruption will experience either no vaginal bleeding or minimal spotting. Abruptions can be hidden, or concealed, where the blood is sitting in the interface between the amnion and the decidua (Figs. 15.1 and 15.2).

> The nurse informs you that after the patient returns from ultrasound she begins to experience vaginal bleeding. She had a category I fetal heart rate tracing prior to ultrasound, and you ask that she be immediately placed on the monitor to assess the tracing. The fetal HR has a baseline of 150/min and moderate variability. Accelerations are present with rare variable decelerations. The tocometer demonstrates irregular contractions. Ultrasound findings are significant for a fundal placenta, grade II, without clear concern for acute hemorrhage or abruption yet with a slightly thickened appearance; there is no placenta previa. There is a normal amniotic fluid volume and the fetus is cephalic, measuring consistent with the patient's estimated date of conception. Physical examination reveals a firm uterine fundus, which is tender to palpation, and scant blood is present in the vaginal vault. The cervix is closed.

> Her lab results are as follows: blood type O positive with a negative antibody screen, KB test is negative, hemoglobin 10.9 g/dL, hematocrit 31%, platelets 222,000/μL and fibrinogen 476 mg/dL. Her liver function tests, amylase, lipase, and urine analysis are within normal limits.

What findings on fetal monitoring are you concerned about, particularly for a placental abruption?
Continuous electronic fetal monitoring is needed for this patient as well as continuous tocometer monitoring. A classic pattern noted on fetal monitoring of a placental abruption shows the uterus

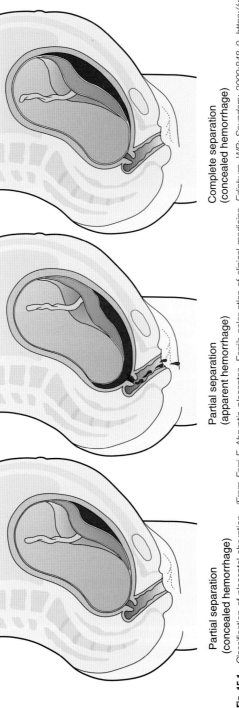

Partial separation
(concealed hemorrhage)

Partial separation
(apparent hemorrhage)

Complete separation
(concealed hemorrhage)

Fig. 15.1 Classification of placental abruption. *(From Ferri F. Abruptio placentae. Ferri's color atlas of clinical medicine. Edinburg, WB: Saunders; 2009:848–9. https://www.clinicalkey.com/#!/content/book/3-s2.0-B9781416049197502620?scrollTo=%233-s2.0-B9781416049197502620-gr1)*

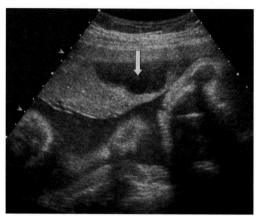

Fig. 15.2 Ultrasound image showing acute placental abruption with a retroplacental hematoma (*arrow*) lifting part of the placenta. *(From Meguerdichian D. Complications in late pregnancy.* Emerg Med Clin N Am. *2012(30)4:919–36. https://www.clinicalkey.com/#!/content/journal/1-s2.0-S073386271200034X?scroll To=%231-s2.0-S073386271200034X-gr1)*

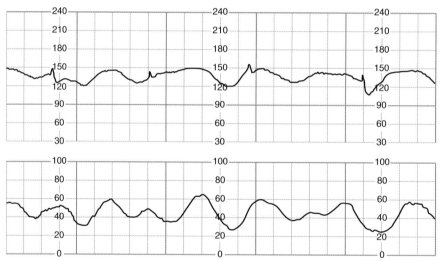

Fig. 15.3 Fetal monitoring concerning for placental abruption, showing uterine tachysystole with repetitive late decelerations. *(From Sibai, Baha M.* Management of acute obstetric emergencies. *Philadelphia: Saunders; 2011:115–23. https://www.clinicalkey.com/#!/content/book/3-s2.0-B978141606270700003X?sc rollTo=%23hl0000906)*

in a hypertonic fashion, with frequent contractions of low amplitude; the fetal heart rate is often tachycardic with decreased variability and late decelerations. The definition of uterine tachysystole, more than five contractions in a 10-minute time period averaged over 30 minutes, can help to diagnose a placental abruption (Fig. 15.3).

> The patient experiences an episode of moderate to heavy vaginal bleeding. Her BP decreases to 80/40 mm Hg and the fetal HR increases to 170/min with decreased variability and intermittent late decelerations. The tocometer also now shows regular low-amplitude contractions (tachysystole).

What is your next step in management?
At this time, delivery is essential due to maternal and fetal instability in the setting of suspected placental abruption. The fetus is in distress (late decelerations with decreased variability of the heart rate), and the mother is demonstrating signs of hemorrhage (hypotension).

> The patient receives general endotracheal anesthesia and undergoes an emergent cesarean delivery. You are able to deliver the fetus without difficulties. The majority of the placenta is detached from the uterus at time of delivery, with regions of fresh hemorrhage. As the placenta is removed you note that the uterus is atonic with brisk bleeding.

How do you diagnose disseminated intravascular coagulation?
Disseminated intravascular coagulation (DIC) originates from an inciting event, which in this scenario is the placental abruption.

CLINICAL PEARL	STEPS 2/3

Triggers for DIC include placental abruption, postpartum hemorrhage, preeclampsia, acute fatty liver, amniotic fluid embolism, and sepsis. The most common of these triggers is placental abruption.

Occurrences such as placental abruption can lead to release of proteolytic enzymes and tissue factor. Cells that line the bed of the placenta at the decidua have a high expressivity of tissue factor. Therefore, when there is trauma at this level, tissue factor is released as the placenta pulls away from the uterus. Moreover, the clot that has been forming from the placental separation consumes coagulation factors, which ultimately results in a type of consumptive coagulopathy. Tissue factor will specifically activate the extrinsic clotting cascade (by activating factor VII), which will ultimately increase generation of thrombin (activated factor II) from prothrombin (factor II).

BASIC SCIENCE PEARL	STEPS 2/3

Thrombin carries the following roles: activating platelets, making fibrin, and activating crucial clotting factors. When thrombin is overproduced in clinical scenarios like DIC, there is excessive fibrin deposition and fibrinolysis. An early laboratory finding of DIC is a low fibrinogen level because fibrinogen (factor I) is being broken down to make more fibrin clots. Fibrinolysis also increases due to excess plasmin production in DIC, and thus the fibrin clot is destructed and an increase in fibrin split products (FSP) and D-dimer can be seen. Moreover, coagulation factors and platelets can decrease profoundly.

BASIC SCIENCE PEARL	STEP 1

Laboratory studies consistent with DIC are:
Low: Fibrinogen, antithrombin III, hemoglobin/hematocrit
High: Fibrin degradation products, D-dimer, PT, INR, aPTT (occasionally), LDH, bilirubin

It is important to recall that baseline coagulation levels are altered in the pregnant patient, which is important when reviewing labs that help to diagnose DIC. Specifically, pregnancy is a procoagulant state with increases in von Willebrand factor; fibrinogen; and factors II, VII, VIII, X and decreases in protein S and resistance to activated protein C and plasminogen activator inhibitor-1.

In the operating room, the anesthesiologist reports the values of her labs, which include fibrinogen 80 mg/dL, hemoglobin 7g/dL, hematocrit 21.1%, FSP 35 mg/L, PT 6.3 seconds, PTT 42.7 seconds, LDH 802 U/L, platelets 46,000/μL.

You have identified that the patient has DIC; intraoperatively, you noted an atonic uterus and were able to perform appropriate measures to achieve hemostasis, including administration of oxytocin and Methergine.

What measures do you need to take to treat her DIC?
When DIC is identified early, it can be more easily reversed. Treatment for DIC varies depending on the event that caused the coagulation disorder. As the inciting event was a placental abruption, the appropriate treatment (delivery) has been performed.

When there is initial concern for extensive bleeding and/or DIC, preemptive interventions should occur. Clear communication is essential among the obstetrician, anesthesiologist, intensivist, and nursing staff. The patient should have appropriate IV access, including at least two large-bore IV lines. A Foley catheter should be placed to monitor strict urine output. With anticipated hemorrhage, the massive transfusion protocol (MTP) should be initiated.

CLINICAL PEARL   **STEPS 2/3**

Hemorrhage is a leading cause of maternal death. Rapid transfusion of large volumes of blood products is required in patients with hemorrhagic shock. Protocol-based management of these patients using a designated MTP have been shown to improve survival using a higher ratio of fresh frozen plasma (FFP) to packed red blood cells (PRBCs) transfusion as compared to the conventional approach. Transfusing fresh whole blood would be ideal; however, the time required to conduct safety tests on whole blood is too lengthy. Therefore, with an MTP, transfusion of PRBCs, coagulation factors, and platelets together maintains the physiological constitution of blood.

MTPs have a predefined ratio of PRBCs, FFP/cryoprecipitate, and platelet units in each pack (e.g., 1:1:1) for transfusion. Once activated, the blood bank ensures rapid delivery of all blood components for resuscitation without delaying delivery pending resulting lab collection, evaluation, or orders from the physician.

MTPs vary by hospital, and it is imperative to be aware of how to activate the protocol at individual hospitals. Given the patient's lab values and critical state, the MTP should be initiated. Some hospitals have criteria that assist in making the decision when the MTP needs to be activated. Typically when the patient has active bleeding in the face of vital signs concerning for shock (i.e., hypotension and tachycardia), the protocol is recommended to be activated.

The blood components included in MTP to treat DIC are FFP, cryoprecipitate, platelets, and PRBCs. FFP and cryoprecipitate are used to replace lost clotting factors. Of note, 1 unit of FFP contains much more volume (250 mL) than cryoprecipitate (35–40 mL). This is important for those patients who you feel need volume repletion along with coagulation factors versus those who may be fluid overloaded yet still need to receive clotting factors. Whether a unit of FFP or cryoprecipitate is given, the fibrinogen will increase by 5–10 mg/dL.

Platelets can be consumed rapidly when administered in the clinical picture of DIC. Generally speaking, one pack of pooled platelets will increase the platelet count by 7000–10,000/μL. PRBCs are transfused to increase the carrying capacity of oxygen and maintain a hematocrit of above 25%. It is also imperative that electrolytes are followed because when hemolysis is occurring and PRBCs are being transfused there can be significant changes in the levels of potassium and calcium. To assist with preventing chelation within the calcium circulatory system, one ampule of calcium can be given after every 5 units of PRBCs.

> The MTP is initiated and the patient receives products in a 1:1:1 ratio of PRBCs to FFP to platelets. Her hemodynamic status improves, and the surgery is completed. Due to the extensive blood loss, her antibiotics are redosed in the operating room, and she is taken to the recovery room in stable condition.

BEYOND THE PEARLS

- Within a coagulation panel you will receive a fibrinogen level, which is the most sensitive lab to predict placental abruption. For example, if the fibrinogen is noted to be less than or equal to 200 mg/dL, the positive predictive value for postpartum hemorrhage is 100% (whereas if the fibrinogen is greater than or equal to 400 mg/dL, the negative predictive value is 70%).
- When there is concern for DIC, 5 mL of blood can be placed in a tube (typically a red top tube) that is not treated with blood thinners such as ethylenediaminetetraacetic acid (EDTA), which is typically a purple top tube. This tube can be taped to the wall and assessed in approximately 8 minutes. If there is not a formed clot, the patient is lacking in fibrinogen and clotting factors. This may be helpful for assessment while waiting for coagulation labs to return.

Case Summary

- A 36-year-old woman presents with new-onset abdominal pain at 33 weeks' gestation. She ultimately experiences vaginal bleeding.
- History and physical examination reveal that the patient has a placental abruption. The fetal heart rate monitoring ultimately shows concern for fetal distress, and emergent delivery via cesarean is necessary.
- Intraoperatively the patient experiences hemorrhage, uterine atony, and DIC. She undergoes resuscitation with transfusion of blood products guided by the hospital's MTP. She is taken to the recovery room in stable condition.

References

Ananth, C. V., Berkowitz, G. S., Savitz, D. A., & Lapinski, R. H. (1999). Placental abruption and adverse perinatal outcomes. *Journal of the American Medical Association, 282*(17), 1646.

Charbit, B., Mandelbrot, L., Samain, E., et al. (2007). The decrease of fibrinogen is an early predictor of the severity of postpartum hemorrhage. *Journal of Thrombosis and Haemostasis, 5*(2), 266–273.

Foley, M. R., Strong, T. H., Jr., & Garite, T. J. (2011). Disseminated intravascular coagulopathy and thrombocytopenia complicating pregnancy. In *Obstetric intensive care manual* (3rd ed.). New York: McGraw-Hill, 39–48.

Glantz, C., & Purnell, L. (2002). Clinical utility of sonography in the diagnosis and treatment of placental abruption. *Journal of Ultrasound in Medicine, 21*(8), 837–840.

Jaffe, M. H., Schoen, W. C., Silver, T. M., et al. (1981). Sonography of abruptio placentae. *American Journal of Roentgenology, 137*(5), 1049–1054.

Oyelese, Y., & Ananth, C. V. (2006). Placental abruption. *Obstetrics and Gynecology, 108*(4), 1005–1016.

Sholl, J. S. (1987). Abruptio placentae: clinical management in nonacute cases. *American Journal of Obstetrics and Gynecology, 156*(1), 40–51.

Taylor, F. B., Jr., Toh, C. H., Hoots, W. K., et al. (2001). Towards definition, clinical and laboratory criteria, and a scoring system for disseminated intravascular coagulation. *Thrombosis and Haemostasis, 86*(5), 1327–1330.

Antonio F. Saad, MD

A 35-Year-Old Woman With Lower Extremity Swelling

A 35-year-old woman presents to labor and delivery triage complaining of lower extremity swelling. Since she left the hospital after an uncomplicated vaginal delivery 2 days ago, her swelling has gotten worse so that she cannot ambulate anymore and now requires a wheelchair. She has been told in the emergency department that the swelling is "normal and part of her recovery from pregnancy."

What are important questions to ask women in the puerperium period with leg swelling?
When evaluating a pregnant/postpartum woman with leg swelling, it is critical to individualize each case presentation. Based on initial history and physical exam, the clinician should decide if further workup is needed. The pregnancy and postpartum period can obscure the diagnosis due to physiological changes that occur during this time, including physiological dyspnea of pregnancy and bilateral leg swelling. The clinician should enquire about family history of blood clots, sudden death, or thrombophilia. The patient should also be asked about the time of onset, location, personal history of blood clots, or recurrent miscarriages. Etiologies for bilateral leg swelling should include physiological changes of pregnancy, but also preeclampsia, postpartum cardiomyopathy, or prior history of cardiac dysfunction. The differential of unilateral leg swelling includes deep vein thrombosis, cellulitis/infectious causes, prior surgery, or prior trauma. Clinicians should also inquire about associated tenderness, exacerbating or relieving factors, and any symptoms of dyspnea, shortness of breath, or other respiratory symptoms. Based on the overall assessment, the smart clinician should build in his or her mind a preclinical probability in order to proceed with further testing.

On further questioning, the patient informs you that the leg swelling initially began a week from her delivery and is worse in her left lower extremity. Patient denies any respiratory symptoms such as dyspnea on exertion or chest pain. She also reports pain that is associated with dorsal flexion and ambulation. The pain initially improved with oral analgesics but is now progressively worse. She also reports a cousin needing to take some kind of "blood thinners."

On physical examination, temperature is 37.1°C (99°F), blood pressure is 130/85 mm Hg, heart rate is 100/min, and respiration rate is 20/min. Cardiac examination is unremarkable. Pulmonary examination is normal. There is bilateral lower extremity pitting edema; swelling is more remarkable in the left lower leg than the right. Skin over the swelling appears normal. Upon dorsal flexion of left foot, patient reports severe tenderness. You also notice pain over the calf when palpated.

What clues in the history and exam will help you to narrow your differential diagnosis?
The patient has bilateral lower extremity edema that was first noted during her pregnancy and worsened in the postpartum period. It is worse on the left side. Heart and lung exams are negative, hence ruling out cardiac etiologies for her peripheral edema. During the exam, pain is elicited by flexion of the left foot (Homan's sign) and palpation of the calf (Pratt's sign). The duration of her symptoms, in conjunction with her other clinical manifestations and exam findings, narrows your differential to deep vein thrombosis (DVT).

CLINICAL PEARL   **STEPS 2/3**

Pregnancy is a state of hypercoagulability secondary to blood stasis in the lower extremity, decreased fibrinolysis, increased hepatic production of coagulation factors, and endothelial injury occurring at time of delivery. The obstetric population has a five times increased odds of developing a thromboembolic disorder compared to the general population. It has become the most common etiology of maternal death in the developed world. The risk for a DVT or pulmonary embolus (PE) is highest in the postpartum period.

What further studies will you order?
Clinical suspicion of DVT needs to be confirmed with imaging studies. Ultrasound Doppler is the initial imaging study to order. If the initial study is negative, further follow-up studies at days 3 and 5 are recommended. Another option is to order an ultrasensitive D-dimer assay. If the test is negative in light of a negative ultrasound, DVT can be ruled out and other etiologies should be pursued. A positive result for D-dimer is not relevant since it is normally high in the obstetrical population (Fig. 16.1).

BASIC SCIENCE PEARL   **STEP 1**

Virchow's triad: Hypercoagulation, Stasis, and Endothelial Injury.

Category	Etiologies
Stasis	Venous stasis, long operating room time, prolonged immobility (as during long travel, hospital immobility), and varicose veins.
Endothelial/vessel injury	Shear stress and hypertension lead to endothelial injury. Other harmful procoagulant factors include bacteria, foreign materials, biomaterials of implants or medical devices, membranes of activated platelets, and membranes of monocytes in chronic inflammation.
Hypercoagulation	Thrombophilias: Coagulation factor V Leiden mutation, coagulation factor II G20210A mutation, deficiency of antithrombin III, protein C or S deficiency. Conditions such as: nephrotic syndrome, severe trauma or burn conditions, cancer, late pregnancy, delivery and postpartum, race, advanced age, hormonal contraceptives, cigarette smoking, and obesity.

BASIC SCIENCE PEARL   **STEP 1**

Alternate causes for increased D-dimer: Advanced age, pregnancy/postpartum, trauma, renal insufficiency, postoperative, cancer, and inflammation/infection.

You order a venous duplex of the lower extremity (Figs. 16.2 and 16.3).

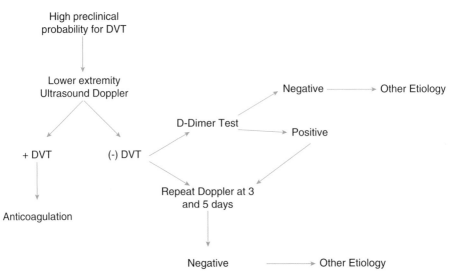

Fig. 16.1   Workup algorithm for deep venous thrombosis (DVT) in the obstetric population.   *(Adapted from Pacheco LD, Saade GR, Hankins GDV. Maternal medicine,* New York, 2015, McGraw-Hill Education.)

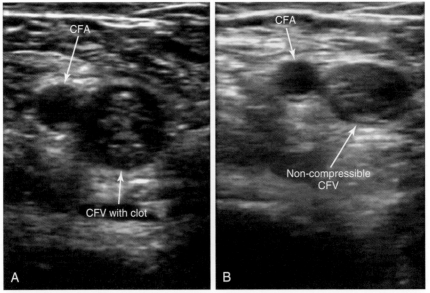

Fig. 16.2   Two-dimensional duplex ultrasound of the common femoral vein with deep venous thrombosis (DVT). A: Without compression. B: With compression (minimally compressible due to DVT). *(From Zaidi G, Tsegaya A. Ultrasonography for deep venous thrombosis.* Crit Care Ultrasound. *2015:60–5. https://www.clinicalkey.com/#!/content/book/3-s2.0-B9781455753574000187?scrollTo=%233-s2.0-B9781455753574000187-f09-05ab-9781455753574)*

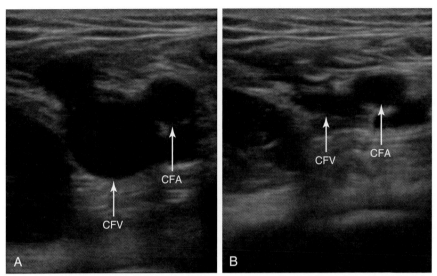

Fig. 16.3   Two-dimensional duplex ultrasound of the common femoral vein without deep venous thrombosis (DVT). A: Without compression. B: With compression; shows complete apposition of the anterior and posterior walls of the vein *(From Zaidi G, Tsegaya A. Ultrasonography for deep venous thrombosis.* Crit Care Ultrasound. *2015:60–5.* https://www.clinicalkey.com/#!/content/book/3-s2.0-B9781455753574000187?sc rollTo=%233-s2.0-B9781455753574000187-f09-05ab-9781455753574)

What are the treatment options?

When the clinical presentation is typical for a DVT, anticoagulation should not be delayed while waiting for results of imaging studies or laboratory results. Therapeutic anticoagulants include either unfractionated heparin (UH) or low molecular weight heparin (LMWH). In the obstetric population, LMWH is currently the first-line agent for both prophylaxis and treatment. The duration of therapy remains controversial but usually when a DVT is diagnosed during pregnancy, full anticoagulation should be continued for the rest of pregnancy and postpartum for a total of at least 3 months.

BASIC SCIENCE/CLINICAL PEARL   STEPS 1, 2, 3

Enoxaparin (LMWH) is the therapy most extensively used in the obstetric population.
   Therapeutic dose: 1 mg/actual weight kg q12h or 1.5 mg/kg q24h subcutaneous
   AntiXa-anti IIa ratio: 4:1
   AntiXa levels (4 hours after third dose) are indicated only for morbid obesity, chronic kidney
   disease, and in patients with mechanical valves: 0.6–1 U/mL (therapeutic).
   Half-life: 4–6 hours
   Renally cleared
   Low incidence of heparin-induced thrombocytopenia and osteoporosis
Unfractionated heparin (UH)
   Therapeutic dose: 80 U/kg load followed by maintenance infusion 18 U/kg intravenous
   AntiXa-anti IIa ratio: 1:1
   Goal partial thromboplastin time (PTT): 6 hours after initiation; between 60–85 seconds or 1.5–2 × normal
   Half-life: 60–90 minutes
   Renally cleared
   Low incidence of heparin-induced thrombocytopenia and osteoporosis

Upon return from her imaging study, the patient reports chest pain and shortness of breath. Her pulse is 120/min, blood pressure is 135/80 mm Hg, respiratory rate is 34/min, and oxygen saturation is 88% on room air. She is placed on oxygen. She is given her therapeutic dose of enoxaparin.

What further workup would you order?

The patient has now developed acute chest symptoms after being diagnosed with acute DVT. Clinical suspicion for a PE should be high. Initial workup should include an EKG, chest X-ray, and an arterial blood gas. Imaging studies should be ordered as soon as possible. If the patient is still pregnant and has a normal chest X-ray, a ventilation perfusion scan should be performed; otherwise computed tomography (CT) angiography should be obtained (Fig. 16.4). In postpartum patients, CT angiography is the study of choice.

CLINICAL PEARL   **STEPS 2/3**

EKG findings with pulmonary embolus:
New right bundle branch block (RBBB, complete or incomplete)
S1Q3T3
Right axis deviation
Sinus tachycardia

CT angiogram confirms your suspicion for PE (Fig. 16.5). Meanwhile, the patient becomes hemodynamically unstable.

What would be your next step of management?

When a patient with acute PE develops sudden systemic hypotension, it is usually secondary to a sudden increase in pulmonary vascular resistance (massive embolus) leading to right ventricular strain/dilation, displacing the interventricular septum toward the left ventricle, decreasing left ventricular end diastolic volume, and ultimately affecting cardiac output. Management should include transfer to the intensive care unit and inotropic/vasopressor support with cautious administration of fluids. Administration of fibrinolytic agents is advised, such as tissue plasminogen activator (t-PA) 100 mg intravenous in 2 hours. Doses of 50 mg have also been shown to be as effective especially in emergent cases. Use of fibrinolytic agents has been shown to improve hemodynamics, but its impact on mortality remains controversial. One should always balance the risks of bleeding versus the benefits of thrombolysis. Patients should not receive thrombolytic therapy if the PE is submassive or if hemodynamics improve with resuscitative measures, vasopressor administration, or support with inotropes.

CLINICAL PEARL   **STEPS 2/3**

Contraindications to thrombolytics:
History of intracranial hemorrhage
Intracranial conditions that increase risk of bleeding (i.e., brain tumor, arteriovenous malformation, or aneurysm)
Active internal bleeding
Severe uncontrolled hypertension
Within 3 months of intracranial or intraspinal surgery or serious head trauma

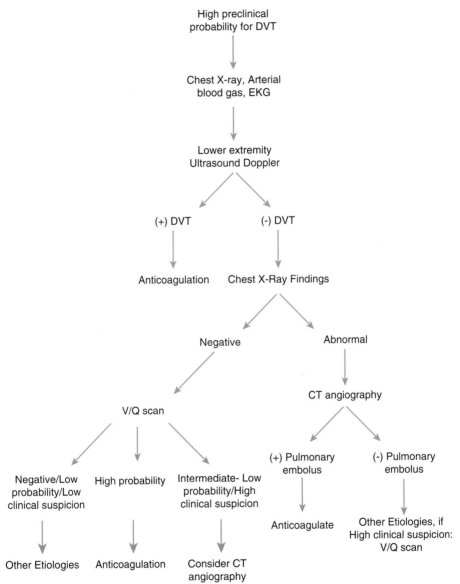

Fig. 16.4   Workup algorithm for pulmonary embolus in the obstetric population. *(Adapted from Pacheco LD, Saade GR, Hankins GDV. Maternal medicine, New York, 2015, McGraw-Hill Education.)*

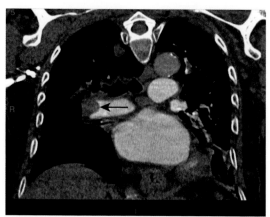

Fig. 16.5 Computed tomography angiogram showing pulmonary embolism. *(From Parks R. Postoperative care and complications. In James Garden O, Andrew Bradbury, John Forsythe, Rowan W Parks, editors: Principles and practice of surgery. 2012, Elsevier, pp 119–26. https://www.clinicalkey.com/#!/content/book/3-s2.0-B9780702043161000098?scrollTo=%233-s2.0-B9780702043161000098-f09-05b-9780702043161)*

Case Summary

- A 35-year-old woman presents with new-onset lower extremity swelling and tenderness and has a past history of recent pregnancy.
- History and physical reveals that the patient has had these symptoms in the past few days and has a positive family history of clotting disorders.
- Initial workup involves an ultrasound Doppler of the lower extremities that confirms a diagnosis of DVT.
- Patient also develops sudden massive PE, confirmed by CT angiography.
- Mainstay of management of DVT/PE involves hemodynamic support and therapeutic UH or LMWH. If hemodynamic instability from massive PE occurs, thrombolytic therapy should be administered.

References

Bates, S. M., Greer, I. A., Middeldorp, S., et al. (2012). VTE, Thrombophilia, antithrombotic therapy, and pregnancy: antithrombotic therapy and prevention of thrombosis, 9th ed. American College of Chest Physicians Evidence-Based Clinical Practice Guidelines. *Chest, 141*(Suppl. 2), e691S–e736S.

Bourjeily, G., Paidas, M., Khalil, H., et al. (2010). Pulmonary embolism in pregnancy. *Lancet, 375*(9713), 500–512.

Cahill, A. G., Stout, M. J., Macones, G. A., et al. (2009). Diagnosing pulmonary embolism in pregnancy using computed-tomographic angiography or ventilation-perfusion. *Obstetrics and Gynecology, 114*(1), 124–129.

Damodaram, M., Kaladindi, M., Luckit, J., et al. (2009). D-dimers as a screening test for venous thromboembolism in pregnancy: is it of any use? *Journal of Obstetrics and Gynaecology, 29*(2), 101–103.

Garcia, D. A., Baglin, T. P., Weitz, J. I., et al. (2012). Parenteral anticoagulants: Antithrombotic therapy and prevention of thrombosis, 9th ed. American College of Chest Physicians Evidence-Based Clinical Practice Guidelines. *Chest, 141*(Suppl. 2), e24S–e43S.

Kearon, C., Akl, E. A., Comerota, A. J., Prandoni, P., et al. (2012). Antithrombotic therapy for VTE disease: Antithrombotic therapy and prevention of thrombosis, 9th ed. American College of Chest Physicians Evidence-Based Clinical Practice Guidelines. *Chest, 141*(Suppl. 2), e419S–e496S.

Malone, P. C., Agutter, P. S. (2008). *The aetiology of deep venous thrombosis: a critical, historical and epistemological survey.* Berlin: Springer, 84.

Verstraete, M., Miller, G. A., Bounameaux, H., et al. (1988). Intravenous and intrapulmonary recombinant tissue-type plasminogen activator in the treatment of acute massive pulmonary embolism. *Circulation, 77*(2), 353–360.

Joses Jain, MD ■ Ellen Mozurkewich, MD

A 31-Year-Old Woman Admitted for Induction of Labor

A 31-year-old G1P0 woman at 37 weeks' gestation is admitted for a scheduled induction of labor due to a pregnancy complicated by oligohydramnios.

What is induction of labor?

Labor induction involves the use of medications or techniques to facilitate uterine contractions and stimulate the process of labor, with the end goal of achieving a vaginal delivery. There are various methods by which induction of labor can be undertaken, including the administration of prostaglandins or oxytocin, amniotomy, mechanical dilation of the cervix, or ancillary outpatient procedures such as membrane stripping.

What are the reasons for inducing labor in a pregnant woman?

Induction of labor may be indicated for a variety of reasons, including situations where the risks of fetal compromise outweigh the benefits of continuing the pregnancy or in the event of potential significant maternal health risks associated with continuing a pregnancy. Some examples of indications for labor induction are listed in Box 17.1. It is important to recognize that any indication for induction is not absolute and must take into account the balance between the potential benefits of an expedited delivery and the potential maternal and fetal risks of continuing pregnancy in addition to the risks of the induction process itself.

CLINICAL PEARL   **STEPS 2/3**

The gestational age at which induction of labor is recommended varies according to each individual patient, but general guidelines exist for the common indications. Although elective induction should not occur before 39 weeks' gestation, there are many clinical situations in which nonelective inductions are recommended prior to 39 weeks as the risks of continuing pregnancy outweigh the potential benefits in these situations. For example, it is recommended that fetuses with oligohydramnios be delivered at 36–37 weeks. Uncomplicated dichorionic-diamniotic twins should be delivered at 38 weeks, monochorionic-diamniotic twins should be delivered at 34–37 weeks, and monochorionic-monoamniotic twins should be delivered at 32–34 weeks.

What are the contraindications to induction of labor?

As with the indications for labor induction, the contraindications must take into consideration the individual clinical scenario. Broadly speaking, the contraindications to labor induction are the contraindications to vaginal delivery. That is, induction of labor is typically

---

INDICATIONS FOR LABOR INDUCTION   **BOX 17.1**

Abruptio placentae
Cholestasis of pregnancy
Chorioamnionitis
Elective[a]
Gestational hypertension
Intrauterine fetal demise
Multiple gestation
Preeclampsia/Eclampsia/HELLP syndrome
Premature rupture of membranes
Postterm pregnancy
Maternal medical conditions (e.g., antiphospholipid syndrome, chronic hypertension, chronic
    lung disease, diabetes mellitus, renal disease)
Fetal compromise (e.g., fetal growth restriction, oligohydramnios, alloimmunization with fetal
    effects)
Fetal conditions requiring immediate intervention at birth (e.g., complex cardiac anomaly
    requiring immediate cardiac catheterization)

---

*[a]Indications for elective induction may include psychosocial indications, distance from hospital, or a risk of rapid
labor. Elective induction should not be performed prior to 39 weeks' gestation due to the increased risk of neonatal morbidity and mortality.*

CONTRAINDICATIONS TO LABOR INDUCTION   **BOX 17.2**

Active genital herpes infection
Complete placenta previa
Invasive cervical cancer
Prior classical or other high-risk cesarean incision
Prior myomectomy entering the endometrial cavity
Prior uterine rupture
Transverse fetal lie
Umbilical cord prolapse
Vasa previa

---

contraindicated in situations that involve maternal and fetal risks that are greater with labor
and vaginal delivery than with cesarean delivery. Some examples of contraindications to labor
induction are listed in Box 17.2.

How can the likelihood of a successful induction be determined?

Factors associated with an increased likelihood of vaginal delivery include multiparity, gestational
age, and the status of the cervix. Currently, the best available clinical predictive tool is the Bishop
pelvic scoring system, which is used to assess the status of the cervix and determine the probability
of a successful induction (i.e., a vaginal delivery). The modified Bishop score is the tool most commonly used in clinical practice in the United States, providing a score based upon four cervical
examination findings: dilatation, effacement, station, and consistency (Table 17.1). An unfavorable cervix is generally defined as a Bishop score of 6 or less, which increases the likelihood that
induction will not result in a successful vaginal delivery. A nulliparous patient undergoing induction of labor with an unfavorable cervix has a twofold higher risk of cesarean delivery compared
to a nulliparous patient in spontaneous labor. A Bishop score of more than 8 is associated with a
similar likelihood of a vaginal delivery whether labor is spontaneous or induced.

TABLE 17.1 ■ **Modified Bishop Scoring System**

Score	Dilatation (cm)	Effacement (%)	Station	Cervical Consistency	Cervical Position
0	Closed	0%–30%	–3	Firm	Posterior
1	1–2	40%–50%	–2	Medium	Midposition
2	3–4	60%–70%	–1, 0	Soft	Anterior
3	5–6	80% or greater	+1, +2	-	-

On physical exam, the estimated fetal weight by Leopold maneuvers is 3500 g. The maternal pelvis appears adequate, but the patient's cervix is noted to be closed, 50% effaced, and –3 station. The fetal heart rate is Category I and the patient is not experiencing uterine contractions.

What is cervical ripening, and how can it be performed?

Cervical remodeling naturally occurs as an important part of normal parturition; it involves enzyme-mediated collagen breakdown, an increase in water content, and other hormone-mediated chemical and structural changes. For an unfavorable cervix, which exists in the absence of these changes, cervical ripening involves the use of medications or techniques to facilitate physical softening of the cervix, in addition to partial thinning (effacement) and dilation. As induction is likely to be ineffective in a woman with an unfavorable cervix, cervical ripening is generally employed prior to induction of labor in order to increase the likelihood of a successful vaginal delivery and decrease the induction-to-delivery time.

Techniques for cervical ripening generally fall into two categories: mechanical dilation methods (e.g., hygroscopic dilators, osmotic dilators (*Laminaria japonicum*), transcervical Foley balloon catheters, double balloon devices, extra-amniotic saline infusion), and cervical ripening agents (e.g., synthetic prostaglandin E_1 and prostaglandin E_2 Fig. 17.1). Misoprostol is a synthetic PGE_1 analogue that can be used for both cervical ripening and induction of labor. PGE_2 preparations include a dinoprostone gel and a dinoprostone vaginal insert. For women undergoing a scheduled induction of labor with an unfavorable cervix, clinical outcomes appear to be similar whether a transcervical balloon catheter or prostaglandin E_1 or E_2 analogue is used for cervical ripening.

CLINICAL PEARL   **STEPS 2/3**

Prostaglandin analogues such as misoprostol have an important role in obstetrics apart from labor induction. Misoprostol is used to prevent and treat postpartum hemorrhage and is most effective for this purpose when administered rectally. Misoprostol binds to myometrial cells causing smooth muscle contraction and hemostasis at the site of placentation. The most common adverse effects are gastrointestinal, including diarrhea and abdominal pain. Carboprost, a prostaglandin F_2 α-analogue, is also available as an intramuscular injection for treating postpartum hemorrhage and can be given in repeat doses at 15- to 90-minute intervals when managing an ongoing hemorrhage.

What are the risks associated with cervical ripening and induction of labor?

The use of both prostaglandin analogues and oxytocin can result in uterine tachysystole with or without fetal heart rate changes. Tachysystole is defined as an average of greater than five uterine contractions in 10 minutes over a 30-minute period Fig. 17.2. This effect is principally dose-related with both misoprostol and oxytocin and can lead to Category II or III fetal heart rate tracings.

Due to the significant risk of uterine rupture, misoprostol should be avoided in women in the third trimester who have had a prior cesarean delivery or any prior major uterine surgery.

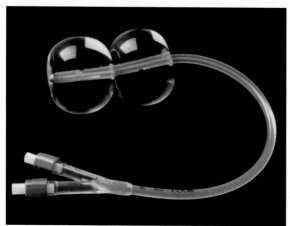

Fig. 17.1 The double-balloon cervical ripening catheter contains silicone material, which can be inflated with 80 mL of fluid. *(From Tsui K, Lin L. Double-balloon cervical ripening catheter works well as an intrauterine balloon tamponade in post-abortion massive hemorrhage. Taiwan J Obstet Gynecol. 2012;51(3):426–9. https://www.clinicalkey.com/#!/content/journal/1-s2.0-S1028455912001349?scrollTo=%231-s2.0-S1028455912001349-gr1)*

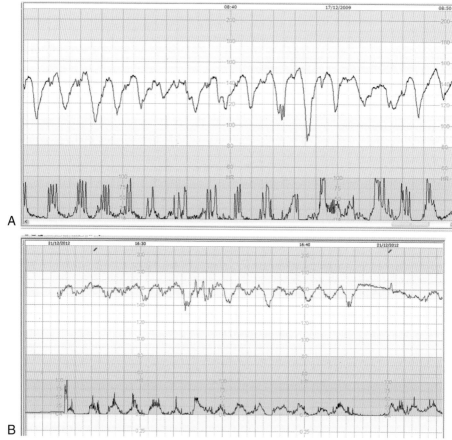

Fig. 17.2 Uterine tachysystole. A: Patient with contraction frequency 8 every 10 minutes. B: Tachysystole induced by prostaglandin administration. *(From Ugwumadu A. Understanding cardiotocographic patterns associated with intrapartum fetal hypoxia and neurologic injury. Best Prac Res Clin Obstet Gynaecol. 2013;27(4):509-36. https://www.clinicalkey.com/#!/search/tachysystole/%7B%22facetquery%22:%5B%22+contenttype:IM%22,%22+contenttype:VD%22%5D%7D)*

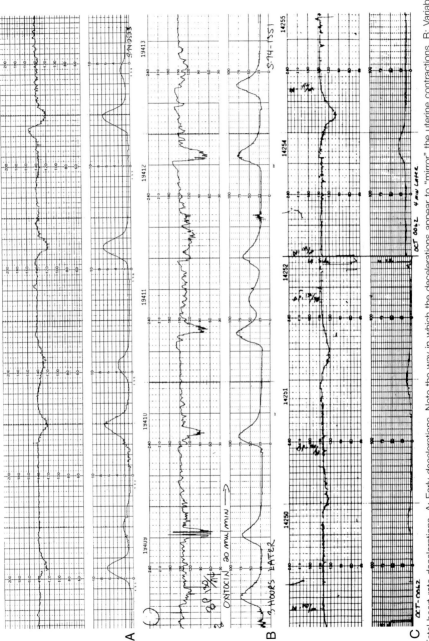

Fig. 17.3 Fetal heart rate decelerations. A: Early decelerations. Note the way in which the decelerations appear to "mirror" the uterine contractions. B: Variable decelerations. C: Late decelerations. Note the timing of the onset, nadir, and recovery of the deceleration, which occur after the onset, peak, and end of the contraction. *(From Hackney D. Estimation of fetal well-being. Fanaroff and Martin's neonatal-perinatal medicine. 2015: 181–95. https://www.clinicalkey.com/#!/content/book/3-s2.0-B9781455756179000130?scrollTo=%2533-s2.0-B9781455756179000130?scrollTo=%6233-s2.0-B9781455756179000130-f013-008-9781455756179)*

Hypotension can occur following rapid oxytocin infusion; this can be avoided by ensuring that a dilute infusion is used, even immediately postpartum. Other rare complications from oxytocin use include uterine rupture and water intoxication. Water intoxication may result if oxytocin is used in high concentrations and infused with large quantities of hypotonic solutions.

What are some important criteria to consider (and document) before labor is induced?
It is important to evaluate the potential risks to both the mother and the fetus prior to induction of labor. A thorough review of the patient's medical and pregnancy history should be undertaken in addition to a detailed assessment of the maternal or fetal condition prompting the induction in order to ensure that the indication is appropriate and to identify any potential contraindications to labor, prostaglandin use, or a vaginal delivery. Preinduction and preoxytocin checklists have been published to assist with this assessment and can be useful tools in this regard.

The gestational age and the method by which it was derived should be reviewed and documented in the patient's chart prior to the start of an induction in order to minimize the potential risk of neonatal morbidity and mortality attributable to incorrect dating. The estimated fetal weight should also be considered, including the potential for dystocia.

At the time of admission, a focused physical examination should include an assessment of the patient's cervical exam findings, a confirmation of the fetal presentation, and an assessment of the fetal heart rate and contraction patterns.

Finally, the indications for induction of labor should be reviewed with the patient and the details involving the induction process, techniques, and risks discussed. This includes the potential need for a cesarean delivery, and a physician capable of performing a cesarean delivery should be readily available during the induction.

> The patient undergoes cervical ripening with 25 µg of vaginal misoprostol. One hour later, her nurse notifies you that the patient is experiencing contractions every minute and the fetal heart rate demonstrates a baseline of 150/min with absent variability and recurrent late decelerations.

How should this patient's tachysystole and abnormal fetal heart rate be managed?
The patient has tachysystole with a Category III fetal heart rate tracing, which is defined as either a sinusoidal heart rate pattern or the presence of absent baseline fetal heart rate variability with recurrent late decelerations, recurrent variable decelerations, or bradycardia. In such cases, routine intrauterine resuscitative measures should be employed, including maternal repositioning, an intravenous fluid bolus, and supplemental oxygen administration. Although this patient is not receiving oxytocin, for patients who are, the infusion should be decreased or discontinued. Subcutaneous terbutaline may also be used in an attempt to resolve the tachysystole and correct the abnormal fetal heart rate tracing. If there is no response to these measures, cesarean delivery should be considered.

CLINICAL PEARL   **STEPS 2/3**

There are four types of fetal heart rate decelerations according to the National Institute of Child Health and Human Development (NICHD), each of which represents a different physiologic occurrence. *Early decelerations* represent a fetal autonomic response to changes in intracranial and/or cerebral blood flow, caused by transient compression of the fetal head. *Late decelerations* represent a transient disruption of oxygen transfer to the fetus resulting in transient hypoxemia and are seen in situations involving uteroplacental insufficiency. *Variable decelerations* represent a transient disruption of oxygen transfer from the environment to the fetus at the level of the umbilical cord and are indicative of cord compression. *Prolonged decelerations* represent a disruption of oxygen transfer from the environment to the fetus at one or more points along the oxygen pathway (Fig. 17.3).

After employing intrauterine resuscitative measures, the tachysystole and fetal heart tracing both resolve. After 1 hour of a Category I tracing, you perform a cervical examination, which reveals a dilatation of 1 cm, effacement 50%, and station –3. You place a transcervical Foley balloon catheter for cervical ripening. Eight hours later, the Foley balloon catheter is spontaneously expelled and the patient's cervical exam demonstrates a dilatation of 4 cm, effacement 60%, and station –1. An amniotomy is performed, and an oxytocin infusion is initiated. Twelve hours later, the patient has received an epidural for analgesia and is experiencing contractions every 2–3 minutes. Her nurse tells you that she is receiving the maximum dose of oxytocin. A cervical examination demonstrates that her cervix is unchanged, with a dilatation of 4 cm, effacement 60%, and station –1.

How is a failed induction diagnosed?

The normal progression of labor for a woman undergoing induction of labor differs significantly from that of a woman undergoing spontaneous labor. As such, allowing a longer period of latent labor before diagnosing a failed induction may reduce the risk of cesarean delivery. A failed induction is generally defined as the failure to generate regular contractions with cervical change after at least 24 hours of oxytocin administration. Artificial rupture of membranes should occur if safe and feasible. If, after rupture of membranes, regular contractions and cervical change do not occur after at least 12 hours of oxytocin administration, the induction may be considered a failure. The time involved in cervical ripening should not be included when determining the length of induction or when diagnosing a failed induction. In this patient's case, it is reasonable to offer a cesarean delivery at this time due to a diagnosis of a failed induction.

BEYOND THE PEARLS

- A labor induction for a nulliparous patient with an unfavorable cervix can be a multiple-day affair that requires patience on the part of the patient and provider. It can be helpful to set this expectation when starting the induction process, especially in situations where multiple cervical ripening techniques are required.
- Amniotomy may be effective as a stand-alone method of labor induction but requires that the cervix be dilated. When performing an amniotomy, the risk of umbilical cord prolapse can be reduced by ensuring that the fetal head is presenting, engaged, and well-applied to the cervix, with no umbilical cord or other fetal part presenting.
- Almost 30% of mothers who gave birth to a singleton infant reported using a nonmedical intervention to try to start labor, including ambulation, sexual intercourse, nipple stimulation, castor oil, and herbal therapies. Unfortunately, these methods and their efficacy have not been thoroughly evaluated.

Case Summary

- A 31-year-old G1P0 woman at 37 weeks' gestation is admitted for a scheduled induction of labor due to a pregnancy complicated by oligohydramnios.
- On physical exam, the patient's cervix is closed, 50% effaced, and –3 station.
- The patient undergoes cervical ripening with 25 µg of vaginal misoprostol. One hour later, the patient is experiencing tachysystole with a Category III tracing.
- After employing intrauterine resuscitative measures, the tachysystole and fetal heart tracing both resolve. A transcervical Foley balloon catheter is placed and spontaneously expelled 8 hours later. The patient's cervical exam demonstrates a dilatation of 4 cm, effacement 60%, and station –1. An amniotomy is performed, and an oxytocin infusion is initiated.
- Twelve hours later, the patient has received an epidural for analgesia and is experiencing contractions every 2–3 minutes on the maximum dose of oxytocin. A cervical examination demonstrates that her cervix is unchanged, with a dilatation of 4 cm, effacement 60%, and station –1. She undergoes a primary cesarean delivery due to a failed induction of labor.

References

Bishop, E. H. (1964). Pelvic scoring for elective induction. *Obstetrics and Gynecology, 24*, 266–268.

American College of Obstetricians and Gynecologists. (2009). ACOG Practice Bulletin No. 107: Induction of Labor. *Obstetrics and Gynecology, 114*(2), 386–397.

Kozhimannil, K. B., Johnson, P. J., Attanasio, L. B., et al. (2013). Use of nomedical methods of labor induction and pain management among U.S. women. *Birth, 40*(4), 227–236.

NICHD Definitions and Classifications: Application to Electronic Fetal Monitoring Interpretation. (2010) *NCC Monograph, 3*(1).

Rouse, D. J., Owen, J., & Hauth, J. C. (2000). Criteria for failed labor induction: prospective evaluation of a standardized protocol. *Obstetrics and Gynecology, 96*(5), 671–677.

Simon, C. E., & Grobman, W. A. (2005). When has an induction failed? *Obstetrics and Gynecology, 105*(4), 705–709.

Spong, C. Y., Berhella, V., Wenstrom, K. D., et al. (2012). Preventing the first cesarean delivery: summary of a joint Eunice Kennedy Shriver National Institute of Child Health and Human Development, Society for Maternal-Fetal Medicine, and American College of Obstetricians and Gynecologists Workshop. *Obstetrics and Gynecology, 120*(5), 1181–1193.

Tucker, S., Miller, L., Miller, D. F., et al. (2009). *Mosby's Pocket Guide to Fetal Monitoring: A Multidisciplinary Approach*. St. Louis: Mosby, 99–125.

Vahratian, A., Zhang, J., Troendle, J. F., et al. (2005). Labor progression and risk of cesarean delivery in electively induced nulliparas. *Obstetrics and Gynecology, 105*(4), 698–704.

Vrouenraets, F. P., Roumen, F. J., Dehing, C. J., et al. (2005). Bishop score and risk of cesarean delivery after induction of labor in nulliparous women. *Obstetrics and Gynecology, 105*(4), 690–697.

Wing D. Induction of Labor with Oxytocin. In: *UpToDate,* Post TW editors. UpToDate, Waltham, MA.

Wing D. (2017). Techniques for ripening the unfavorable cervix prior to induction. In: *UpToDate*. Post TW editors. UpToDate. Waltham, MA.

Shaina R. Eckhouse, MD

A 35-Year-Old Pregnant Woman With Abdominal Pain

Abdominal pain during pregnancy is a common reason for a general surgery consultation. However, it is uncommon for pregnant women to require surgery for abdominal pain secondary to a nonobstetrical diagnosis. In fact, only 1 in every 500–700 pregnant women require general surgical procedures during pregnancy. Acute appendicitis is the most common general surgical problem affecting pregnant women, while the second and third most common general surgery diagnoses are gallbladder disease and small bowel obstructions, respectively. Acute appendicitis carries significant risk to both the mother and the fetus if there is a delay in diagnosis and subsequent treatment. Furthermore, an expeditious and accurate diagnosis may be difficult due to the altered anatomy and physiology of a pregnant patient. Therefore, the overarching theme guiding management of general surgery diagnoses in pregnant women, including acute appendicitis, is "earlier diagnosis means better prognosis," as stated by Sir Zachary Cope in 1921. The case presented here is of a pregnant woman with abdominal pain from acute appendicitis.

> A 27-year-old G4P3 woman now at 20 weeks of estimated gestational age presents to the emergency department with a history of worsening abdominal pain. The patient reports nausea, but she denies fever or emesis. She reports taking ibuprofen with no improvement in the abdominal pain. She has no significant past medical history. She delivered her last child by cesarean delivery.

What are the imperative questions to ask in the patient who presents with abdominal pain?
The most important questions relate to understanding the patient's abdominal pain. Initially, it is crucial to evaluate the timeline for the development of abdominal pain. Typically, patients with general surgery pathology present with abdominal pain as their first symptom. Emesis before the onset of abdominal pain is more likely related to a nonsurgical diagnosis, such as viral gastroenteritis. Therefore, not only understanding the timing of abdominal pain but also the timeline of the patient's symptoms is of the utmost importance in creating your differential diagnosis. Next, it is important to characterize the quality of the abdominal pain. Does the abdominal pain refer to any other areas of the abdomen? Does the pain limit the patient's activities, such as standing up straight or walking normally? What makes the abdominal pain better, and what makes the abdominal pain worse? Last, it is important to ask about associated symptoms.

How does the clinical picture develop in a patient with appendicitis?
Classically, appendicitis presents initially with vague visceral abdominal pain in the periumbilical or epigastric region. As the inflammatory process in the appendix worsens, the parietal peritoneum becomes involved, and somatic pain develops at that location. Typically, the somatic pain associated with acute appendicitis occurs in the right lower quadrant. However, if the appendix is not in a classic position, pelvic pain, right flank pain, or even right upper quadrant pain can occur. As pregnancy progresses, the appendix is displaced superiorly, which can alter the pain experienced by the patient. As the patient's uterus enlarges in the second and third

trimester, the abdominal pain of appendicitis may develop in the mid-abdomen, the right upper quadrant, and in the epigastrium. Furthermore, it is important to ask about associated symptoms and the duration of these associated symptoms. Fever is only present in acute appendicitis about 40% of the time. Commonly, anorexia, nausea, and emesis follow the development of abdominal pain. These three symptoms are commonplace in pregnancy; therefore, the presence of anorexia, nausea, and emesis are not particularly helpful in diagnosing appendicitis. Either diarrhea or constipation can be reported. An appendix located lower in the abdomen into the pelvis can cause local irritation to the rectum, which then leads to loose stools. Urinary symptoms may develop due to appendiceal inflammation in close proximity to the bladder. With the displacement of the appendix upward due to the gravid uterus, urinary symptoms and changes in bowel habits occur less frequently.

BASIC SCIENCE PEARL   **STEP 1**

The appendix is a diverticulum of the cecum measuring about 10 cm in length and 3–5 mm in diameter. Its blood supply derives from the appendiceal artery, a terminal branch of the ileocolic artery. The appendix is thought to have some immunologic function as it secretes immunoglobulin A, a mucosal surface antibody.

BASIC SCIENCE PEARL   **STEP 1**

The pathophysiology of acute appendicitis is initiated by obstruction of the appendiceal lumen, which is most commonly caused by fecaliths. Luminal obstruction of the appendix can also occur from lymphoid hyperplasia, malignancy, foreign bodies, and, rarely, parasitic infections.

Obstruction of the appendiceal lumen with persistent mucosal secretions leads to venous congestion and tissue ischemia or infarction. This results in bacterial translocation and overgrowth that results in a suppurative and inflammatory process leading to acute appendicitis. With time, uncomplicated appendicitis left untreated can lead to phlegmon formation, gangrenous appendicitis, and subsequent perforation of the appendix with eventual abscess formation if left untreated.

What should be considered in your differential diagnosis?

The differential diagnosis in pregnant women with abdominal pain, which includes acute appendicitis, is extensive and covers many different medical specialties (Table 18.1).

CLINICAL PEARL   **STEP 2/3**

Because abdominal pain can be caused by gastrointestinal, genitourinary, gynecologic, obstetric, and vascular pathologies, a carefully taken history and physical examination can aid in narrowing the differential diagnosis to only a few disease processes.

On further questioning, the patient reports her pain started in the periumbilical region 24 hours ago, but has now localized to the right side of her abdomen. Initially the pain was dull and colicky, but it progressed to a sharp and constant pain. The patient further states that she feels weak and has no appetite. She denies any changes in her stool habits. On review of systems, the patient denies any genitourinary or gynecologic symptoms.

TABLE 18.1 ■ **Differential Diagnosis for Abdominal Pain**

Gastrointestinal	Acute appendicitis
	Diverticulitis
	Inflammatory bowel disease
	Gastroenteritis
	Gallbladder disease
	Acute hepatitis
	Pancreatic disease
	Bowel obstruction
	Gastroesophageal reflux disease
	Peptic ulcer disease
	Meckel's diverticulitis
Genitourinary	Nephrolithiasis
	Urinary tract infection
	Pyelonephritis
	Urinary retention
Gynecologic	Ovarian torsion
	Ruptured ovarian cyst
	Tubo-ovarian abscess
	Ovarian vein thrombophlebitis
	Pelvic inflammatory disease
	Salpingitis
	Mittelschmerz
	Endometriosis
	Fibroid degeneration
Obstetric	Labor
	Ectopic pregnancy
	Miscarriage
	Placental abruption
	Intra-amniotic infection
	Pregnancy-related liver disease
	Uterine incarceration
	Pubic symphysis separation
Vascular	Arterial dissection
	Arterial aneurysm
	Mesenteric ischemia
Other	Psoas abscess
	Abdominal wall hernia
	Rectus sheath hematoma
	Sickle-cell crisis
	Abdominal compartment syndrome
	Foreign body
	Unrecognized visceral injury
	Trauma

On physical examination, the patient's heart rate is 94/min, blood pressure is 115/79 mm Hg, respiration rate is 16/min, and oxygen saturation is 97% on room air. Cardiac and pulmonary examinations are normal. When examining the abdomen, the patient is found to have a gravid abdomen with her uterus palpable at the level of the umbilicus. She has rebound tenderness at McBurney's point, but she has a negative Rovsing's sign, psoas sign, and obturator sign. A rectal exam is negative for pain.

How can the physical exam findings change in the setting of appendicitis in a pregnant female?
As pregnancy progresses, the anatomy inside the abdomen changes as the uterus enlarges. During the first trimester, the uterus remains within the pelvis. Shortly after the pregnancy progresses into the second trimester, the uterus becomes intra-abdominal. By weeks 22–23, the gravid uterus is at

TABLE 18.2 ■ Classic Physical Exam Findings of Acute Appendicitis

McBurney's point tenderness	Rebound tenderness approximately 2 cm medial to the anterior superior iliac spine towards the umbilicus
Rovsing's sign	Right lower quadrant pain elicited by deep palpation of the left lower quadrant
Psoas sign	Abdominal pain on extension of the right hip with patient lying on left side caused by irritation of the psoas muscle by a retrocecal appendix
Obturator sign	Abdominal pain on internal rotation of the right hip caused by inflammation of obturator internus by pelvic appendix
Dunphy's sign	Increased abdominal pain with coughing
Markle's sign	Abdominal pain in the right lower quadrant elicited when a standing patient drops from standing on toes to heels with a jarring landing

the level of the umbilicus. As the uterus gets bigger with a maturing fetus, the appendix becomes displaced. The growing uterus makes it difficult to localize abdominal pain as the appendix may be in an atypical position, such as in the right upper quadrant or epigastrium. If the appendix is displaced posteriorly, the development of peritoneal signs can be masked or delayed. Peritoneal signs can be further masked by abdominal wall laxity. Nevertheless, there are specific physical exam findings that aid in the diagnosis of acute appendicitis. Please see Table 18.2 for a list of these findings.

What laboratory changes are associated with appendicitis?
When diagnosing acute appendicitis, it is important to check blood work. In a female, whether pregnant or not, the blood work checked should include a complete blood count (CBC), a basic metabolic panel (BMP), a urinalysis, and a β-human chorionic gonadotropin (β-hCG). With appendicitis, more than 80% of nonpregnant patients have a leukocytosis. Furthermore, a BMP may demonstrate labs consistent with mild dehydration. For example, the blood urea nitrogen (BUN) and creatinine levels may be mildly increased, and the bicarbonate level may be mildly decreased. Also microscopic hematuria and pyuria may occur in about 20% of patients where the inflammatory process in the appendix irritates the bladder, which is in close proximity.

The laboratory changes just described are less apparent in a pregnant woman. A mild leukocytosis is normal during pregnancy. As the pregnancy progresses, the white blood cell count can rise to as high as 20,000–25,000 cells per μL or more by the time of delivery. Trying to differentiate a leukocytosis related to pregnancy versus appendicitis can be challenging. Moreover, the BUN and creatinine levels are mildly decreased in pregnancy; therefore, testing is less likely to develop laboratory changes consistent with dehydration in the pregnant patient. Last, abnormalities on the urinalysis are less likely in the pregnant patient. This is especially evident as the uterus enlarges in the second and third trimesters, which further displaces the appendix superiorly and away from the bladder.

> Lab work is sent on the patient, and she is found to have a white blood cell count of 18,000 cells per μL with a left shift, a BUN of 30, a creatinine level of 1.2, a total bilirubin of 1.2, and a bicarbonate level of 20. The patient has a urine sample sent, and she is noted to have both microscopic hematuria and pyuria.

What imaging studies are useful in diagnosing appendicitis?
With laboratory data being less helpful during pregnancy, expeditiously confirming the diagnosis of acute appendicitis with imaging is key. In the nonpregnant patient, the radiologic test of choice is computed tomography (CT) scanning. However, diagnosing appendicitis during pregnancy poses a dilemma to the clinician, where the risk of appendiceal rupture from a delay in diagnosis must be considered against the risk of exposing the fetus to ionizing radiation secondary to a CT

TABLE 18.3 ■ **Comparison of Imaging Modalities**

Benefits	Risks
Ultrasound • Traditionally first-line imaging in pregnant patients • Noninvasive • No radiation or contrast • Widely available • Low cost	• Limited by body habitus and bowel gas pattern • Increasing inability to image the appendix as pregnancy progresses • Low sensitivity • Ultrasonographer dependent
Magnetic Resonance Imaging (MRI) • Cross-sectional imaging without radiation • High sensitivity and specificity • Reduces the negative appendectomy rate	• Less available • Requires experienced MRI technicians • More difficult to interpret for radiologists • Potential fetal effects of usage of gadolinium (unless ordered without contrast)
Computed Tomography (CT) • Cross-sectional imaging • High sensitivity and specificity • Reduces the negative appendectomy rate • First-line imaging modality in nonpregnant patients	• Ionizing radiation is associated with effects to the fetus including teratogenesis and increased risk of malignancy (but are dose dependent)

scan. Thus, the three imaging studies considered during pregnancy are abdominal ultrasound, magnetic resonance imaging (MRI), and, less commonly, CT scan.

Abdominal ultrasonography is considered the imaging modality of choice in pregnancy because it is the least invasive imaging study and can be quickly performed. Acute appendicitis is confirmed on ultrasound by the presence of a noncompressible tubular structure that blindly ends with a diameter of at least 6 mm. If the appendix is normal, then ultrasound can be useful to evaluate the reproductive organs and kidneys. On average, abdominal ultrasound confirms the diagnosis of appendicitis about 40% of the time during early pregnancy. The usefulness of ultrasound diminishes with progression of pregnancy. By the late second and third trimesters, the appendix may not be visualized up to 60–80% of the time. A normal or inconclusive ultrasound of the appendix with no other findings should trigger further imaging to evaluate the broad differential diagnosis of abdominal pain in pregnancy.

In the setting of a normal or inconclusive abdominal ultrasound, a noncontrasted MRI is the next diagnostic imaging test to perform because it has a high sensitivity and a high specificity for confirming the presence of acute appendicitis. MRI will demonstrate an enlarged and thickened appendix of greater than 6 mm in diameter with peri-appendiceal inflammation and fluid. A perforated appendix may be associated with a phlegmon or rim-enhancing fluid collection adjacent to the appendix. Nevertheless, MRI requires specialty-trained technicians to perform the study and experienced radiologists to read the study. Furthermore, MRI is not ubiquitously available. In these situations, CT scanning should be considered in consultation with an obstetrician. As previously mentioned, a CT scan is the imaging test of choice to diagnose appendicitis in a nonpregnant patient, and the findings are similar to those described for MRI. Newer CT scan protocols can be utilized to minimize the ionizing radiation exposure to the fetus to as low as 2 rads. Some CT scan protocols still reach 5 rads when a full abdominal and pelvic study is performed. In 2011, Society of American Gastrointestinal and Endoscopic Surgeons (SAGES) guidelines reported that low radiation CT protocols can be used judiciously during pregnancy. However, the ionizing radiation utilized to perform CT scans comes with raised risk to the fetus. In the first trimester, teratogenic side effects can occur with ionizing radiation. Throughout pregnancy, a risk also exists for childhood malignancy when a pregnant female and her fetus are exposed to ionizing radiation. Table 18.3 lists the risks and benefits of each imaging modality.

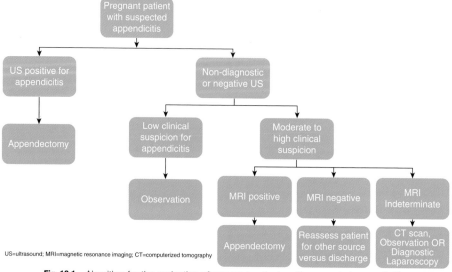

Fig. 18.1   Algorithm for the evaluation of pregnant patients with suspected appendicitis.

The patient's history, physical examination, and laboratory work up are concerning for the general surgery diagnosis of acute appendicitis versus a possible acute cholecystitis. The gravid uterus makes it more difficult for the emergency medicine physician to differentiate these two diagnoses without imaging. Therefore, an abdominal ultrasound is ordered to further evaluate the patient, and consultations to general surgery and obstetrics is called. The abdominal ultrasound is inconclusive. The general surgery, obstetric, and emergency medicine physicians all agree to order a STAT MRI. The MRI demonstrates an enlarged and thickened appendix measuring 10mm in diameter with peri-appendiceal inflammation. The gallbladder is normal.

Diagnosing acute appendicitis in a pregnant patient.

As previously mentioned, "early diagnosis means better prognosis."[4] Therefore, it is important to coalesce your history, physical exam, laboratory values, and imaging into a treatment plan. The patient described underwent a full work up and has been diagnosed with acute appendicitis. Fig. 18.1 depicts an algorithm that can be utilized in the evaluation of pregnant women with suspected appendicitis.

What is the treatment of choice for a pregnant female with appendicitis?

Once acute appendicitis is diagnosed in a pregnant female, the treatment of choice is an emergent appendectomy. A delay in surgery can increase the risk of appendiceal rupture, which has up to a 35% risk of fetal mortality. Thus, early treatment is of the utmost importance. The two surgical approaches used to perform an appendectomy are open or laparoscopic. In a pregnant patient, multiple small studies and systematic reviews have looked at whether open or laparoscopic surgery is safer. With the evolution of minimally invasive surgery and the continued improvement in laparoscopic techniques, a laparoscopic approach has become the more popular approach. SAGES, the largest society for laparoscopic surgeons, has written two position papers supporting the safety of laparoscopic appendectomy in the pregnant patient. Furthermore, several retrospective studies have demonstrated low rates of preterm labor (6%–10%) and low risk for fetal demise (4%–6%) with a laparoscopic approach in patients with nonruptured appendicitis.

Prior to starting the operative procedure, there are multiple perioperative considerations that must be addressed. First, the patient should receive preoperative antibiotics targeted toward Gram-negative rods and anaerobic bacteria, the common bacteria associated with appendicitis. The patient should also be aggressively rehydrated to avoid hypotension perioperatively. Also, sequential compression devices (SCDs) should be placed prior to surgery and continued after surgery to decrease the risk of thromboembolic events because pregnancy increases the risk of venous thromboembolism. Last, fetal monitoring should be discussed with the consulting obstetrician. Intraoperative fetal monitoring is typically considered if the fetus is viable based on estimated gestational age.

Once on the operating room table, positioning the patient should be optimized based on the age of the pregnancy. For instance, a supine position is safe in the first and early second trimesters. However, as the patient's pregnancy progresses, the inferior vena cava (IVC) can be compressed by the gravid uterus. Therefore, after 15–17 weeks' gestation, a modified left lateral decubitus position, where the patient's left side is elevated by 20–30 degrees, should be utilized to avoid IVC compression.

When performing a laparoscopic appendectomy in a pregnant patient, the technique for insufflation of the abdomen and trocar placement has to be carefully considered. Surgeon comfort and preference is an important consideration. The larger the uterus, the higher the trocars should be placed within the abdomen to avoid injury to the uterus and to increase the ease of performing an appendectomy.

> The patient underwent an uncomplicated laparoscopic appendectomy. She tolerated her diet without difficulty. She is discharged on post operative day one with close follow up in one week with her surgeon and obstetrician.

Case Summary

- A 35-year-old G4P3 woman presents with acute-onset abdominal pain and nausea. She is currently 20 weeks pregnant without any gynecologic, obstetric, or urinary symptoms.
- History and physical exam are concerning for acute appendicitis, which is the most common cause of abdominal pain in pregnancy requiring a general surgery abdominal operation.

However, the patient does not demonstrate any of the classical findings of appendicitis on physical exam or laboratory work-up. Radiologic imaging is ordered to confirm the diagnosis.

- The treatment of choice for acute appendicitis in a pregnant woman is an emergent appendectomy. Prior to surgery, the patient is hydrated with intravenous fluids and given antibiotics that will cover both Gram-negative and anaerobic bacteria.
- There are multiple small series examining whether surgery should be performed open or laparoscopically. With the advancement of minimally invasive surgery, laparoscopic appendectomy is now considered safe.

References

Aggenbach, L., Zeeman, G. G., Cantineau, A. E., et al. (2015). Impact of appendicitis during pregnancy: no delay in accurate diagnosis and treatment. *International Journal of Surgery, 15*, 84–89.

Awad, Z. T. E., & Steven, W. (2007). Laparoscopic appendectomy. In M. D. Josef, & E. Fischer (Eds.), *Mastery of surgery* (pp. 1434–1438). Philadelphia, PA: Lippincott Williams & Wilkins.

Bouyou, J., Gaujoux, S., Marcellin, L., et al. (2015). Abdominal emergencies during pregnancy. *Journal of Visceral Surgery, 152*(Suppl. 6), S105–S115.

Cheng, H. T., Wang, Y. C., Lo, H. C., et al. (2015). Laparoscopic appendectomy versus open appendectomy in pregnancy: a population-based analysis of maternal outcome. *Surgical Endoscopy, 29*(6), 1394–1399.

Diegelmann, L. (2012). Nonobstetric abdominal pain and surgical emergencies in pregnancy. *Emergency Medicine Clinics of North America, 30*(4), 885–901.

Flexer, S. M., Tabib, N., & Peter, M. B. (2014). Suspected appendicitis in pregnancy. *Surgeon, 12*(2), 82–86.

Freeland, M., King, E., Safcsak, K., et al. (2009). Diagnosis of appendicitis in pregnancy. *American Journal of Surgery, 198*(6), 753–758.

Guidelines Committee of the Society of American Endoscopic, G. S., & Yumi, H. (2008). Guidelines for diagnosis, treatment, and use of laparoscopy for surgical problems during pregnancy: this statement was reviewed and approved by the Board of Governors of the Society of American Gastrointestinal and Endoscopic Surgeons (SAGES), September 2007. It was prepared by the SAGES Guidelines Committee. *Surgical Endoscopy, 22*(4), 849–861.

Lowry, S. F. H., & John, J. (2007). Acute Appendicitis. In M. D. Josef, & E. Fischer (Eds.), *Mastery of surgery* (pp. 1430–1433). Philadelphia, PA: Lippincott Williams & Wilkins.

Lurie, S., Rahamim, E., Piper, I., et al. (2008). Total and differential leukocyte counts percentiles in normal pregnancy. *European Journal of Obstetrics, Gynecology, and Reproductive Biology, 136*(1), 16–19.

McGory, M. L., Zingmond, D. S., Tillou, A., et al. (2007). Negative appendectomy in pregnant women is associated with a substantial risk of fetal loss. *Journal of the American College of Surgeons, 205*(4), 534–540.

Miloudi, N., Brahem, M., Ben, A., et al. (2012). Acute appendicitis in pregnancy: specific features of diagnosis and treatment. *Journal of Visceral Surgery, 149*(4), e275–e279.

Pearl, J., Price, R., Richardson, W., et al. (2011). Guidelines for diagnosis, treatment, and use of laparoscopy for surgical problems during pregnancy. *Surgical Endoscopy, 25*(11), 3479–3492.

Puskar, D., Bedalov, G., Fridrih, S., et al. (1995). Urinalysis, ultrasound analysis, and renal dynamic scintigraphy in acute appendicitis. *Urology, 45*(1), 108–112.

Sadot, E., Telem, D. E., Arora, M., et al. (2010). Laparoscopy: a safe approach to appendicitis during pregnancy. *Surgical Endoscopy, 24*(2), 383–389.

Soper, N. J. (2011). SAGES' guidelines for diagnosis, treatment, and use of laparoscopy for surgical problems during pregnancy. *Surgical Endoscopy, 25*(11), 3477–3478.

Tehrani, H. Y., Petros, J. G., Kumar, R. R., et al. (1999). Markers of severe appendicitis. *The American Surgeon, 65*(5), 453–455.

Vu, L., Ambrose, D., Vos, P., et al. (2009). Evaluation of MRI for the diagnosis of appendicitis during pregnancy when ultrasound is inconclusive. *The Journal of Surgical Research, 156*(1), 145–149.

Walker, H. G., Al Samaraee, A., Mills, S. J., et al. (2014). Laparoscopic appendicectomy in pregnancy: a systematic review of the published evidence. *International Journal of Surgery, 12*(11), 1235–1241.

Wilasrusmee, C., Sukrat, B., McEvoy, M., et al. (2012). Systematic review and meta-analysis of safety of laparoscopic versus open appendicectomy for suspected appendicitis in pregnancy. *The British Journal of Surgery, 99*(11), 1470–1478.

Eva E. Szabo, MD

A 32-Year-Old Woman With Severe Postpartum Headache

A 32-year-old G2P2 woman presents to the obstetric emergency room with a severe headache. She had delivered a healthy newborn 4 days prior with epidural analgesia. Her labor was induced for preeclampsia with severe features. She was discharged home the previous day. Her husband has to return to work tomorrow, and she will have no help at home. She is very concerned that she will be unable to care for her infant and her 2-year-old child.

What is the first step in evaluating the patient with a postpartum headache?
The most important questions to ask are the time of onset and the location and quality of the pain. It is important to find out what brings the pain on and if there are any exacerbating or relieving factors. Ask about radiation and the presence of any associated symptoms such as nausea, vomiting, visual or auditory changes, and extremity weakness or numbness, fever, swelling, and abdominal pain.

On further questioning, the patient describes pain in the frontal and occipital area. It comes on within a few minutes every time she stands and radiates to her neck. She complains of neck stiffness, photophobia, tinnitus, and nausea. The headache started that morning, soon after she woke up. It gradually increased until she had to lie down. The headache subsided, but when she arose, it soon returned. The patient is also concerned that her back is still sore after the epidural placement. She says the epidural catheter was difficult to place and the anesthesiologist had to make several passes. The anesthesiologist did see her the next day and said everything looked normal, there was a little bruising at the site, but there was no complication.

What clues in the presentation and history point toward postdural puncture headache (PDPH)?
The postural nature of the headache is the strongest diagnostic indicator of PDPH. PDPH usually occurs within a couple of days of dural puncture, but it can present immediately after dural puncture or the onset can be delayed up to 5 days. The patient received epidural labor analgesia 4 days ago, and she describes multiple attempts at placement of the epidural catheter. It is possible that the epidural needle accidentally punctured the dura mater during repeated attempts.

What are the diagnostic criteria by the International Headache Society?
The International Headache Society's latest headache classification system provides the following definition:
"Headache occurring within five days of a lumbar puncture, caused by cerebrospinal fluid (CSF) leakage through the dural puncture. It is usually accompanied by neck stiffness and/or subjective hearing symptoms. It remits spontaneously within two weeks, or after sealing of the leak with autologous epidural lumbar patch.

Diagnostic criteria:

A. Any headache fulfilling criterion C
B. Dural puncture has been performed
C. Headache has developed within five days of the dural puncture
D. Not better accounted for by another ICHD-3 diagnosis"

Why is it important to elicit a history of headache?

Headache is very common in the postpartum period. The patient may present with the recurrence of her existing chronic headache, or it can be a new-onset headache. Most headaches are benign, but severe intracranial pathology also has to be considered. Many patients present with a recurrence of their known headache. Migraines are common headaches in young women. The headache caused by a migraine may improve during pregnancy, but it can recur in the postpartum period. The pain is described as severe, unilateral, and throbbing, and it may be associated with nausea or light and sound sensitivity. It can be preceded by an aura. An aura is a focal neurologic symptom that may include visual and other sensory, and also verbal or motor disturbances. For example, a visual aura (the most common) may present with a small area of visual loss (scotoma), a bright spot, flashing light, or shimmering, geometric patterns in the field of vision. A sensory aura may occur as a tingling sensation in the face or extremities. The pain is throbbing in nature, and it does not improve in the recumbent position; on the contrary, it may get worse. Tension headache is also very common in this population. The pain is usually bilateral, not as severe, and not positional. Your patient mentioned that her labor was induced for preeclampsia. This headache can also be a symptom of preeclampsia with severe features that present in the postpartum period.

Your patient tells you that she has a history of migraine headaches, but this headache feels somewhat different and it did not respond to her usual medication. Her migraines are usually one-sided, unlike this headache. Her migraine responds well to sumatriptan and does not get worse in the upright position. She tried sumatriptan anyway but got minimal relief. She also took a pill that contained acetaminophen with caffeine but did not get relief.

How does this information help you form a differential diagnosis?

The patient has a known primary headache, which can have a similar presentation and is more common than PDPH. It is not uncommon for migraine headache to recur in the postpartum period. But her migraine usually responds to sumatriptan; this headache did not. The patient did have epidural analgesia, and, while there is no confirmation of a known dural puncture at this time, the postural nature of the headache supports the diagnosis of PDPH. PDPH is the most common complication of epidural analgesia. In this case, her reported symptoms are concerning for PDPH, which is caused by the loss and continued leakage of spinal fluid if the dura mater was punctured during placement of the epidural catheter. It is important to review the anesthetic record for this complication. In addition, other etiologies that could present with a similar headache in the postpartum period have to be considered. There are also secondary headaches that can have a similar presentation. A patient can have more than one type of headache, which further complicates the diagnosis.

CLINICAL PEARL   **STEPS 2/3**

The risk of unintentional dural puncture with an epidural needle during epidural catheter placement is 1%–2% in the obstetric population. This number is higher in teaching institutions. More than half of these patients will experience PDPH because of the large size of an epidural needle. The risk of developing a PDPH from spinal anesthesia with much smaller, atraumatic (pencil point) needles, which have a conical tip, is much lower.

What is the anatomy of the spinal tract?

The dural sac contains the CSF, which surrounds and supports the brain and the spinal cord. The space external to the dura mater is the epidural space, which contains fat, venous plexuses, and the nerve roots. The local anesthetic injected into the epidural space spreads and blocks conduction of nerve impulses in the nerve roots. When the epidural space is located using a special epidural needle, the bevel of the needle is located within the epidural space; however, if the tip of the needle inadvertently pierces the dura mater, CSF will leak out through the puncture hole. This is called a "wet tap" (Figs. 19.1 and 19.2).

What other types of headaches have to be considered?

Headaches are common in the postpartum period, but the most common headaches, like migraine and tension headache, are not positional. Although in this case everything points toward PDPH, there are a few other pathologies that can initially present with a headache that has a postural component to it. The differential diagnosis for other postural headaches includes potentially life-threatening pathologies such as hemorrhage and thrombosis. Subdural hemorrhage can be a complication of dural puncture itself. Subdural hemorrhage may be caused by tearing of the bridging veins from the surface of the brain to the dural sinuses when the brain's weight is not supported by adequate CSF volume. Cortical vein or sinus thrombosis can also present with a postural headache. It can present after delivery in the setting of the hypercoagulable state associated with pregnancy and the immediate

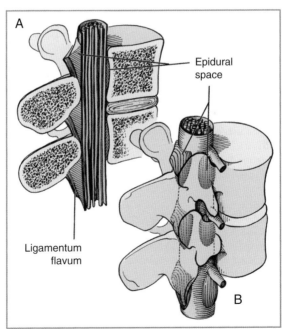

Fig. 19.1 Anatomy of the epidural space. A: Sagittal section of the epidural space demonstrates that the contents of the epidural space depend on the level of the section. B: Three-dimensional drawing of the epidural space shows the discontinuity of the epidural contents. However, this potential space can be dilated by the injection of fluid into the epidural space. *(Redrawn from Stevens RA. Neuraxial blocks. In Brown DL, editor. Regional anesthesia and analgesia. Philadelphia: WB Saunders; 1976: 323.* https://www.clinicalkey.com/#!/content/book/3-s2.0-B9781455748662000122?scrollTo=%233-s2.0-B9781455748662000122-f012-002-9781455748662)

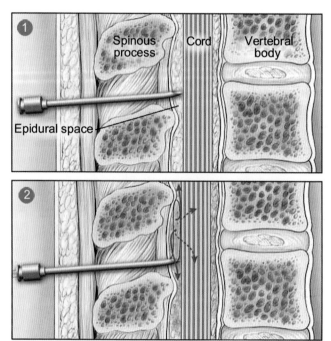

Fig. 19.2 Epidural analgesia is achieved by placing a catheter into the lumbar epidural space. *(From Chow L, Farber M, Camann W, et al. Anesthesia in the pregnant patient with hematologic disorders.* Hematol Oncol Clin N Am. *2011;425–43.* https://www.clinicalkey.com/#!/content/journal/1-s2.0-S0889858811000050?scrollTo=%231-s2.0-S0889858811000050-gr2)

postpartum period, but it can also be a complication of dural puncture itself. Preeclampsia is also associated with headache and intracranial hemorrhage. A dural puncture in these patients can confuse the diagnosis. Headache caused by pneumocephalus can also complicate the picture if air is used to identify the epidural space and is accidentally injected when the dura mater is punctured. Meningeal irritation by intracranial air causes a headache very similar to PDPH but is usually less severe and resolves quickly. The same patient can then develop PDPH, too.

On physical examination, her blood pressure is 130/85 mm Hg, heart rate is 80/min, respiratory rate is 16/min, and temperature is 36.5°C (97.7°F). Cardiac and pulmonary exam are normal. Her documented weight is 98 kg (216 lb) and her height is 152 cm (5 ft). She is in no apparent distress, lying supine, with the light off. Neurologic exam is normal. She states that her headache is better now.

You consult the anesthesiologist. The anesthetic record reveals difficult placement due to the depth of the epidural space (8 cm) requiring multiple attempts. However, no mention is made of a dural puncture.

How does a history of a difficult epidural placement support your presumed diagnosis of PDPH?

Risk factors for developing PDPH include female gender, younger age, large needle size, and number of dural punctures. Your patient is a young female; the epidural needle is 17 or 18 gauge, which is large; and it took several attempts to place the catheter. The patient is morbidly obese (body mass index of 42), which explains the larger than average depth of the epidural space. In obese patients, the bony landmarks (spinous processes) are difficult to palpate, and, with increasing thickness of the adipose layer, needle placement becomes more difficult. PDPH is highest on the differential based on the strong positional component of the headache, the associated symptoms, and the information provided by the anesthesia record. Although a "wet tap" is not described, the record reveals multiple attempts. It is possible to puncture the dura mater and not see CSF return in the syringe during rapid, repeated advancement and withdrawal of the needle. With multiple attempts, the risk increases.

BASIC SCIENCE PEARL	STEP 1

The dura mater is composed of layers of collagen fibers. When the dura mater (and adherent arachnoid mater) is punctured with a needle, some CSF will be lost. The continued leakage of CSF and diminished CSF pressure leads to the headache. Epidural needles are much larger than spinal needles; therefore the hole created in the dura mater is larger and takes longer to heal.

What is the pathophysiology of PDPH?

There are two presumed mechanisms leading to headache. One is the traction on meningeal structures by the brain in the upright position. The average adult has 150 mL of CSF, which surrounds and supports the brain and the spinal cord. The volume of the CSF is diminished by the persistent loss of CSF through the puncture if it is not matched by production of CSF. Depending on the size of the defect and the rate of CSF loss, the onset of the headache may be immediate when assuming the upright position, but it may be delayed by a few minutes, up to 15 minutes. The other theory is that of compensatory cerebral vasodilation, which would cause a pain similar to migraine. Assuming that the intracranial volume (the sum of brain and spinal cord, CSF, and blood volume) has to be constant, cerebral vasodilation (increased blood volume) compensates for the decreasing volume of CSF.

How do you treat this patient who complains of severe headache?

PDPH should initially be treated conservatively, with analgesics; opioid analgesics may be necessary in severe headache. The oral route is preferred. Intravenous (IV) hydration and IV analgesics are not usually necessary unless the patient has severe nausea and vomiting. Bed rest provides symptomatic relief but prolonged bed rest is not recommended due to the risk of thromboembolic complication in the immediate postpartum period. Aggressive hydration has not been shown to decrease the incidence of PDPH.

There are other pharmacologic treatments, but very little evidence exists to support their use. Caffeine has been recommended based on its cerebral vasoconstrictor properties. Intravenous caffeine 500 mg was commonly used but large doses of caffeine have side effects, such as palpitations and dysrhythmias; therefore the routine use of caffeine is no longer recommended. However, patients used to drinking large amounts of caffeinated drinks may get a caffeine withdrawal headache if they stop suddenly.

Serotonin agonists commonly used to treat migraine have also been used for their vasoconstrictive properties based on the presumed pathomechanism of vasodilation, but evidence does not support their routine use. There are several small studies discussing other potential pharmacologic agents, such as gabapentin, cosyntropin, or epidural morphine.

Since your patient has tried oral analgesics and sumatriptan without relief, you offer her an epidural blood patch (EBP). After discussing the risks and benefits, she agrees because she is unable to perform the necessary tasks of caring for her newborn and her other child at home because of the severity of the headache.

CLINICAL PEARL   **STEPS 2/3**

EBP is the gold standard for treating severe PDPH.

What is an EBP, and how is it performed?

The patient's own blood is injected into the epidural space, close to the puncture site, usually just below it. The blood will spread cephalad and presumably "patch" the dural defect. The goal is to inject 20 mL. The lower back is prepped in the usual way, and the epidural space is located using an epidural needle. The blood is drawn from the hand or arm in a sterile fashion, then incrementally injected into the epidural space.

How does EBP work?

There are two possible mechanisms by which the injection of blood can relieve the pain. The first is the increase in intracranial pressure. The injected blood will compress the dural sac and shift CSF toward the brain. It is also possible that the compensatory vasodilation is reversed at this time. This hypothesis is supported by the almost immediate relief of pain experienced by some patients. The blood will also form a clot, sealing the puncture and allowing it to heal. Injection of a colloid or crystalloid is less effective; they will also increase the pressure, but they do not block the leak.

What are the risks and benefits of an EBP?

The procedure has the same inherent risks as the original epidural placement that resulted in the dural puncture. Depending on what the reason for the initial "wet tap" was, there may be an increased risk of causing another dural puncture. The risk of infectious complication, nerve root or spinal cord damage, or epidural hematoma is very low. There is also the risk of inadvertently injecting blood into the intrathecal space (into the CSF) causing meningeal irritation. Even though the risk of severe complication is low, a thorough evaluation has to precede the procedure. Some headaches are not severe, and the symptoms will resolve with conservative management within 2 weeks. On the other hand, severe PDPH requires invasive management. If untreated, it can lead to more severe complications such as subdural hemorrhage, persistent cranial nerve palsies, or chronic headache. At least two-thirds of patients experience relief of their symptoms after a blood patch. If the pain recurs within a few days, the procedure can be repeated.

> The anesthesiologist performs the blood patch without further complications. Two days later, the patient returns with the same complaints. She has a recurrence of her headache and it is debilitating.

What is your differential diagnosis at this point?

Her symptoms resolved after the blood patch. She resumed her usual activities, took care of the baby and the household. Now her symptoms returned and are very similar to the ones earlier. A positional headache in this setting points toward the recurrence of her PDPH. However, the previously discussed, less common causes have to be considered again. The physical exam has to be repeated.

> On exam, there are no new findings; the neurologic exam is benign. You consult the anesthesia team again. They perform a blood patch the second time. The patient has immediate relief of her symptoms. You observe her for a couple hours, and then discharge her home.

What would you do if she returned in a few days with a recurrence of the headache?
Further neurologic workup is indicated at this point. Even though there are case reports of patients requiring three blood patches, it is rare. Even if the symptoms are consistent with PDPH, neuro-imaging is indicated to rule out other, more serious, pathology.

CLINICAL PEARL   **STEPS 2/3**

Other potentially life-threatening diagnoses have to be considered if a second EBP fails.

BEYOND THE PEARLS

- Unintentional dural puncture is the most common complication of labor epidural analgesia; it should not be considered a "minor" complication.
- PDPH causes significant delays in hospital discharge.
- PDPH decreases patient satisfaction, often leading to lawsuits.
- Most of these headaches resolve with time, but serious long-term complications, including life-threatening complications such as intracranial hemorrhage, can occur.
- EBP is the only effective treatment, but it has a risk of severe complications.
- The optimal timing of the EBP and the optimal volume of blood are still under debate, but it seems prudent to wait 2–3 days before repeating an EBP.
- The obstetrician has an important role in identifying postpartum patients who may have PDPH. PDPH may present after hospital discharge.

Case Summary

- A 32-year-old G2P2 woman with a history of migraine headaches presents with postpartum headache. She underwent labor induction for preeclampsia with severe features. She had a difficult labor epidural placement.
- Symptoms of a typical postural headache are consistent with a postdural puncture headache even though dural puncture was not recognized at the time of the procedure.
- She is treated with an EBP, but her symptoms recur.
- After the second blood patch, her symptoms resolve.

References

Carlswärd, C., Darvish, B., Tunelli, J., et al. (2015). Chronic adhesive arachnoiditis after repeat epidural blood patch. *International Journal of Obstetric Anesthesia*, *24*(3), 280–283.

Choi, P. T., Galinski, S. E., Takeuchi, L., et al. (2003). PDPH is a common complication of neuraxial blockade in parturients: a meta-analysis of obstetrical studies. *Canadian Journal of Anaesthesia*, *50*(5), 460–469.

Headache Classification Committee of the International Headache Society. (2013). The international classification of headache disorders, 3rd edition (beta version). *Cephalalgia*, *33*(9), 629–808.

Ilkhchoui, Y., Szabo, E. E., Gerstein, N. S., et al. (2014). Cerebral venous thrombosis complicating severe preeclampsia in the postpartum period: a diagnostic challenge. *Journal of Clinical Anesthesia*, *26*(2), 143–146.

Paech, M. J., Doherty, D. A., Christmas, T., et al. (2011). Epidural Blood Patch Trial Group. The volume of blood for epidural blood patch in obstetrics: a randomized, blinded clinical trial. *Anesthesia and Analgesia*, *113*(1), 126–133.

Riley, C. A., & Spiegel, J. E. (2009). Complications following large-volume epidural blood patches for postdural puncture headache. Lumbar subdural hematoma and arachnoiditis: initial cause or final effect? *Journal of Clinical Anesthesia*, *21*(5), 355–359.

Sachs, A., & Smiley, R. (2014). Post-dural puncture headache: The worst common complication in obstetric anesthesia. *Seminars in Perinatology*, *38*(6), 386–394.

Van de Velde, M., Schepers, R., Berends, N., et al. (2008). Ten years of experience with accidental dural puncture and post-dural puncture headache in a tertiary obstetric anaesthesia department. *International Journal of Obstetric Anesthesia*, *17*(4), 329–335.

Sangeeta Jain, MD ■ Joey England, MD

A 25-Year-Old Woman With Obesity in Pregnancy

A 25-year-old Caucasian G2P0 woman presents at 10 weeks' gestation for prenatal care. She has had one spontaneous miscarriage in the past. She and her partner are very excited about this pregnancy. They have been trying to conceive for almost 1 year. She works as an administrative assistant, and her partner works as a supervising engineer at an oil refinery. They have been together for the past 2 years. The history of miscarriage was with same partner 1 year ago.

On presentation to prenatal care, what is the first assessment?
A detailed history and physical examination should be performed for all patients presenting for obstetric care.

The patient describes her gynecologic history as significant for irregular menses that occur every 1–2 months. She will have bleeding for 5 days without passing clots, and she utilizes approximately three to four pads or tampons daily during that time. She has been sexually active since the age of 17 with two partners and has had all normal Pap smears. She had one infection with chlamydia that was treated at 17 years of age. She denies smoking and illicit drug use. She drank an occasional glass of wine in the evenings prior to knowing she was pregnant. Family history is significant for diabetes and chronic hypertension (CHTN); both her parents have CHTN. Her mother, sister, and maternal grandmother have diabetes. She denies family history of major congenital anomalies, mental delay, cancer, or blood clots.

The patient's vital signs are collected. She has a height of 1.6 m (5'3") and a weight of 91.6 kg (202 lb) with a body mass index (BMI) of 36 kg/m². Her temperature is 36.6°C (98°F), blood pressure is 122/78 mm Hg, heart rate is 89/min and respiratory rate 20/min. On physical exam she appears overweight but otherwise healthy. She has a normal cardiopulmonary, abdominal, breast, and pelvic examination. Her lower extremities do not demonstrate tenderness or edema.

CLINICAL PEARL   **STEPS 2/3**

The occurrence of abnormal uterine bleeding including metrorrhagia (menses occurring at irregular intervals) and menorrhagia (heavy menstrual bleeding) is associated with obesity. Additionally, polycystic ovary syndrome may be diagnosed; this can involve noncyclic bleeding, hyperandrogenic signs, and characteristic ovarian appearance on ultrasound.

Upon review of this preliminary history and physical exam, what is the greatest risk factor for this pregnancy? How prevalent is it among women in the United States?

Obesity is the greatest risk factor for this pregnancy. Thirty-six percent of women 20 years of age and older are obese. This number increases to 64% when overweight and obese categories are combined. Among Caucasians, 66.7% were considered overweight or obese, 34.3% were considered obese, and 5.7% were considered to have extreme obesity. Among African-Americans, 76.7% were considered overweight or obese, 49.5% were considered obese, and 13.1% were considered to have extreme obesity. Among Hispanics, 78.8% were considered overweight or obese, 39.1% were considered obese, and 5% were considered to have extreme obesity. In 2013, obesity was estimated to affect more than 2 billion individuals worldwide.

What are the goals during her first prenatal visit?

After obtaining a thorough history with a focus on comorbid medical conditions, a physical examination should be performed and prenatal laboratories collected, including an early glucose challenge test (GCT). The early GCT will screen for pregestational diabetes. The GCT should be repeated (if negative) at the usual 24- to 28-week time frame as in patients undergoing routine prenatal care. Patients with a history of bariatric surgery should undergo a 1-week paneling of fasting and 2-hour postprandial fingersticks for glucose levels in lieu of GCT. GCT may cause dumping syndrome because a high carbohydrate intake can lead to osmotic diarrhea, distension, and hypovolemia. Hypovolemia occurs as fluid shifts from the intravascular space to the enteric intraluminal space. During this visit, the patient should be scheduled for a nutrition consult and encouraged to exercise. Pregnancy is an ideal time for behavior modification due to frequent medical provider supervision and increased patient motivation to optimize her health and the health of her baby. She should be encouraged to start exercising to achieve the goal of moderate-intensity exercise for approximately 30 minutes daily on most days of the week. Walking, swimming, stationary cycling, and low-impact aerobics are safe to initiate during pregnancy. If performed regularly prior to pregnancy, strength training can be included.

> The patient's prenatal lab results are within normal limits including a normal GCT of 120 mg/dL.

What are complications of obesity during pregnancy?

Obesity is associated with increased risk for spontaneous miscarriage, fetal congenital anomalies, gestational diabetes, preeclampsia, acute fatty liver disease, sleep apnea, anesthesia complications, and cardiac dysfunction. Increased fetal risks from maternal obesity are stillbirth, and congenital anomalies.

> The patient advances to 21 weeks gestational age and undergoes a detailed anatomy ultrasound revealing an estimated fetal weight of 450 g (84th percentile), normal amniotic fluid, and without structural abnormalities. At each prenatal visit, her BMI and weight gain are addressed, and she has a repeat GCT performed at 28 weeks with a value of 150 mg/dL. Due to the elevated 1-hour GCT, she undergoes a confirmatory 3-hour GCT. The results are fasting, 94 mg/dL; 1-hour, 182 mg/dL; 2-hour, 150 mg/dL; and 3-hour, 132mg/dL. She is relieved that although one value (the 1-hour) was elevated, the remaining values were within normal limits and she does not meet criteria for diagnosis of gestational diabetes.

CLINICAL PEARL   **STEPS 2/3**

Screening for gestational diabetes is performed between 24 and 28 weeks' gestation. A 1-hour 50 g oral GCT (Glucola) is administered. If blood glucose levels are higher than 140 mg/dL at 1 hour, suspect gestational diabetes. Diagnosis is confirmed after a 3-hour 100 g oral GCT yields two abnormal values:
>95 mg/dL fasting
>180 mg/dL at 1 hour
>155 mg/dL at 2 hours
>140 mg/dL at 3 hours

Intrapartum, patients with obesity are at increased risk for failed induction, cesarean delivery, postpartum hemorrhage, postoperative wound infection, endometritis, and venous thromboembolism. There is increased risk of delivery of an infant that is large for gestational age. Also increased are the rates of shoulder dystocia, Erb's palsy, clavicular fracture, and low Apgar scores.

In the postpartum period, early termination of breastfeeding, increased risk of anemia, depression, and metabolic dysfunction is seen. If glucose intolerance was present during pregnancy, assessment for type 2 diabetes should be performed 6 weeks after delivery. A plan for weight reduction should be developed for the patient.

What are the recommendations for weight gain during pregnancy in obese women?
The Institute of Medicine guidelines for weight gain during pregnancy are based on BMI on entry to care. In overweight women with BMIs of 25–29.9, the recommended range of total weight gain is 6.8–11.3 kg (15–25 lb). In obese women with BMIs 30 or above, 4.9–9 kg (11–20 lb) (0.2 kg/0.5 lb per week in second and third trimesters) is recommended. They do not give recommendations for individual classes of obesity. Prepregnancy weight loss is recommended for best pregnancy and long-term outcome. Limited data showed that, in women with BMIs of greater than 35 kg/m², minimal or lack of weight gain during pregnancy had no adverse effect on the newborn.

In the third trimester, the fundal height is difficult to assess during her prenatal visit, so the patient undergoes a growth ultrasound revealing an appropriately grown fetus measuring at the 70th percentile for gestational age. She is scheduled for an anesthesiology consultation prior to delivery and undergoes an uncomplicated spontaneous vaginal delivery at term.

For patients with obesity, what type of skin incision is preferred during a cesarean delivery?
The optimal skin incision has not been decided upon. Options include supraumbilical, vertical, and transverse skin incisions. The Maternal-Fetal Medicine Units Network performed a secondary analysis of vertical versus transverse cesarean delivery incisions. Vertical skin incision was associated with a lower wound complication rate, but there was concern regarding the study's observational nature and selection bias. The supraumbilical incision has been preferred in some patients with a large panniculus. Some studies have reported an association between the supraumbilical incision and increased rates of classical hysterotomy (due to restricted intraoperative exposure) and longer operative times. Randomized clinical trials are needed to answer this question.

Are there any long-term implications of obesity on the women's health?
Obesity-related infertility is prevalent worldwide. After delivery, obese women are at increased risk for type 2 diabetes, hypertension, cardiovascular disease, and stroke. Certain cancers, especially

endometrial cancer, is associated with obesity; in women who lose weight, their risk for endometrial cancer decreases.

What has been the impact of bariatric surgery on the health of a woman of reproductive age?

The U.S. Centers for Disease Control and Prevention (CDC) reports a rate of 30% of obesity among reproductive-age women. After introduction of bariatric surgery, by 2006, 200,000 surgeries were performed in the United States. Of those, 80% were for females, and 65% of those were younger than 50 years of age.

What is bariatric surgery? What are the types and their risk and benefit profiles?

Bariatric surgery is weight loss surgery performed for obese individuals who have failed weight loss attempts and have normal psychological screening. There are several types:

- *Restrictive procedures* such as the lap band: A small and simple surgery where a band is placed around the stomach close to the gastroesophageal junction. The band can be adjusted with the help of a connecting port located in subcutaneous tissue close to the stomach. Complications of this surgery include band slippage (13.9%), band erosion (3%), and port access problems (5%).
- *Restrictive surgery* such as the sleeve gastrectomy: A narrow gastric sleeve is created by stapling the stomach vertically, and the fundus and greater curve of the stomach are removed from the abdomen. Complications include leakage (2%) or gastric luminal narrowing due to stenosis of the sleeve.
- *Malabsorptive procedures* such as Roux-en-Y gastric bypass: A more extensive procedure in which stomach and duodenum are bypassed. There is decreased nutrient absorption. Complications include bowel obstruction (1%), anastomotic leaks (1%–2%), stomal stenosis (2%–14%), and marginal ulcers (2%–10%). Small bowel obstruction resulting from internal herniation has a lifetime incidence of up to 10% in patients who underwent Roux-en-Y gastric bypass.

CLINICAL PEARL   **STEPS 2/3**

In the United States, the Roux-en-Y gastric bypass is considered the gold standard for bariatric surgery and entails division of the upper stomach to create a small gastric pouch (15–30 mL) connected to a 100 to 150 cm limb of jejunum (the Roux limb). Food thus bypasses the majority of the stomach, the duodenum, and the proximal jejunum. Because of the limited size of the stomach, the patient is limited in the amount of food she can consume.

CLINICAL PEARL   **STEPS 2/3**

Signs and symptoms of small bowel obstruction from internal herniation may mimic symptoms of pregnancy and include nausea, vomiting, abdominal/ epigastric pain, constipation, abdominal distension, tympanic abdominal percussion, and hyperperistalsis on abdominal auscultation.

A recent meta-analysis reported that bariatric surgery reduces the incidence of gestational diabetes by half as compared with obese patients. Similarly, the risk for preeclampsia may be decreased significantly after bariatric surgery.

The American College of Obstetricians and Gynecologists (ACOG) recommends avoiding pregnancy for 12–24 months after bariatric surgery due to rapid weight loss and concern for nutritional deficits. Folic acid supplementation is recommended at a higher dosage of 4 mg daily (although with limited data) due to increased risk of folic acid deficiency after bariatric surgery. During pregnancy, monitoring of nutritional status is recommended, with lab evaluations including complete blood count (CBC) and iron, ferritin, calcium, and vitamin D levels every trimester. Some studies associated bariatric surgery with fewer large for gestational age infants and more small for gestational age infants. In a population-based study ($n = 298$) following previous bariatric surgery there was a similar rate of perinatal death, congenital malformations, and Apgar scores.

CLINICAL PEARL   **STEPS 2/3**

Folic acid deficiency during pregnancy is associated with neural tube defects. The proposed mechanism is enhanced cell proliferation for neural tube closure directly or involvement in the epigenetic regulation of gene expression that controls neural closure. Neural tube closure occurs within the first 4 weeks of embryonic life (by 6 weeks' gestation); due to the many unplanned pregnancies, folic acid supplementation is recommended for all women of reproductive age.

BEYOND THE PEARLS

- Despite frequent provider recommendation, bed rest is rarely indicated during pregnancy and may lead to harm including deconditioning and venous thromboembolism.
- Absolute contraindications to aerobic exercise in pregnancy include restrictive lung disease, cervical insufficiency, preterm labor or rupture membranes, preeclampsia, persistent vaginal bleeding, and significant maternal heart disease.

Case Summary
- A 25-year-old G2P0 woman presents at 10 weeks' gestation for prenatal care; her medical history is significant for obesity with a BMI of 36 kg/m^2.
- During her prenatal care she undergoes a thorough history and physical examination, routine prenatal labs, and an early GCT, which is normal. Her anatomy ultrasound is normal at 21 weeks. Throughout her pregnancy her weight gain is monitored, and repeat GCT is performed at 28 weeks' gestation.
- She undergoes anesthesia evaluation prior to delivery and has an uncomplicated spontaneous vaginal delivery.

References

American College of Obstetricians and Gynecologists. (2009). Practice bulletin no. 105: Bariatric surgery and pregnancy. *Obstetrics and Gynecology, 113*(6), 1405–1413.

American College of Obstetricians and Gynecologists. (2013). Practice bulletin no. 136: Management of abnormal uterine bleeding associated with ovulatory dysfunction. *Obstetrics and Gynecology, 122*(1), 176–185.

American College of Obstetricians and Gynecologists. (2015). Practice bulletin no. 156: Obesity in pregnancy. *Obstetrics and Gynecology, 126*(6), e112–e126.

Anderson, N. H., McCowan, L. M., Fyfe, E. M., et al. (2012). The impact of maternal body mass index on the phenotype of pre-eclampsia: a prospective cohort study. An International Journal of Obstetrics & Gynaecology, *119*(5), 589–595.

Arnolf, M., Jiang, L., Stefanick, M. L., et al. (2016). Duration of adulthood overweight, obesity, and cancer risk in the women's health initiative: a longitudinal study from the united states. *PLoS Medicine, 13*(8), e1002081.

Brocato, B. E., Thorpe, E. M. Jr., Gomez, L. M., et al. (2013). The effect of cesarean delivery skin incision approach in morbidly obese women on the rate of classical hysterotomy. *Journal of Pregnancy.* Article ID 890296. http://dx.doi.org/10.1155/2013/890296.

Catalano, P. M. (2007). Management of obesity in pregnancy. *Obstetrics and Gynecology*, *109*(2), 419–433.

Galazis, N., Docheva, N., Simillis, C., et al. (2014). Maternal and neonatal outcomes in women undergoing bariatric surgery: a systematic review and meta-analysis. *European Journal of Obstetrics, Gynecology, and Reproductive Biology*, *181*, 45–53.

Greene, N. D., Stanier, P., & Moore, G. E. (2011). The emerging role of epigenetic mechanisms in the etiology of neural tube defects. *Epigenetics*, *6*(7) 875–883.

Lashen, H., Fear, K., Sturdee, D. W. (2004). Obesity is associated with increased risk of first trimester and recurrent miscarriage: matched case control study. *Human Reproduction*, *19*(7), 1644–1646.

Lemon, L. S., Naimi, A. I., Abrams, B., et al. (2016). Prepregnancy obesity and the racial disparity in infant mortality. *Obesity (Silver Spring)*, *24*(12), 2578–2584.

Ng, M., Fleming, T., Robinson, M., et al. (2014). Global, regional, and national prevalence of overweight and obesity in children and adults during 1980-2013; a systematic analysis for the Global Burden of Disease Study 2013. *Lancet*, *384*(9945), 766–781.

National Institute of Diabetes and Digestive and Kidney Diseases. Overweight and obesity statistics. https://www.niddk.nih.gov/health-information/health-statistics/Pages/overweight-obesity-statistics.aspx.

Nocca, D., Krawczykowsky, D., Bomans, B., et al. (2008). A prospective multicenter study of 163 sleeve gastrectomies: results at 1 and 2 years. *Obesity Surgery*, *18*(5), 560–565.

Patel, J. A., Patel, N. A., Thomas, R. L., et al. (2008). Pregnancy outcomes after laparoscopic Roux-en-Y gastric bypass. *Surgery for Obesity and Related Diseases*, *4*(1), 39–45.

Sheiner, E., Levy, A., Silverberg, D., et al. (May. 2004). Pregnancy after bariatric surgery is not associated with adverse perinatal outcome. *American Journal of Obstetrics and Gynecology*, *190*(5), 1335–1340.

Stothard, K. J., Tennant, P. W., Bell, R., et al. (2009). Maternal overweight and obesity and the risk of congenital anomalies: a systemic review and meta-analysis. *Journal of the American Medical Association*, *301*(6), 636–650.

Tixier, H., Thouvenot, S., Coulange, L., et al. (2009). Cesarean section in morbidly obese women: supra or subumbilical transverse incision? *Acta Obstetricia et Gynecologica Scandinavica*, *88*(9), 1049–1052.

Vannevel, V., Jans, G., Bialecka, M., et al. (2016). Internal herniation in pregnancy after gastric bypass: a systematic review. *Obstetrics and Gynecology*, *127*(6), 1013–1020.

Weiss, J. L., Malone, F. D., Emig, D., et al. (2004). Obesity, obstetric complications and cesarean delivery rate: a population based screening study. *American Journal of Obstetrics and Gynecology*, *190*(4), 1091–1097.

CASE 21

Noelle Niemand, MD ■ Joey England, MD

A 33-year-Old Woman With Postpartum Vaginal Edema

A 33-year-old G1P1 woman underwent spontaneous vaginal delivery of a 4 kg (8 lb 14 oz) female infant 1 hour ago. She now complains of vaginal swelling. The patient tells you her swelling is inside her vagina, accompanied by pain, 6/10 in severity, worsened by movement.

What is your differential diagnosis?

Diagnostic considerations in a postpartum patient with vaginal swelling include vulvar edema, vulvar hematoma, vaginal hematoma, and retroperitoneal hematoma. Location will often determine clinical presentation, blood loss, and treatment decisions. Vulvar hematomas result from injuries to branches of the pudendal artery and can be further classified by the anterior or posterior pelvic triangle.

BASIC SCIENCE PEARL	STEP 1

In the anterior triangle, bleeding is confined by the perineal membrane preventing expansion into the ischiorectal fossa, superiorly by the levator ani, and limited from spread onto the thigh by Colle's fascia and the fascia lata. Bleeding in the posterior triangle is limited by the anal fascia.

The central tendon of the perineum prevents spread across the midline. These hematomas may occur after an episiotomy or perineal lacerations during delivery (see Fig. 21.1). Trauma to vessels supplying the vaginal and paravaginal regions are not limited by fascia and can lead to a large accumulation of blood. These hematomas result from delivery-related soft tissue damage and are commonly associated with forceps delivery. A retroperitoneal hematoma is a rare, serious complication of delivery and is due to injury of branches of the internal iliac artery. This can occur with trauma, injury of the uterine artery during cesarean delivery, extension of a paravaginal hematoma, or uterine rupture. Hemorrhage can be very severe and cause immediate hypovolemic shock. Most hematomas will present within 24 hours of delivery. The diagnosis is based on characteristic symptoms and findings on physical examination (Table 21.1).

On initial physical exam, she has vaginal swelling that is consistent with a right posterior wall vaginal hematoma approximately 2 cm in size. Examination of the vulva, cervix, and rectum is normal. Her abdomen is soft and nontender to palpation. The fundus of her uterus is firm and approximately 2 cm above her umbilicus. She has a temperature of 37.1°C (98.8° F), a heart rate of 90/min, and a blood pressure of 120/68 mm Hg. Her oxygen saturation is 99% on room air.

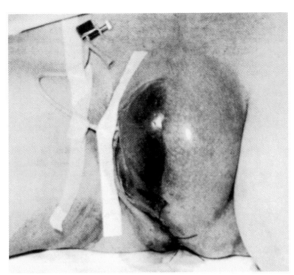

Fig. 21.1 Large vulvar hematoma. *(From Francois K, Foley M. Anetpartum and postpartum hemorrhage. In: Obstetrics: Normal and problem pregnancies. 2017:395–424. https://www.clinicalkey.com//?_escaped_ fragment_=/#!/content/book/3-s2.0-B9780323321082000184?scrollTo=%23hl0001243)*

TABLE 21.1 ▪ Common Locations for Puerperal Hematomas With Corresponding Vascular Injuries

Puerperal Hematoma	Vascular Injury
Vulva	Branches of the pudendal artery (inferior rectal, perineal, posterior labial, urethral, clitoral, and vestibule)
Vaginal/paravaginal	Branches of the uterine artery
Retroperitoneum	Branches of the hypogastric (internal iliac) artery.

CLINICAL PEARL   **STEPS 2/3**

The incidence of puerperal hematoma ranges from 1 in 300 to 1 in 1000 deliveries. Reported risk factors include nulliparity, forceps delivery, episiotomy, infant weight of greater than 4000 g, clotting disorder, and inadequate laceration/episiotomy repair.

What is the initial management?

Thorough examination to determine the size and location of the hematoma should be performed (Fig. 21.2). If it cannot be adequately visualized, imaging studies should be employed. Analgesia and an ice pack are offered due to the vaginal pain. Depending on the extent of the vaginal hematoma, it may or may not require surgical drainage. If not expanding, the hematoma can simply be observed. If expanding, packing should be placed with continued monitoring. Vaginal hemostatic balloon devices have been utilized to achieve hemostasis in patients with vaginal hematomas following vaginal delivery (Fig. 21.4).

Initial vaginal packing fails to prevent expansion, and the hematoma is now 10 cm.

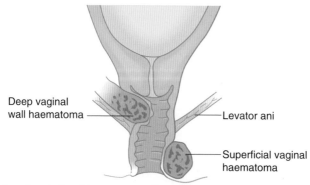

Deep vaginal wall haematoma

Levator ani

Superficial vaginal haematoma

Fig. 21.2 The sites of vaginal wall hematomas. *(From Vacca A. Management of delivery. In:* Essential obstetrics and gynaecology. *2013:183–98. https://www.clinicalkey.com//?_escaped_fragment_=/#!/searc h/Vaginal%2520hematoma/%7B%22facetquery%22:%5B%22+contenttype:IM%22,%22+contenttype:VD% 22%5D%7D)*

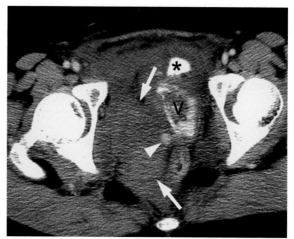

Fig. 21.3 Puerperal genital hematoma from a vaginal wall injury caused by an episiotomy in a 26-year-old woman. Contrast-enhanced computed tomography (CT) image shows intravenous contrast material extravasation and a large hematoma *(arrows)* in the right perivaginal space. Note the intravenous contrast material extravasation *(arrowhead)* adjacent to the vagina *(V)*. The presence of contrast media in the bladder is noted *(asterisk)*. *(From Lee N, Kim S, Lee J, et al. Postpartum hemorrhage: Clinical and radiologic aspects.* Eur J Radiol. *2010;74:50–9. https://www.clinicalkey.com//?_escaped_fragment_=/#!/content/journal/1-s2.0-S0720048X0900268X?scrollTo=%231-s2.0-S0720048X0900268X-gr16)*

How would you manage the patient now?

Since expansion has continued despite conservative methods, exploration should be undertaken. Blood products should be available, and a surgical team should be assembled. If the patient does not have regional anesthesia in place, anesthesia consultation for pain control should be established. Larger, expanding vaginal hematomas require surgical intervention. If apparent, the bleeding artery should be identified and ligated. The cavity can be closed and a vaginal pack or tamponade device placed usually for at least 12 hours. A transurethral catheter should be placed until after edema subsides and removal of vaginal packing.

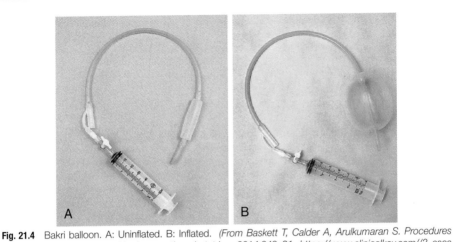

Fig. 21.4 Bakri balloon. A: Uninflated. B: Inflated. *(From Baskett T, Calder A, Arulkumaran S. Procedures and techniques. In: Munro Kerr's operative obstetrics. 2014:242–81. https://www.clinicalkey.com//?_esca ped_fragment_=/#!/content/book/3-s2.0-B9780702051852000281?scrollTo=%233-s2.0-B978070205185 2000281-f028-010ab-9780702051852)*

CLINICAL PEARL	STEPS 2/3

Morbidity associated with puerperal hematomas includes transfusion complications, coagulopathy, infection, anemia, reformation of the hematoma, venous thromboembolism, scarring, and prolonged hospitalization.

Despite repair and absence of ongoing bleeding the patient's vital signs continue to deteriorate. She has a heart rate of 130/min and a blood pressure of 80/50 mm Hg. Her oxygen saturation is 96% on room air.

What would your management be now? What is the most likely cause of worsening hemodynamic instability?

With hemodynamic instability, ensure large-bore intravenous access is in place and begin resuscitation with crystalloid and blood transfusion. Close monitoring of the patient's vital signs and urine output (with placement of a Foley catheter if not already in place) are essential to follow the patient's clinical status and response to resuscitative efforts. Laboratory evaluation should include a complete blood count, fibrinogen level, prothrombin time, and partial thromboplastin time to determine current levels and presence of a bleeding diathesis.

The patient likely has a retroperitoneal hematoma that had not been identified. Imaging would confirm this, but, in the setting of rapid decompensation, exploratory laparotomy is indicated. Computed tomography (CT), ultrasonography, and magnetic resonance imaging (MRI) have been described to identify the hematoma location and extent (Fig. 21.3). A massive transfusion protocol (MTP) should be initiated instead due to the patient's hypotension and tachycardia. Next, identification and ligation of the bleeding vessel should be undertaken if obvious and/or ligation of the internal iliac artery. If ipsilateral ligation fails to resolve bleeding, bilateral ligation should be performed.

If the patient is hemodynamically stable and interventional radiology is readily available, artery embolization is an alternative to surgical repair. Selective arterial ligation allows for selective occlusion of bleeding vessels, which may be valuable in circumstances of aberrant pelvic vasculature. Case series have reported successful pregnancies following this procedure, allowing for possible preservation of future fertility. Complications of selective arterial embolization include fever, infection, ischemic pain, vascular perforation, and tissue necrosis. Complications have been reported in 3%–6% of cases.

In the setting of hemodynamic instability, an MTP is initiated. The patient is taken to the OR and undergoes exploratory laparotomy. She is noted to have bleeding into the right retroperitoneal space. Ligation of the right hypogastric artery ligation is performed with no further expansion noted. Patient is taken to the recovery room awake and in stable condition. Her postoperative recovery is uneventful. Vital signs, urine output, and labs are closely monitored over the next several days. She is discharged home on postoperative day 3.

BEYOND THE PEARLS

- Retroperitoneal packing is a technique used by trauma surgeons to tamponade hemorrhage and can be utilized to control bleeding in the obstetrical patient. Through a laparotomy the fascia is divided and the space of Retzius is accessed. Two to three laparotomy sponges are placed in the retroperitoneal space bilaterally, below the pelvic brim in the true pelvis. The packing should be removed or exchanged at 24–48 hours.
- The use of drains has been reported; however, data are insufficient to support their routine use.
- Blood loss is nearly always more than the clinical estimate. Patients with preeclampsia in the postpartum period may appear normotensive with marked hypovolemia, or the initial catecholamine release from hemorrhage may initially lead to hypertension.

Case Summary

- A 33-year-old woman presents after spontaneous vaginal delivery with vaginal swelling.
- History and physical examination reveals that the patient has a posterior vaginal hematoma. Conservative measures are undertaken, but the patient develops an expanding hematoma.
- She undergoes exploratory laparotomy with control of bleeding through hypogastric artery ligation.
- She has an uneventful recovery course.

References

Alexander, J. M., & Wortman, A. C. (2013). Intrapartum Hemorrhage. *Obstetrics and Gynecology Clinics of North America, 40*(1), 15–26.

Cunningham, F., Leveno, K., Bloom, S., et al. (2014). Obstetrical hemorrhage. In *Williams Obstetrics* (24th ed.) (p. 780).

Gizzo, S., Saccardi, C., Patrelli, T., et al. (2013). Bakri balloon in vaginal-perineal hematomas complicating vaginal delivery: a new therapeutic approach. *Journal of Lower Genital Tract Disease, 17*(2), 125–128.

Sentilhes, L., Gromez, A., Clavier, E., et al. (2009). Predictors of failed pelvic arterial embolization for severe postpartum hemorrhage. *Obstetrics and Gynecology, 113*(5), 992–999.

Smith, W. R., Moore, E. E., Osborn, P., et al. (2005). Retroperitoneal packing as a resuscitation technique for hemodynamically unstable patients with pelvic fractures: report of two representative cases and a description of technique. *Journal of Trauma and Acute Care Surgery, 59*(6), 1510–1514.

You, W. B., & Zahn, C. M. (2006). Postpartum hemorrhage: abnormally adherent placenta, uterine inversion, and puerperal hematomas. *Clinical Obstetrics and Gynecology, 49*(1), 184–197.

Zahn, C. M., Hankins, G. D., & Yeomans, E. R. (1996). Vulvovaginal hematomas complicating delivery. Rationale for drainage of the hematoma cavity. *The Journal of Reproductive Medicine, 41*(8), 569–574.

Maria I. Villegas Kastner, MD ■ Oscar A. Viteri, MD

A 16-Year-Old Girl With Diabetic Ketoacidosis in Pregnancy

A mother brings her 16-year-old daughter to the emergency room (ER). Since this morning she seems lethargic and refuses to eat or drink. According to the mother, she has been complaining of decreased appetite, nausea, and abdominal pain for the past 2 days.

When evaluating a patient at the ER or any other clinical setting, identify the most significant problem or major complaint and work the differential diagnosis around it; in this case, decreased consciousness (lethargy).

What is most likely causing this patient's lethargy?

The evaluation of a patient with altered mental status can be complex. A thorough history and physical examination can give clues to the etiology. Identifying the presence of sudden focal neurological deficits or signs of increased intracranial pressure (papilledema, projectile vomiting, and the "worst headache of my life," etc.) are important clues pointing to ischemic events, hemorrhagic events, or structural damage (compression). On the other hand, the absence of focalization should direct the differential toward substance abuse, drug adverse effects, infectious causes (meningitis, encephalitis), or metabolic disorders (hypo- or hyperglycemia, hyponatremia, uremia, hepatic encephalopathy, etc.). While cerebrovascular accidents and infections have an abrupt onset, metabolic disturbances and intoxication present more insidiously and with a slow deterioration in consciousness.

What other important questions or findings will help in our differential?

Exposure to sick contacts, travel history, living in dormitories (increased risk of meningococcal meningitis), immunosuppression therapies, and symptoms like fever, rash, petechiae, photophobia, and headache elicited with neck movements are clear hints for meningeal irritation and infectious causes.

A family or personal history of diabetes or a current triad of polyuria, polydipsia, and weight loss should raise suspicion for it and its complications: hypoglycemia or hyperglycemia, hyperglycemic hyperosmolar state (HHS), and diabetic ketoacidosis (DKA).

Other metabolic derangements and electrolyte imbalances to consider are hyponatremia following severe dehydration and uremic encephalopathy, particularly in kidney or liver failure.

Last, a social history of use and abuse of drugs, mood disorders, or lack of family support can be indicative of intoxication.

CLINICAL PEARL   **STEPS 2/3**

At all times perform finger stick blood glucose. It is fast and will narrow the possible etiologies. Remember, the brain and red blood cells are the only ones that cannot synthetize glucose by themselves; they require a continuous supply in order to avoid irreversible damage (cellular lysis); hence hypoglycemia is the first etiology to be ruled out because it is easy to correct, and failure in treatment can be fatal.

On further questioning, the patient's responses are slow but coherent; she lives with her family and denies any substance abuse, exposure to sick contacts, or history of travel. She denies past medical history; however, she complains of weight loss, nausea, increased thirst, and urinary frequency, which she attributes to a history of a urinary tract infection (UTI) 1 month ago as she didn't complete her treatment. Since yesterday, she presents with fever, and her abdominal pain has increased. She denies any other symptoms. Additionally, she states a history of irregular menses; her last menstrual period was approximately 4 months ago.

The description of a young patient with weight loss, polydipsia, and polyuria is suggestive of an initial presentation of diabetes mellitus (DM), possibly type 1. Furthermore, the presence of nausea, starvation, abdominal pain, and the possibility of infection (fever and a past history of UTI) are precipitating factors for DKA.

BASIC SCIENCE PEARL   **STEP 1**

The fruity odor of DKA is the result of the decarboxylation and conversion of acetoacetic acid into acetone, which produces the characteristic smell similar to nail polish remover.

On physical examination, her body mass index (BMI) is 22 kg/m², her temperature is 38.8°C (102°F), blood pressure is 80/60 mm Hg, heart rate is 120/min, respiratory rate is 24/min, and oxygen saturation is 95% on room air. The patient is diaphoretic and lethargic. Her oral mucosa is dry with a fruity odor, and her breathing is rapid and shallow. She has a normal neurologic and cardiopulmonary exam. Her abdomen is soft and tender to deep palpation with costovertebral tenderness.

Laboratory results are pending. Blood glucose by finger stick is 450 mg/dL, and a urine pregnancy test is positive. The patient was not aware of her pregnant state.

With the information provided, what is the likely diagnosis?
This is a young pregnant female with decreased mental status, severe dehydration, and symptoms of diabetes. Her severe hyperglycemia and breathing pattern are highly suggestive of DKA (Table 22.1).

TABLE 22.1 ■ **Diagnostic Criteria for Diabetic Ketoacidosis (DKA)**

- Hyperglycemia ≥300 mg/dL (350–500 mg/dL)
- Increased anion gap metabolic acidosis (pH <7.30; anion gap >14 mEq/L)
- Ketosis (positive serum and urine ketones)

Nevertheless DKA in pregnancy is extremely rare; it presents in 0.5%–3% of all pregnant women with diabetes and is more common in previously known patients with diabetes. Thirty percent of women had undiagnosed preexisting diabetes until presenting with DKA.

The presence of hypotension, tachycardia, fever, and a history suggestive of UTI/pyelonephritis should raise suspicion not only for an acute episode of decompensated diabetes but for systemic inflammatory response syndrome (SIRS) and sepsis.

What is the clinical presentation of DKA?

DKA develops in the background of a patient presenting with the classic diabetic triad that acutely deteriorates over a period of hours to days with progressive neurologic decline from full alertness to stupor. Common complaints are nausea, vomiting, and severe abdominal pain, the latter presenting in approximately 50% of the cases and exacerbated by delayed gastric emptying and ileus resultant from the metabolic imbalance. In the gravid patient, intractable nausea, vomiting, and dehydration can aggravate the condition, triggering uterine contractions and developing DKA at a faster rate and to lower levels of glycemia. This condition is known as *euglycemic ketoacidosis* (defined as, *in the absence of pronounced hyperglycemia, severe ketoacidosis with bicarbonate* (HCO_{3-}) *<10 mEq/L).*

On physical examination, signs of volume depletion, a distinctive fruity odor, and the elaborated Kussmaul respiration pattern can be observed. Fever can be present with infection.

BASIC SCIENCE AND CLINICAL PEARL   **STEPS 1/2/3**

Decrease in plasma bicarbonate (HCO_3-) or a rapid increase in acid production (ketones, lactic acid, etc.) will lead to an acid–base and electrolyte imbalance resulting in metabolic acidosis. In an effort to compensate the increasing acidosis, the excess of hydrogen (H^+) production will stimulate the respiratory center chemoreceptors, causing hyperventilation. The increase in the respiratory rate will expel the carbon dioxide and raise the pH. As the acidosis becomes more severe, the initial rapid and shallow breathing pattern worsens to "Kussmaul breathing."

CLINICAL PEARL   **STEPS 2/3**

When assessing a woman of reproductive age, always perform a pregnancy test. The diagnostic approach, differential diagnosis, and management might differ in those in whom pregnancy is confirmed. Pregnancy has also been described as a precipitating factor of DKA.

Once a thorough physical evaluation is completed and the cardiopulmonary and mental status assessed and stabilized, laboratory evaluation is undertaken including urinalysis, urine culture, basic metabolic panel, serum bicarbonate, blood gases, and complete blood count (CBC) (Table 22.2). HHS presents with greater alteration of sensorium (stupor, coma), glucose levels greater than 600 mg/dL, plasma osmolarity greater than 320 mOsm/kg (normal is 280 mOsm/kg), and absence of ketosis. Furthermore, HHS is more common in those with type 2 diabetes. On the other hand, DKA classically presents with glucose levels of approximately 350–500 mg/dL, dehydration, ketosis, and acidosis (metabolic).

Mild leukocytosis can be normal in pregnancy; however, it may be the result of stress-induced hypercortisolemia or infection-related, especially if markedly elevated.

A pH of less than 7.30 and bicarbonate level of less than 15 mEq/L, are indicative of metabolic acidosis. Elevated anion gap (AG) metabolic acidosis can be caused by DKA.

BASIC SCIENCE AND CLINICAL PEARL   **STEPS 1/2/3**

An elevated AG is the result of the acidosis generated by the increased production and accumulation of unmeasured organic acids like ketone bodies (3-β–hydroxybutyrate [3-HB], acetoacetate, and lactic acid). Values greater than 14 mEq/L are often seen in DKA.
  The AG is calculated as follows:
  Serum sodium (Na^+) − [serum chloride (Cl^-) + bicarbonate (HCO_3-)].

With ketonuria, serum ketones should be measured (3-HB). To monitor improvement, serum 3-HB measurement is preferred (ketonuria may persist >36 hours due to slow elimination rate).

Hyponatremia may be present due to the shift of fluids from the intracellular to the extracellular space (in efforts to decrease plasma osmolality caused by severe hyperglycemia). Serum potassium levels may appear deceptively normal or even elevated secondary to pronounced hyperglycemia. However, total body potassium K^+ concentration is severely depleted, and it can lead to serious rhythm disturbances; therefore an electrocardiogram (EKG) should be ordered.

BASIC SCIENCE PEARL   **STEP 1**

Insulin drives K^+ into the cell. As insulin is being administered to the patient with DKA, K^+ reenters the cell and causes hypokalemia.

In severe metabolic acidosis, the cells exchange potassium for hydrogen (H^+); in other words, the cell takes all the acid and shifts the K^+ from the intracellular to the extracellular space as a compensatory mechanism to decrease the degree of acidosis.

Once the patient is stable and initial treatment has started, a formal obstetrical ultrasound can be obtained to determine gestational age.

Direct diagnostic tests to determine fetal acidosis are not available; nevertheless, an indirect assessment by fetal heart rate monitoring (after viability of 24 0/7 weeks) can be performed. Ultrasound and other fetal tests ought to be reserved if fetal well-being is in question after the mother's volume status and metabolic derangements have been corrected.

TABLE 22.2 ■ **Initial Laboratory and Diagnostic Tests**

Electrocardiogram (EKG)	Sinus Tachycardia. (HR: 120/minute)
Leukocyte count	16.900 /μL (16.9 × 10 ⁹)
Leukocyte differential	85% neutrophils, 8 % bands
Serum glucose	475 mg/dL
Hemoglobin A1C	7.0%
BUN	28 mg/dL
Serum creatinine	1.1 mg/dL
Serum HCO_3^-	11 mEq/L
Blood gases	pH: 7.24, HCO_3:11 mEq/L, CO_2:16
Electrolytes	Na^+: 130 mEq/L, K^+: 5.1 mEq/L, Cl^+: 100 mEq/L
β -hydroxybutyrate	1.3 mmol/L (<0.4–0.5 mmol/L)
Urinanalysis	Ketones ++, Glucose +, Nitrites +, Bacteria +++, Leukocyte esterase ++

What are the precipitating factors for the development of DKA?

Several conditions such as undiagnosed diabetes, infection, poor insulin compliance, insulin pump failure, acute major illness (pancreatitis, myocardial infarction, sepsis, etc.), and drugs that affect carbohydrate metabolism are among the events that have been reported as triggering factors for DKA.

Pregnancy has also been established as a precipitating factor. Indeed, its inherent physiologic adaptations promote a diabetogenic state that, combined with several other factors frequently seen in pregnancy, like nausea, emesis, UTIs, and the use of glucocorticoids, can trigger an acute episode of ketoacidosis at a faster rate.

BASIC SCIENCE PEARL	STEP 1

Glucocorticoids alter carbohydrate metabolism, decreasing the peripheral uptake of glucose and stimulating hepatic gluconeogenesis resulting in increased in glucose levels and glycogen storage.

What is the mechanism for the development of DKA?

DKA is the result of the relative or absolute lack of insulin production in the β cells of the pancreas. In the absence of insulin the peripheral uptake of glucose is diminished and perceived by the cell as a lack of substrate, forcing it to seek alternative sources of energy (muscle and adipose tissue breakdown). In response to this perceived hypoglycemia a counter regulatory mechanism is activated and increases the release of glucagon, epinephrine, cortisol, and growth hormone leading to gluconeogenesis, glycogenolysis, and decreased peripheral uptake of glucose along with massive breakdown of triglycerides into glycerol and fatty acids; the latter are then oxidized in the liver and converted to ketone bodies (acetoacetic acid, 3-HB, and acetone). The accumulation exceeds the buffering capacity of bicarbonate to neutralize the excess hydrogen and leads to a high AG metabolic acidosis that is exacerbated by the lactic acid production (from decreased tissue perfusion and hypovolemia).

What are the implications of acidosis (DKA) on the fetus?

Pregnancy by itself is a well-known precipitating factor of DKA, and its presence in the mother is synonymous with acidosis and hypoxemia in the fetus as the uteroplacental flow soon becomes affected. The depletion of the intravascular volume due to the marked osmotic diuresis leads to a redistribution of the maternal cardiac output and diminishes the perfusion and oxygenation of the uteroplacental unit, perpetuating the acidotic state in both the mother and the fetus. Moreover, the maternal decrease in 2-3 diphosphoglycerate (DPG) shifts the oxygen-hemoglobin dissociation curve to the left, increasing the affinity of maternal hemoglobin for oxygen and decreasing oxygen delivery to the fetus.

BASIC SCIENCE PEARL	STEP 1

Four principal factors shift the oxygen-hemoglobin dissociation curve to the right: increased carbon dioxide, increased 2-3DPG, rise in temperature, and acidosis, all with the purpose of decreasing the affinity of oxygen (O_2) to hemoglobin so it facilitates the delivery of O_2 to tissues in periods of stress or high demand. However, the opposite of these conditions will shift it to the left, exacerbating hypoxemia.

As glucose and ketoacids readily cross the placenta, the same maternal pathophysiologic effects can occur in the fetus. Specifically, elevated glucose, osmotic diuresis with hypovolemia, and fetal acidosis with fetal arrhythmias due to hypokalemia can occur. Thus the rate of fetal loss without treatment is high.

Fetal well-being can be assessed indirectly through external fetal monitoring and biophysical profile (BPP). It is not uncommon that these tests may be abnormal during an acute episode of DKA. Fetal hypoxemia will reveal variations in fetal heart rate tracing; absent accelerations, late decelerations (placental insufficiency), and minimal or absent variability often can be seen (Fig. 22.1).

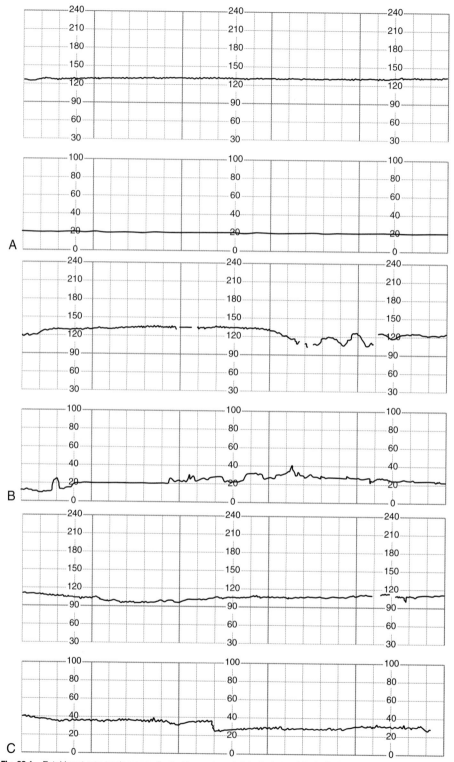

Fig. 22.1 Fetal heart rate tracing complicated by maternal diabetic ketoacidosis (DKA). A: Fetal heart rate (FHR) tracing demonstrating absent accelerations and absent variability. B: Nonreassuring FHR tracing after correction of metabolic acidosis. C: Ominous FHR tracing recorded approximately 30 minutes prior to fetal demise. *(From Sibai BM. Management of acute obstetric emergencies. Philadelphia, PA: Elsevier Saunders, 2011; 194:137–42. https://www-clinicalkey-com.ezproxyhost.library.tmc.edu/#!/content/book/3-s2.0-B9781416062707000120)*

Is DKA a mandatory indication for delivery?

No. The successful correction of the maternal metabolic imbalance and her prompt stabilization frequently improves the fetal heart rate pattern and other abnormalities. An emergent cesarean section in the setting of acute decompensation increases maternal morbidity and mortality as well as the rate of preterm delivery and adverse fetal outcomes.

What is the prognosis for the mother and the fetus?

Even though DKA during pregnancy is rare, it is still a very serious complication of diabetes. An inadequate diagnosis and delay in treatment carries increased morbidity (acute renal insufficiency, acute respiratory distress syndrome, cerebral edema, etc.) and mortality for both mother and fetus. Studies have reported a mortality rate of 5%–15% for the mother and as high as 57% for the fetus, particularly in women in whom DKA was the initial presentation of diabetes.

What is the treatment for DKA?

DKA management includes (1) correcting the severe volume depletion by aggressive fluid replacement and stabilizing the hemodynamic status, (2) decreasing the hyperglycemic state by administering intravenous insulin, (3) correcting acidosis and electrolyte imbalance, and (4) identifying and treating any underlying conditions or precipitating factors (Fig. 22.2).

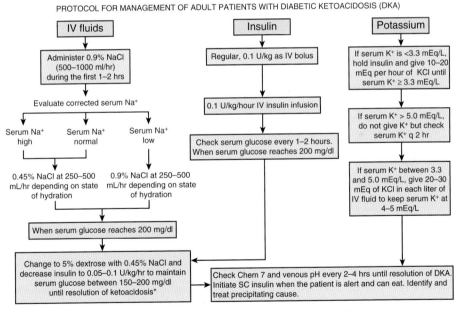

Fig. 22.2   Treatment algorithm. *(From Jameson JL.* Endocrinology: adult & pediatric. *7th edition.* Philadelphia: Saunders, 2016; 2687: 809 chapter 46, 805–15. *https://www-clinicalkey-com.ezproxyhost.library.tmc.edu/#!/content/book/3-s2.0-B9780323189071000469?scrollTo=%23f0015)*

How do we know if the patient is getting better?

Laboratory monitoring is required every hour initially and can be decreased in frequency with improvement in the patient's clinical response. DKA is considered to be resolved if ketoacids have been cleared from the serum and the subsequent closure of the AG is observed.

Once volume and insulin replacement were started, the patient improved. Antibiotics were initiated for the UTI, and IV fluids were continued until hemodynamic stability and oral tolerance was achieved. A formal ultrasound was performed confirming an intrauterine pregnancy at approximately 20 weeks' gestational age with active cardiac activity. The patient improved over her hospital stay and was discharged home with an insulin regimen, nutrition advice, insulin education, and a follow-up clinic visit.

BEYOND THE PEARLS

- A SOFA score of 2 or more reflects an overall mortality risk of approximately 10% in a general hospital population with suspected infection.
- Patients with septic shock can be clinically identified by a vasopressor requirement to maintain a mean arterial pressure of 65 mm Hg or greater and a serum lactate level greater than 2 mmol/L (>18 mg/dL) in the absence of hypovolemia. This combination is associated with hospital mortality rates of greater than 40%.
- Although diabetic ketoacidosis (DKA) mainly presents in type 1 diabetes, it can also be seen in type 2 diabetes and gestational diabetes (GDM). An increase in its incidence is expected as the rate of obesity and the prevalence of type 2 diabetes increase.

Case Summary

- A 16-year-old girl presents with altered mental status secondary to metabolic imbalance. Her history and physical examination reveals signs and symptoms of DKA.
- Laboratory evaluation confirmed the presence of ketoacidosis as well as an early pregnancy and urinary infection, both precipitating factors for DKA.
- Aggressive fluid replacement therapy was started immediately, as well as insulin. The patient was hemodynamically stabilized, and antibiotics were initiated for her urinary infection. Fetal surveillance was deferred since her obstetric ultrasound revealed a 20-week pregnancy.
- The patient recovered and was scheduled for a follow-up prenatal clinic visit.

References

Carroll, M. A., & Yeomans, E. R. (2005). Diabetic ketoacidosis in pregnancy. *Critical Care Medicine, 33*(10), S347–S353.

Jameson, J. L. (2016). *Endocrinology: adult & pediatric* (7th ed.). Philadelphia, PA: Elsevier Saunders, 2687. 77, 809.

Marcdante, K., & Kliegman, R. (2015). *Nelson essentials of pediatrics* (7th ed.). Philadelphia, PA: Elsevier/ Saunders, 634–642. Chapter 184.

Parker, J. A., & Conway, D. L. (2007). Diabetic ketoacidosis in pregnancy. *Obstetrics and Gynecology Clinics of North America, 34*(3), 533–543.

Schneider, M. B., Umpierrez, G. E., Ramsey, R. D., et al. (2003). Pregnancy complicated by diabetic ketoacidosis: maternal and fetal outcomes. *Diabetes Care, 26*(3), 958–959.

Sibai, B. M., & Viteri, O. A. (2014). Diabetic ketoacidosis in pregnancy. *Obstetrics and Gynecology, 123*(1), 167–178.

Sibai, B. M. (2011). *Management of acute obstetric emergencies* (Vol. 194). Philadelphia, PA: Elsevier Saunders, 137–142.

Singer, M. (2016). The new sepsis consensus definitions (Sepsis-3): the good, the not-so-bad, and the actually-quite-pretty. *Intensive Care Medicine, 42*(12), 2027–2029.

CASE 23
Sangeeta Jain, MD

A 38-Year-Old Woman With Abnormal Quad Screen

A 38-year-old woman presents to the clinic for a routine prenatal visit. She is at 18 weeks' gestation. She had a quad screen drawn in the clinic 2 weeks ago, and you received the results reporting a risk of 1:51 for Down syndrome. She is dated by a 10-week ultrasound; she has a healthy 13-year-old son born by normal vaginal delivery.

The patient is a middle-school teacher and is very much into healthy eating and lifestyle. She enjoys yoga exercises and takes long walks in the woods on weekends. Earlier she had declined screening for aneuploidy or genetic counseling but later agreed to a second-trimester quad screen. She and her partner are happy to accept the baby as it is.

What is prenatal genetic screening? What are its objectives?

Prenatal genetic screening is designed to assess whether a patient is at increased risk of having a fetus affected by a genetic disorder; it is commonly applied for trisomy 21 (Down syndrome), trisomy 18 (Edwards syndrome), and trisomy 13 (Patau syndrome). The purpose is to provide the patient and her obstetrician with enough information about any health problems that could affect the baby to allow them to make informed decisions about pregnancy management. If a positive screening test results, it still cannot predict the severity of complications from trisomy 21.

What is aneuploidy? What are some common aneuploidies for which patients are offered screening?

Aneuploidy is defined as one or more extra or missing chromosomes in the cells. The most common aneuploidies are autosomal trisomies, particularly trisomy 21, which is seen in 1 in 800 live births. Screening is routinely also done for trisomy 13 and trisomy 18.

Compare the various genetic screening methods during pregnancy

The *first-trimester screen* consists of a serum screen and a nuchal translucency (NT) measurement, both of which are done between 10 weeks and 13 weeks 6 days of gestation. The serum screen measures levels of β-human chorionic gonadotropin (β-hCG) and pregnancy-associated plasma protein A (PAPP-A) in maternal serum. NT is the normal fluid-filled subcutaneous space under the skin at the back of the fetal neck. It is performed when the crown-rump length of the fetus measured by ultrasound is between 38 and 84 mm. An NT of 3 mm or greater is considered abnormal. NT has to be measured with great accuracy because a difference of 0.5 mm can reduce the sensitivity of the test by 18%. Together with a serum screen, this test has 84% sensitivity for the detection of Down syndrome with a 5% false-positive rate.

TABLE 23.1 ■ Positive Predictive Value (PPV) of the Noninvasive Prenatal Test (NIPT) Varies With Maternal Age

Age (years)	PPV for Trisomy 21	PPV for Trisomy 18
25	33	13
40	87	68

The *second-trimester serum screen*, called the *quad screen*, consists of measuring free or total hCG, inhibin-A, estriol, and α-fetoprotein (AFP) in maternal serum at 15–22 weeks' gestation. Age, ethnicity, weight, presence of diabetes, and plurality are factors taken into consideration when calculating risk. Accurate pregnancy dating is very important for the sensitivity of this test, which is 81% with a 5% false-positive rate for detecting Down syndrome. Typically, with increased risk for Down syndrome, there is an elevated hCG and inhibin-A with low AFP and estriol. In trisomy 18, all four analytes are low. The quad screen also offers the advantage of screening for neural tube defects, in which the AFP level is typically elevated.

The *cell free fetal DNA test*, also called the noninvasive prenatal test (NIPT), can be performed at any time after 10 weeks of gestation. It evaluates short segments of fetal DNA in maternal blood. The fetal DNA is released into maternal blood from placental cells undergoing apoptosis and comprises 3%–13% of total free DNA in maternal blood. This amount increases throughout gestation and is cleared from maternal circulation within hours after childbirth. It can be used to screen for a variety of fetal conditions such as aneuploidy, Rhesus (Rh) status, fetal gender, and paternally derived autosomal dominant genetic abnormalities. Its detection rate for Down syndrome is 99% with a false-positive rate of less than 0.5%. The detection rate for trisomies 18 and 13 is lower (Table 23.1). If test results report "too little fetal DNA to report," the pregnancy should be managed as increased risk.

What are integrated, sequential, and contingent screenings?

In *integrated screening*, a pregnant woman undergoes the first-trimester screen followed by the quad screen. She receives a single result in the second trimester. The detection rate for Down syndrome is 96%.

In *sequential screening*, a pregnant woman undergoes the first trimester screen and receives the results. This may be followed by the quad screen. However, after the patient receives the results of the first-trimester screen, she may opt to have diagnostic testing with chorionic villus sampling (CVS) or a screening test with NIPT instead of waiting to undergo amniocentesis later in the second trimester. The detection rate for Down syndrome is 93%. The advantage of this approach is that women at highest risk benefit from earlier detection of an affected fetus, whereas women at lower risk benefit from the high detection rate and low false-positive rates of second-trimester screening.

In *contingent screening*, a pregnant woman undergoes the first-trimester screen. If there is an elevated risk, she is offered NIPT or CVS. If the result is low risk, no further tests are offered. If the result is intermediate, a quad screen is offered. The detection rate for Down syndrome is 88%–94%.

What is the management plan for the patient?

After a screening test is designated high risk, the patient will be offered genetic counseling and an ultrasound for a detailed anatomic survey. The genetic counselor meets with the patient and partner to go through their family history and past obstetrical history in great detail and advises them of their risks for having a baby with aneuploidy. She describes and offers them diagnostic testing with an amniocentesis. The amniocentesis is the definitive test to determine the baby's chromosomal status.

CLINICAL PEARL   **STEPS 2/3**

Chorionic villus sampling (CVS) is the sampling of placental villi as a means of prenatal genetic testing; it can be performed between 10 weeks and 13 weeks 6 days of gestation. The approach may be transabdominal or transcervical under ultrasound guidance (Fig. 23.1).

Amniocentesis is the sampling of amniotic fluid for prenatal genetic testing; it can be performed after 15 weeks' gestation after fusion of the amnion and chorion (Fig. 23.2).

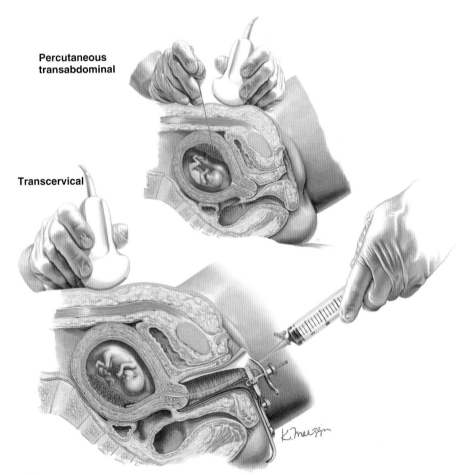

Percutaneous transabdominal

Transcervical

Fig. 23.1 Chorionic villus sampling procedure. *(From Smith R. Chorionic villus sampling. In:* Netter's obstetrics and gynecology. *2008: 590–1. https://www.clinicalkey.com/#!/content/book/3-s2.0-B9781416056829502419?scrollTo=%233-s2.0-B9781416056829502419-fx1)*

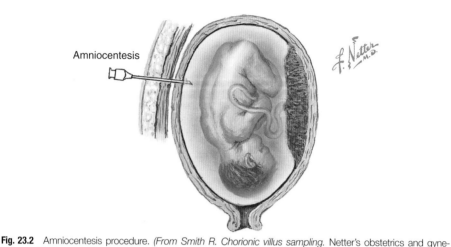

Amniocentesis

Fig. 23.2 Amniocentesis procedure. *(From Smith R. Chorionic villus sampling.* Netter's obstetrics and gynecology. *2008: 572–4. https://www.clinicalkey.com/#!/content/book/3-s2.0-B9781416056829502328?scroll To=%233-s2.0-B9781416056829502328-fx1)*

CLINICAL PEARL   **STEPS 2/3**

The American College of Obstetricians and Gynecologists (ACOG) states that invasive diagnostic testing should be available to all women, regardless of age or risk.

The patient is counseled that pregnancies complicated by Down syndrome are at increased risk for miscarriage and stillbirth. Additionally, infants may have characteristic facial features, learning disabilities, seizures, childhood leukemia, and early onset of Alzheimer disease. In developed countries, survival may be to 60 years of age.

Ultrasound can detect approximately 50%–60% of all congenital anomalies. Some anomalies are associated with Down syndrome more frequently, such as the presence of a thickened nuchal fold, an absent nasal bone, an endocardial cushion defect of the heart, intestinal atresia, pyelectasis, an absent middle phalanx of the fifth digit in the upper extremities, echogenic bowel, cystic hygroma, and a short femur or humerus. These are referred to as "soft markers of aneuploidy."

If considering an isolated finding, which ultrasound anomaly is associated with maximum likelihood for Down syndrome in the fetus?

Ultrasound exam's sensitivity for Down syndrome is about 50%–60%. Among the markers of aneuploidy, nuchal fold thickening is associated with the greatest likelihood ratio for Down syndrome (11–18.6 with 50% sensitivity). The likelihood ratio of echogenic bowel is 5.5–6.7.

The patient's ultrasound shows a ventricular septal defect; how would this finding affect further management?

Although the finding of a ventricular septal defect (VSD) is not characteristic of Down syndrome, it is the most common congenital cardiac defect and would increase the risk for aneuploidy further. The patient should be offered NIPT or diagnostic testing with amniocentesis, and the benefits and risks of amniocentesis discussed. If the patient chooses the NIPT, it must be clarified that it is not a diagnostic test like amniocentesis; instead it is a screening test.

BASIC SCIENCE PEARL	STEP 1

Congenital VSD occurs as a result of incomplete septation of the ventricles. Embryologically, the interventricular septum has a membranous and a muscular portion. Most defects are perimembranous (at the junction of the membranous and muscular portions). VSDs are the most common congenital cardiac defect, occurring in 1 in 500 live births.

The patient declines amniocentesis but undergoes NIPT. The NIPT results are low-risk for aneuploidy.

What are the risk factors for Down syndrome in the fetus?

Risk factors associated with having a fetus with Down syndrome include advanced maternal age, a parental translocation involving chromosome 21, a previous child with a trisomy, significant ultrasound findings, and a positive screening test result.

What is the significance of an increased NT finding in the first trimester?

Increased NT increases the risk for genetic syndromes, congenital cardiac defects, abdominal wall defects, and diaphragmatic hernias, even if normal chromosomes are found by karyotyping. Hence ultrasound should be performed to include a detailed anatomic survey and a fetal echocardiogram should be accomplished in the second trimester.

What is a cystic hygroma?

The finding of increased NT along the whole length of the fetus with visible septations is called cystic hygroma (Fig. 23.3).

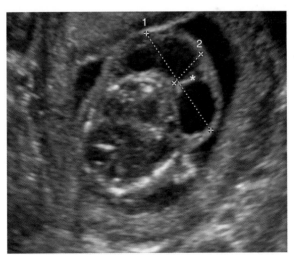

Fig. 23.3   Axial view of a septated cystic hygroma in the early second trimester. The nuchal ligament (*asterisk*) is identified. *(From Arigita M, Bennasar M, Puerto B et al. Cystic hygroma. Obstet Imaging. 2012: 370–2. https:// www.clinicalkey.com/-!/search/cystic%2520hygroma/%7B%22facetquery%22:%5B%22+contenttype:IM %22,%22+contenttype:VD%22%5D%7D)*

BASIC SCIENCE PEARL   **STEP 1**

Cystic hygroma is a congenital malformation resulting from lymph accumulation in the fetal neck. It may be septated or without septation.

It is associated with a 50% likelihood of fetal aneuploidy such as trisomy 21, Turner's syndrome, and trisomy 18. The other 50% may have congenital cardiac defects, diaphragmatic hernia, skeletal dysplasia, or other genetic syndromes. Less than 20% of these pregnancies will result in a healthy, term, live-born infant.

With its high sensitivity and specificity, why can't NIPT replace invasive diagnostic tests?
The NIPT has its limitations:
- It has the potential for false-positive and false-negative results.
- The screening test cannot distinguish between fetal and maternal DNA: a positive test could represent placental mosaicism, a resorbed twin, a maternal malignancy, or maternal aneuploidy.
- Its positive predictive value (PPV) in the general population (younger women) is lower because the prevalence of aneuploidy is lower.
- The test cannot distinguish aneuploidy derived from translocation or nondisjunction, and this will affect the counseling the patient receives in regards to recurrence risk.
- The test does not provide information regarding risk for neural tube defects in the fetus.
- The residual risk of a chromosomal abnormality after a normal NIPT result is 2%.

How does multifetal gestation affect the screening test's performance?
The accuracy of the screening test in a multiple gestation pregnancy is limited compared to when performed for a singleton gestation. Data are available for twins but not for higher order pregnancies. In dizygotic twins, the women's risk for aneuploidy is increased; in monozygotic twins, it is similar to the mother's age-adjusted risk.

The NT is measured in each twin. The first-trimester screen has a detection rate of 75% for Down syndrome. The second-trimester screening of a twin gestation can identify 50% of fetuses affected with Down syndrome. Because of limited evidence, NIPT is not recommended for screening in multifetal gestation.

The patient undergoes a fetal echocardiogram, which confirms a small VSD without other cardiac defects. She is counseled that, as a neonate, the pediatrician will closely follow the baby due to this finding. However, in the absence of aneuploidy or other cardiac abnormalities, the prognosis is very good given its small size.

BEYOND THE PEARLS

- All women should be offered the option of aneuploidy screening for genetic disorders, regardless of maternal age.
- Women with a negative screening test should not be offered additional screening tests for aneuploidy because this will only increase their potential for a false-positive test result.
- As an isolated finding, an increased nuchal skinfold thickness confers the highest risk of aneuploidy. An isolated echogenic intracardiac focus carries the lowest risk.
- Women with an abnormal NT measurement should be offered ultrasound for a detailed anatomy survey regardless of normal chromosomes.
- Of the soft markers, third-trimester ultrasound follow-up is only indicated for isolated pyelectasis, echogenic bowel, or short femur or humerus.

Case Summary

- A 38-year-old woman presents to the clinic for a routine prenatal visit. Her quad screen reveals a risk of 1:51 for Down syndrome.
- The patient undergoes a detailed anatomic survey revealing a VSD. She receives extensive genetic counseling, declines the amniocentesis procedure, and opts for NIPT, which shows a low risk for abnormalities.
- She is further counseled regarding the anticipated excellent prognosis for her baby.

References

American College of Obstetricians and Gynecologists. (2007). ACOG Practice Bulletin No. 88. Invasive prenatal testing for aneuploidy. *Obstetrics and Gynecology, 110*(6), 1459–1467.

American College of Obstetricians and Gynecologists. (2016). Practice bulletin no. 162: Prenatal diagnostic testing for genetic disorders. *Obstetrics and Gynecology, 127*(5), e108–e122.

Agathokleous, M., Chaveeva, P., Poon, L. C., et al. (2013). Meta-analysis of second trimester markers for trisomy 21. *Ultrasound in Obstetrics and Gynecology, 41*(3), 247–261.

Verheecke, Amant F., Wlodarska, I., et al. (2015). Presymptomatic identification of cancers in pregnant women during noninvasive prenatal testing. *JAMA Oncology, 1*(6), 814–819.

Evans, M. I., Van Decruyes, H., & Nicolades, K. H. (2007). Nuchal translucency measurements for first trimester screening: the price of inaccuracy. *Fetal Diagnosis and Therapy, 22*(6), 401–404.

Glasson, E. J., Sullivan, S. G., Hussain, R., et al. (2002). The changing survival profile of people with Down syndrome: implications for genetic counseling. *Clinical Genetics, 62*(5), 390–393.

Malone, F. D., Ball, R. H., Nyberg, D. A., et al. (2005). First-trimester septated cystic hygroma: prevalence, natural history and pediatric outcome. *Obstetrics and Gynecology, 106*(2), 288–294.

Nicolaides, K. H., Heath, V., & Cicero, S. (2002). Increased fetal nuchal translucency at 11–14 weeks. *Prenatal Diagnosis, 22*(4), 308–315.

Norton, M. E., Jelliffe-Pawlowski, L. L., & Currier, R. J. (2014). Chromosome abnormalities detected by current prenatal screening and noninvasive prenatal testing. *Obstetrics and Gynecology, 124*(5), 979–986.

Nussbaum, R., McInnes, R. R., & Willard, H. F. (2016). Principles of clinical cytogenetics and genome analysis. In *Thompson and Thompson genetics in medicine* (pp. 57–74). Philadelphia, PA: Elsevier.

Spencer, K., & Nicolaides, K. H. (2003). Screening for trisomy 21 in twins using first trimester ultrasound and maternal serum biochemistry in a one-stop clinic: a review of three years experience. *British Journal of Obstetrics and Gynaecology, 110*(3), 276–280.

Taylor-Phillips, S., Freeman, K., Geppert, J., et al. (2016). Accuracy of non-invasive prenatal testing using cell free DNA for detection of Down, Edwards and Patau syndromes: a systemic review and meta-analysis. *BMJ Open, 6*(1), e010002.

Luis A. Izquierdo, MD

A 17-Year-Old Woman With a History of Sickle-Cell Disease Presenting With Bone Pain

A 17-year-old woman G2P 0010, of African-American descent, presents to obstetrical testing and triage at 24 weeks of gestation. She has a history of sickle-cell disease (SCD) and complains of generalized pain, which is more pronounced in both wrists. She is jaundiced and anemic. She does not feel any chest discomfort or pain. She denies abdominal pain. She had a similar episode 1 year ago while she was traveling to Santa Fe, New Mexico (greater than 6,000 feet above sea level) and developed a urinary tract infection (UTI). Her pain is unbearable, and she wants to feel better by the time her baby is born.

Why is it important to ask about and address the past history, ethnicity, family history, and transfusion history of pregnant patients?

Around 5% of the global population carries a genetic mutation for hemoglobinopathies. These include the sickle hemoglobinopathies and the thalassemias. SCD is one of the most common hereditary diseases. SCD is most prevalent in individuals of African descent, but is also seen in those from the Caribbean, the Middle East, the Mediterranean, India, and Central and South America. It is important to be aware that because of increasing rates of immigration patients of different ethnicities can be seen in your service.

All blood transfusions carry risks for transfusion reactions, infections, and lung injury; in SCD, the most serious consequence is the risk of developing alloimmunizations and a delayed hemolytic transfusion reaction. The blood phenotypes C and E and the Kell group antigens should be compatible.

BASIC SCIENCE/CLINICAL PEARL   **STEPS 1/2/3**

SCD is a group of autosomal recessive disorders involving abnormal hemoglobin (hemoglobin S or Hb S). Hb S is different from the normal hemoglobin A (Hb A) due to a single nucleotide substitution of thymine for adenine in the β-globin gene; this in turn causes a substitution of valine for glutamic acid in the number 6 position of the β-globin polypeptide. These changes allow for sickle hemoglobin to polymerize when it is deoxygenated, triggering injury to the red cell membrane, hemolysis, multiple organ failure, and have devastating consequences for patients and their families. Individuals with heterozygous Hb S are those assigned the diagnosis of sickle-cell trait. Those individuals with Hb SS (homozygous Hb S) have sickle-cell anemia (Table 24.1).

The pain continues to worsen, 8/10 in severity. In the past, this pain has been alleviated by nonsteroidal antiinflammatory agents and opioids. She remembers that in the last similar pain episode she was given narcotics, oxygen by mask, and intravenous fluids (IVF's). She has a history of being diagnosed in the past with SCD with Hb SS and has been followed by the pediatric hematology clinic.

TABLE 24.1 ▨ **Hematologic Features of Sickle Hemoglobinopathies**

Disorder	Heterozygous State	Homozygous State	DNA Analysis
Hb S	Hb A, Hb S, Hb A$_2$	Hb S, Hb F (1%–15%), Hb A$_2$	PCR: Dde 1 digestion PCR, ASO- dot blot
Hb S/β- Thalassemia	-	If β^0 thalassemia, severe sickle cell anemia; if β$^+$ thalassemia, less severe	PCR: Dde 1 digestion PCR, ASO- dot blot

Modified from old JM. (2016). Prenatal diagnosis of the hemoglobinopathies. In: A. Milunsky, & J. M. Milunsky (Eds.), *Genetic disorders and the fetus: diagonis, prevention, and treatment* (7th ed.) (pp. 718–754). Hoboken (NJ): Wiley Blackwell.

What clues in the history and physical point to the diagnosis of SCD crisis?

Patients with SCD have chronic anemia and an average hemoglobin level of 6–9 g/dL. The other major clinical features include recurrent, unpredictable episodes of bony pain, which occur throughout life. Adult pain more typically occurs in the long bones or in the trunk. The frequency of these episodes varies from less than one episode per year, to more than one episode per month (Table 24.2).

SCD is a multiorgan disorder and can incur additional complications such as increased risk of stroke, renal dysfunction, pulmonary hypertension, retinal disease, leg ulcers, cholelithiasis, and avascular necrosis.

BASIC SCIENCE/CLINICAL PEARL   **STEPS 1/2/3**

Clinical acumen is required to diagnose SCD vaso-occlusive crisis because laboratory assessment is very nonspecific. Fortunately, most women with hemoglobinopathies are known to have the condition before they become pregnant. The most accurate diagnostic test is hemoglobin electrophoresis. As clinicians, we need to determine whether these painful crises are a vaso-occlusive episode, a crisis associated with an infection, malingering, or possibly a surgical or obstetric complication.

As many as one-third of adult vaso-occlusive crises are associated with infections. It is particularly common in young patients to see pneumococcal infections and gram-negative sepsis with *Escherichia coli* and *Salmonella* infections. The most frequent types of infections are pneumonia, UTIs, puerperal endomyometritis, and osteomyelitis.

The patient expresses the concern of having an affected child because her husband is also from an Afro-Antillean background.

How would you treat this patient?

When a patient with SCD desires pregnancy, a multidisciplinary approach should be developed to create a reproductive plan. The patient and her partner should undergo genetic counseling to determine the risk of the child inheriting SCD (Figure 24.1). During preconception visits, update immunizations, screen for alloimmunizations, counsel about smoking cessation, optimize hemoglobin levels, and optimize medications.

It is recommended that patients undergo fetal ultrasound during the first trimester for viability and confirmation of the estimated date of confinement and again at 20 weeks for a fetal

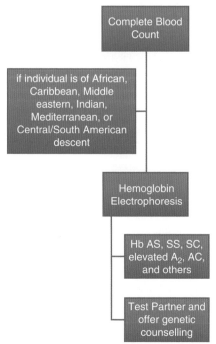

Fig. 24.1   Evaluation for sickle hemoglobinopathy during pregnancy.

TABLE 24.2 ■ Signs and Symptoms of Sickle-Cell Crisis

Vaso-occlusive Group	1. Sudden attacks of pain in the abdomen, chest, vertebrae, and extremities
	2. Obstructive microcirculation of the bones or joints
	3. Obstructed microcirculation of the chest and lungs (acute chest syndrome)
	4. Obstructive microcirculation of the liver, spleen, and kidneys
	5. Affected central nervous system
Hematologic	Anemia, reticulocytopenia, aplastic crisis

anatomical survey. After 20 weeks, fetal growth should be followed-up with ultrasounds every 4 weeks due to the association of SCD with fetal growth restriction.

> Now that we have admitted the patient to a high-risk pregnancy service, her family is worried about the potential complications that these pregnancies carry to the mother.

How should you counsel the patient's family?

Pregnancy in women with SCD has become more common as a direct result of improved survival from the advances in medical care and generalized interventions that begin at birth. These interventions include newborn screening, antibiotic prophylaxis with penicillin, immunizations against encapsulated bacteria, and the administration of hydroxyurea.

Improved fetal and maternal outcomes may also be in part a result of advances in antenatal and obstetric care.

BASIC SCIENCE/CLINICAL PEARL	STEPS 1/2/3

Pregnancy in women with SCD is complicated not only by maternal condition, characterized by years of chronic organ damage, but by the specific physiologic changes and adaptations that are inherent to pregnant patients. There are adaptations required by the hematological, cardiovascular, renal, and respiratory systems.

In a normal pregnancy, a 50% blood volume increase triggers the cardiovascular system response to create a hyperdynamic state. The glomerular filtration rate increases. There is an increased minute ventilation as the respiratory system responds with a mild respiratory alkalosis. The maternal adaptation to pregnancy often compounds or exacerbates the underlying chronic organ damage initially created by SCD.

Pregnancy in SCD is associated with an increased incidence of painful episodes. There is an increase in antenatal hospitalizations. There is an increase in pulmonary complications, infections, thromboembolic events, and antepartum bleeding, and there is an increased risk of preeclampsia and pregnancy-induced hypertension. The fetal morbidity is increased due to fetal growth restriction and an increased rate of preterm labor and delivery.

Will the patient get a blood transfusion?

The only general modalities available in the treatment of SCD in pregnancy are supportive care and the judicious use of transfusions. Understanding the features that precipitate painful sickle-cell crisis provides the rationale for our current therapy with fluids to reduce intracellular hemoglobin concentrations, correct acidosis when present, reduce fever, and increase the oxygen concentration of inspired air.

The most important therapy is some form of partial exchange transfusion to decrease the amount of Hb S in the circulation.

Some investigators have argued against the use of prophylactic transfusions to pregnant patients with SCD. Small randomized trials do not show any clear benefit of prophylactic transfusion in the treatment of this condition when compared to selective transfusion.

Therapeutic transfusions are indicated in patients who have particularly severe disease manifestation or for symptomatic patients who are unresponsive to conservative management (Box 24.1).

INDICATIONS FOR THERAPEUTIC BLOOD TRANSFUSIONS	BOX 24.1

Hemodynamic instability
Acute stroke
Acute chest syndrome (ACS)
High-output cardiac failure
Multiorgan failure
Symptomatic anemia
Severe refractory pain
Reticulocytopenia

CLINICAL PEARL	STEPS 2/3

Acute chest syndrome (ACS) is seen in 7%–20% of pregnancies with SCD. It is characterized by a new infiltrate on chest x-ray in association with respiratory signs and symptoms. It is difficult to distinguish ACS from pneumonia, and it can coexist with infection and is associated with high morbidity and mortality. Hypoxia is an early sign of ACS, and pregnant women who develop hypoxia should be assessed for this complication by clinical examination, blood gas monitoring, and chest x-ray.

How do we manage SCD pain?

Engage an aggressive pain relief program. This is accomplished by utilizing opioid dosing; that is, morphine/hydromorphone every 2–3 hours or by continuous opioid infusion (morphine/hydromorphone) with patient-controlled analgesia demand dosing every 20 minutes. Opioids should not be weaned until after 24 hours of adequate pain relief.

> The patient is admitted to the hospital and receives aggressive IV hydration and pain control with morphine PCA. Her evaluation for infectious processes is negative including normal vital signs, normal physical exam, and negative urinalysis with culture. She is discharged from the hospital after a 36-hour observation period and feels much improved.

Will the patient require a cesarean delivery?

There is not a definite advantage in terms of maternal or perinatal outcomes in delivering these patients by cesarean. Vaso-occlusive crisis during labor offers an additional challenge to the provider. During labor the patient should remain in left lateral decubitus position and receive oxygen via face mask. Monitoring of the mother and the fetal heart rate is crucial. Urinary catheters, as well as intrauterine catheters should be used with caution because of their association with infections.

The use of general anesthesia can result in significant postpartum sickling complications. If cesarean delivery is indicated, regional anesthesia is preferred unless an obstetric emergency occurs.

What are the postpartum recommendations for patients with SCD?

Sickle-cell crisis can be decreased in the postpartum period if measures are taken to avoid hypovolemia, infection, and acidosis. Early detection and treatment of UTIs and endomyometritis is important to prevent new vaso-occlusive events. There is also an increased risk of pulmonary edema and thromboembolic disorders in this period. It is important that, during this period, sequential compression devices and/or prophylactic anticoagulation are utilized.

What type of contraception can be utilized in patients with SCD?

There is limited evidence on the safety and effectiveness of hormonal contraception in women with SCD. Progestogens are effective and safe in patients with SCD. They also may decrease the frequency and severity of painful crisis. There is reluctance to prescribe combined oral contraceptives in SCD because of the association with increased thrombosis. First-line recommendations are injectable contraceptives (medroxyprogesterone acetate), progesterone intrauterine contraceptive devices, and/or implantable contraceptives.

Box 24.2 presents a summary of the management of sickle-cell crisis.

MANAGEMENT GUIDELINES FOR SICKLE-CELL CRISIS   **BOX 24.2**

1. Relieve symptoms and try to achieve a Hb A concentration of greater than 50%.
2. Hospitalize patient in a high-risk pregnancy unit.
3. Begin electronic fetal monitoring.
4. Begin hydration after ruling out congestive heart failure (1 L Ringer's lactate over 2 hours, continuing with 125 mL per hour).
5. Avoid central venous pressure line.
6. Begin morphine sulfate by standard IV infusion or patient-controlled administration pump.
7. If infection is diagnosed, the appropriate antibiotics should be started.
8. Schedule early anesthesia consultation.

Adapted from Clark SL, Cotton DB, Hankins GDV, Phelan JP. (1992). Critical care obstetrics.

BEYOND THE PEARLS

- For a hematocrit of less than 15%, direct transfusion is always preferable. For a hematocrit of greater than 15%, an exchange transfusion can be considered.
- Women with sickle-cell trait are at increased risk of UTI and therefore should have a urine culture performed at the initial prenatal visit and once in each following trimester, with treatment of asymptomatic bacteriuria.
- A higher median daily dose of opioids during pregnancy is associated with more severe neonatal abstinence syndrome.

Case Summary

- A 17-year-old woman of African-American descent, presents to obstetrical testing and triage at 24 weeks of gestation with generalized pain, most severe in bilateral wrists.
- The patient is admitted to the high-risk pregnancy service and undergoes IVF hydration, receives morphine, and is given counseling regarding her disease. She is discharged from the hospital in stable condition with a planned follow-up in her prenatal clinic.

References

American College of Obstetricians and Gynecologists. (2007). ACOG Practice Bulletin no. 78. Hemoglobinopathies in pregnancy. *Obstetrics and Gynecology, 109*(1), 229–237.

Boga, C., & Ozdogu, H. (2016). Pregnancy and sickle cell disease: a review of the current literature. *Critical Reviews in Oncology/Hematology, 98*, 365–374.

Clark SL, Cotton DB, Hankins GDV. (1992). *Critical care obstetrics*. Boston, MA: Blackwell Scientific Publications.

Hathaway, A. R. (2016). Sickle cell disease in pregnancy. *Southern Medical Journal, 109*, 554–556.

Howard, J., & Oteng-Ntim, E. (2012). The obstetric management of sickle cell disease. *Best Practice & Research Clinical Obstetrics and Gynecology, 26*(1), 25–36.

Kuo, K., & Caughey, A. B. (2016). Contemporary outcomes of sickle cell disease in pregnancy. *American Journal of Obstetrics and Gynecology, 215*(4), 505.e1–505.e5.

Malinowski, A. K., Shehata, N., D'Souza, R., et al. (2015). Prophylactic transfusion for pregnant women with sickle cell disease: a systematic review and meta-analysis. *Blood, 126*(21), 2424–2435.

Naik, R. P., & Haywood, C. Jr. (2015). Sickle cell trait diagnosis: clinical and social implications. *Hematology/the education program of the American Society of Hematology. American Society of Hematology, 160*–167.

Okusanya, B. O., & Oladapo, O. T. (2013). Prophylactic versus selective blood transfusion for sickle cell disease in pregnancy (review). *Cochrane Database of Systematic Reviews, 12*, CD010378.

Parrish, M. R., & Morrison, J. C. (2013). Sickle cell crisis and pregnancy. *Seminars in Perinatology, 37*(4), 274–279.

Rogers, D. R., & Molokie, R. (2010). Sickle cell disease in pregnancy. *Obstetrics and Gynecology Clinics of North America, 37*(2), 223–227.

Shirel, T., Hubler, C. P., Shah, R., et al. (2016). Maternal opioid dose is associated with neonatal abstinence syndrome in children born to women with sickle cell disease. *American Journal of Hematology, 91*(4), 416–419.

Bradley D. Holbrook, MD

A 28-Year-Old Woman With Valvular Heart Disease in Pregnancy

A 28-year-old woman presents for a new obstetric visit to establish care at 11 weeks' gestation. Her medical history is unremarkable. Notable in her family history is a bicuspid aortic valve in her mother.

What are critical questions to ask any patient with a personal or family history of cardiac disease?

When obtaining the patient's history, attention should be paid to the presence or absence of any current cardiac symptoms, including chest pain, shortness of breath, palpitations, swelling, or easy fatigability (although the latter two are quite common in pregnancy!). It is also critical to inquire about functional status and any impairment in the activities of daily living.

If the patient has a personal history of cardiac disease, it is important to determine the age at diagnosis and the symptoms leading to the diagnosis. You should also obtain detailed information regarding any valve or cardiac procedures she may have had performed previously. Records from prior cardiology visits and echocardiography reports should be obtained.

CLINICAL PEARL   STEPS 2/3

Remember that patients may not think of things in medical terms. They may not refer to minimally invasive procedures as surgeries, so asking specifically about any procedures they may have had (in this case, a cardiac procedure through a wire inserted in the groin) is very helpful.

In patients with a positive family history of cardiac disease, questioning should focus on the individual's relationship to the patient, the age of diagnosis, symptoms leading to the diagnosis, age of death, and any repairs performed.

CLINICAL PEARL   STEPS 2/3

The patient may have family members with a cardiac condition that was never diagnosed. You should ask about any family members with a history of sudden unexplained death, or any death at a younger age. If they have a family member with such a history, further questioning is necessary, including sometimes speaking with older family members who have more information regarding details of the individual.

You perform a physical exam. Her temperature is 37.1°C (98.8°F), blood pressure is 118/72 mm Hg, heart rate is 96/min, respiration rate is 20/min, and oxygen saturation is 94% on room air. Cardiac exam reveals a systolic murmur best auscultated at the right second intercostal space. The gravid uterus is not palpable abdominally. Fetal heart tones are auscultated at 140/min. The remainder of the physical exam is unremarkable.

CLINICAL PEARL   **STEPS 2/3**

The gravid uterus becomes palpable just above the pubic symphysis at approximately 12 weeks' gestation and should reach the umbilicus at approximately 20 weeks. From 20 weeks on, the measurement from the pubic symphysis to the top of the fundus in centimeters approximates gestational age in weeks. This is measured at each prenatal visit to follow fetal growth.

CLINICAL PEARL   **STEPS 2/3**

A normal fetal heart rate is between 110 and 160/minute.

What is the differential diagnosis of a systolic murmur?
Potential causes of a systolic murmur include:
- Increased flow across the semilunar valves (flow murmur)
- Aortic or pulmonary valve stenosis or obstruction
- Mitral or tricuspid valve prolapse
- Mitral or tricuspid valve regurgitation
- Ventricular septal defects

What cardiac exam findings will be altered during pregnancy?
As the gravid uterus enlarges, the heart will shift upward, anteriorly, and to the left. However, this is rarely appreciated on physical exam. There is also a modest increase in the heart rate by approximately 10/minute. Blood pressure will slowly lower throughout the first and second trimesters before climbing back to normal prepregnancy values by the third trimester. It is important to note that pregnant women become easily fatigued with minimal exertion, and this may become apparent during history-taking or even on physical exam.

On auscultation of the heart of a pregnant woman, significant changes will be present. These are usually first seen toward the end of the first trimester and can continue throughout pregnancy and into the early postpartum period. The heart sounds tend to all become louder. The first heart sound (S1) becomes widely split, and a third heart sound (S3) is often heard. Systolic ejection murmurs are very commonly heard due to increased flow across the semilunar valves.

Do heart murmurs during pregnancy require a workup?
Heart murmurs are extremely common during pregnancy, with an estimated 90% of women having an auscultable heart murmur—usually a systolic ejection murmur— at some point during gestation. An isolated finding of a systolic ejection murmur in a pregnant woman requires no further workup (meaning no symptoms of heart disease, no personal or family history of heart disease, and no other abnormal findings on physical exam). However, this patient's family history of a bicuspid aortic valve should raise some concern, and further testing is indicated. Any diastolic murmur also requires a workup; while this type of murmur may be physiologic in rare cases, a pathologic condition cannot be ruled out without further information.

What workup should be performed to evaluate a concerning heart murmur in pregnancy?
Following a thorough history and physical, the first step in working up a concerning heart murmur should be echocardiography.

> You order an outpatient echocardiogram. This reveals a bicuspid aortic valve with resultant moderate aortic stenosis. Left ventricular ejection fraction is normal, but there is some early evidence of left ventricular diastolic dysfunction. There is no dilation of the aortic root. All other findings are within normal limits.

How common is aortic stenosis in pregnancy, and what are the common causes?
In the developed world, aortic stenosis in women of reproductive age is usually due to a congenital bicuspid aortic valve. The incidence of a bicuspid aortic valve is estimated at 2% of the general population. In developing nations, aortic stenosis is commonly caused by rheumatic heart disease.

Should you be concerned about aortic stenosis in pregnancy?
Aortic stenosis has the potential to significantly complicate pregnancy because the increase in cardiac output during pregnancy leads to a higher pressure left ventricle. A severely obstructed outflow limits the increase in cardiac output that needs to occur and thus can lead to heart failure. In rare cases, the increase in pressure across the valve can even lead to an aortic dissection. Aortic dissection is extremely rare but is more likely to occur if the aortic root is dilated to greater than 40 mm or if there is a coexisting coarctation of the aorta.

There are three main complications which may arise in pregnancies complicated by maternal aortic stenosis:
- The possibility of inheritance (i.e., having a fetus with a bicuspid aortic valve)
- The possible development of functional impairment due to the lesion (left heart failure)
- The possibility of aortic complications such as aortic dilation or dissection

The rates of preterm delivery and perinatal mortality are not increased in pregnancies complicated by maternal aortic stenosis as compared to the general population; however, rates of intrauterine growth restriction (IUGR) and small for gestational age (SGA) are increased in women with moderate to severe aortic stenosis.

How can pregnancy outcomes with aortic stenosis be predicted?
Aortic stenosis can be classified into stages based on valve characteristics, flow velocities, and patient symptoms. It is generally considered mild if the patient is asymptomatic and there are either no, or minimal, changes on echocardiography. Mild aortic stenosis usually has excellent outcomes in pregnancy.

However, if the patient develops symptoms of heart failure, evidence of diastolic dysfunction, or significant flow abnormalities, she would be considered to have moderate to severe disease. This more advanced disease can be quite problematic and lead to ventricular arrhythmias or even heart failure during pregnancy.

Among all pregnant patients with congenital aortic stenosis, arrhythmias will be present in 2%–3%, and symptoms of heart failure in approximately 7%. However, among pregnant women with severe aortic stenosis, 25% will develop arrhythmias and 10%–44% will develop heart failure. Severe cardiovascular morbidity such as myocardial infarction, stroke, or maternal mortality will occur in 2.5% of patients.

What workup should be performed for a pregnant patient with aortic stenosis?
The physical exam just described will be important in establishing a baseline and ruling out any early complications such as an arrhythmia or pulmonary edema. The patient should then be sent

for electrocardiography (EKG) and an echocardiogram. Echocardiography generally provides excellent views of the heart and valves, but imaging distal to the valves may require magnetic resonance imaging (MRI). This should be done if there are any concerns about a coarctation, dilated aortic root, or other aortopathies.

Due to the possibility of inheritance, the fetus should also have a fetal echocardiogram to evaluate for the presence of a bicuspid aortic valve or for other abnormalities.

> You order an EKG, which shows a heart rate of 98/min. Normal sinus rhythm is seen but with voltage findings suggesting a left axis deviation.

What cardiac testing will be altered in pregnancy?
As noted earlier, the growing uterus causes the heart to shift upward, anteriorly, and to the left. This results in a slight enlargement of the cardiac silhouette on chest radiograph (CXR). An EKG may also demonstrate left axis deviation as well as a mild increase in heart rate.

> A fetal echocardiogram is performed, which shows the heart to be normal in size, situs, and position. There is no evidence of major structural cardiac anomalies; however, evaluation of the valves shows a bicuspid aortic valve.

What is the familial inheritance risk of a bicuspid aortic valve?
A bicuspid aortic valve has a variable inheritance pattern, with an estimated inheritance of 4%–9%. If the patient has a first-degree relative with a bicuspid aortic valve, she should be evaluated with echocardiography. Any pregnant patient with a known bicuspid valve should have fetal echocardiography performed. On the other hand, if a fetus is found to have a bicuspid valve in a mother whose aortic valve has not previously been evaluated, maternal echocardiography is indicated.

How should a pregnant patient with aortic stenosis be managed during pregnancy?
The first step after performing the preceding workup will be immediate referral to a cardiologist. In conferring with the cardiologist, a plan for the pregnancy can be jointly agreed upon. This plan will almost certainly include serial maternal echocardiography. If there is evidence of aortic root dilation, she will likely require repeat echocardiography every 2–4 weeks throughout the pregnancy. If no dilation, the decision may be to repeat the echocardiogram every few months or once a trimester.

If the echocardiogram shows severely diminished left ventricular function with an ejection fraction less than 30%, there is a high likelihood of adverse outcome. Termination of pregnancy should be offered/recommended with surgical repair prior to any future attempts at pregnancy.

Is surgical repair of aortic stenosis recommended during pregnancy?
Surgery to repair a stenotic aortic valve is generally not recommended during pregnancy. The maternal risks are overall similar to that of nonpregnant women undergoing the same procedure, with a mortality risk of 3%–5%. In contrast to this, fetal outcomes are extremely poor, with a fetal mortality rate approaching 30%–40%. For this reason, intervention during pregnancy is only recommended if the patient exhibits evidence of New York Heart Association (NYHA) class 3 or 4 heart failure (Table 25.1), if there is hemodynamic deterioration, or if an aortic dissection occurs. If repair during pregnancy becomes necessary, it should be performed in a tertiary care center, under the care of a multidisciplinary team involving cardiologists, cardiothoracic surgeons, maternal–fetal medicine specialists, and cardiac anesthesiologists.

TABLE 25.1 ■ **New York Heart Association Functional Classification**

Class	Limitation	Symptoms
1	None	Ordinary physical activity does not cause undue fatigue, palpitation, or dyspnea.
2	Slight	No symptoms at rest. Ordinary physical activity leads to fatigue, palpitations, or dyspnea.
3	Marked	No symptoms at rest. Less than ordinary physical activity leads to fatigue, palpitations, or dyspnea
4	Severe	Symptoms of heart failure at rest. Unable to perform any physical activity without discomfort.

Adapted from The Criteria Committee of the New York Heart Association, 1994.

Surgical repair *prior* to pregnancy is recommended in patients with symptomatic aortic stenosis. Additionally, in asymptomatic patients with severe disease, surgical repair should also be considered prior to pregnancy.

> The patient sees a cardiologist, and, given her moderate disease with no dilation of the aortic root, the plan is made for serial echocardiography once per trimester with close follow-up in your clinic. At 39 weeks 4 days gestation, the patient presents to labor and delivery complaining of regular, strong contractions and leakage of fluid. Exam reveals her membranes to be ruptured and her cervix dilated to 4 cm.

How should women with aortic stenosis be delivered?
In nearly all cases of pregnant women with aortic stenosis, vaginal delivery is preferred. However, this decision should be individualized and should be discussed by a multidisciplinary team that includes maternal–fetal medicine specialists, cardiologists, and anesthesiologists.

> Following her delivery, the patient is followed by cardiology. Over time, her aortic stenosis slowly worsens to the point that it is recommended she have a valve replacement. She undergoes a minimally invasive valve replacement. Two years following this procedure, she is again contemplating pregnancy and comes to you for a preconceptional counseling visit.

What is the role of a preconceptional counseling visit in women with valvular heart disease?
Ideally, patients with valvular heart disease will present for preconceptional counseling with a maternal–fetal medicine specialist as well as their cardiologist. In practice, this rarely occurs. This preconceptional visit and workup is crucial for a number of reasons:
- A full workup is essential in identifying any issues that could be resolved before pregnancy.
- This workup can also determine the extent of the lesion and thus provide more information to the physicians and the patient to be able to appropriately weigh the risks of attempting pregnancy. A candid discussion of these risks is much easier to do before a patient is actually pregnant (especially due to the emotionally and politically charged issues relating to termination of pregnancy). It also allows for possible surgical repair prior to attempting pregnancy.
- Evaluation prior to pregnancy allows for the establishment of baseline values before the hemodynamic and other physiologic changes of pregnancy occur.
- This visit also allows for time to change medications to those that are safe during pregnancy.

If the patient does not present for preconceptional counseling, a full workup should be performed as soon as possible.

Following her preconceptional visit with both you and her cardiologist, it is felt that it is safe for her to become pregnant. A few months later, she comes to you after a positive pregnancy test. You follow her in the same way you did during her first pregnancy with the exception of her mechanical valve.

How should mechanical valves be monitored during pregnancy?

Pregnant patients with mechanical valves are at high risk of adverse outcomes and should be treated as such. Pregnancy is a hypercoagulable state and thus pregnant women with prosthetic valves *must* be on therapeutic anticoagulation, with levels followed to ensure appropriate anticoagulation. Without therapeutic anticoagulation, there is a risk of maternal mortality of approximately 25%. Additionally, repeat transthoracic echocardiography should be performed if the patient develops any concerning symptoms (dyspnea, fatigue, chest pain, shortness of breath, etc.).

What anticoagulant should be used in pregnant women with prosthetic valves?

All women with mechanical valves who are pregnant should receive low-dose aspirin in addition to another agent. The choice of the other agent is much less clear because there is no ideal regimen.

In women with mechanical valves, taking warfarin throughout pregnancy has been shown to have the lowest rate of thromboembolic events, estimated at less than 4%. On the other hand, unfractionated heparin (UFH) throughout pregnancy has a very high rate of thromboembolic events, approximately 33%. Low-molecular-weight heparin (LMWH) is usually preferred over UFH due to fewer bleeding complications, less bone loss, and lower risk of thrombocytopenia. The rate of thromboembolic complications in these women when taking LMWH is also much lower, estimated at approximately 9%.

At the same time, warfarin is a known teratogen, and a pattern of malformations termed "warfarin embryopathy" has been identified. When taken in the first trimester, warfarin can affect development of the bones and cartilage, including stippled epiphyses and nasal and limb hypoplasia. These risks seem to be highest when warfarin is taken between weeks 6 and 12, and with higher doses. At doses of 5 mg/day or less, the risk of malformations is less than 3%, while doses above this level lead to a risk of 8% or greater.

BASIC SCIENCE/CLINICAL PEARL	**STEPS 1/2/3**
Please remember that in clinical obstetrics we use menstrual dating, which will be roughly 2 weeks farther along than embryonic dating. This means that 6 weeks gestation is only 2 weeks after the missed menstrual period.	

Warfarin also freely crosses the placenta and will anticoagulate the fetus. There is some evidence suggesting that this may lead to minor neurologic deficits, possibly due to microhemorrhages in the developing brain. Furthermore, fetal anticoagulation increases the risk of intracranial hemorrhage from passage through the birth canal. For all these reasons, warfarin is usually avoided in pregnancy in nearly every condition except mechanical heart valves.

BASIC SCIENCE/CLINICAL PEARL	**STEPS 1/2/3**
Warfarin freely crosses the placenta. Heparins, including LMWHs, do not.	

Most experts recommend using warfarin for anticoagulation of women with mechanical heart valves during the second and third trimesters. There is great disagreement on the ideal regimen for anticoagulation during the first trimester, and no randomized trials exist upon which to guide treatment. Some recommend switching to LMWH during the first trimester and then resuming warfarin later in pregnancy.

In the end, either option is valid. Each option and its benefits and risks should be explained, and the patient should be allowed to make the decision of which risks she is willing to accept.

TABLE 25.2 ■ Management of Anticoagulation for Pregnant Women With Mechanical Heart Valves

First Trimester (conception - 13w 6d)	
Low-dose aspirin PLUS:	
Warfarin	**Heparin**

• Safer for the mother
• ~10% risk of fetal malformations
• Usually recommended for doses ≤5 mg
	• Lower risk of fetal malformations
	• But less safe for the mother
	  • 33% risk of maternal thromboembolic event with unfractionated heparin (9% with low-molecular-weight heparin)
	  • 15% risk of death with unfractionated heparin
	• Target anti–Xa level: 0.8–1.2

Second Trimester (14w 0d–27w 6d)	
Low-dose aspirin PLUS warfarin	
Third Trimester (28w 0d–delivery)	
Low-dose aspirin • Discontinue 1 week prior to delivery Warfarin • Discontinue at 36 weeks (sooner if likely to deliver early) and convert to heparin or low-molecular-weight heparin	

Adapted from Nishimura et al, Circulation, 2014.

How should other valvular diseases in pregnancy be managed?

The World Health Organization (WHO) classification of maternal cardiovascular risk is fairly simple and is an excellent predictor of risk. This classification is presented in Table 25.3.

BEYOND THE PEARLS

- A number of cardiac lesions can affect pregnant women. Management of these conditions must be individualized based on the patient's cardiac anatomy and function, repairs that have been performed, and symptoms/functional status. Consultation with cardiology and anesthesiology, as well as maternal–fetal medicine, is critical in managing the patient's pregnancy, her labor and delivery, and the postpartum period.
- Swelling and fatigue are common symptoms in normal pregnancy. Findings that should raise your level of concern for possible cardiac etiology would include:
  - The presence of these symptoms early in pregnancy
  - A known heart lesion, with or without repair
  - A positive family history
  - Cardiac abnormalities on fetal imaging
- In cases of severe maternal disease, the benefits of treatment often outweigh the possible adverse fetal effects of treatment. This may include medications, imaging modalities, or surgical interventions.
- In nearly all cardiac lesions in pregnancy, vaginal delivery is preferred to cesarean delivery (unless obstetric reasons exist to perform a cesarean delivery). Rare exceptions to this would include:
  - a patient with advanced heart failure who is hemodynamically unstable and does not respond to treatment
  - a patient continuing to take warfarin at the time of delivery (due to increased risk of fetal intracranial hemorrhage)
- Continuous warfarin use throughout pregnancy in women with prosthetic valves has been associated with better maternal outcomes but may lead to fetal malformations, especially at higher doses.

TABLE 25.3 ■ **Modified World Health Organization Classification of Maternal Cardiovascular Risk**

Class	Definition	Recommendations	Specific Conditions
1	Maternal mortality: No increased risk Maternal morbidity: No increased risk or mildly increased risk	None	• Isolated atrial or ventricular ectopic beats • Uncomplicated pulmonary stenosis • Small PDA • Mild mitral valve prolapse • Successfully repaired simple lesions: 　• ASD/VSD 　• PDA 　• Anomalous pulmonary 　• venous return
2	Maternal mortality: Small increased risk Maternal morbidity: Moderate increased risk	None	• Unrepaired ASD/VSD • Repaired major tetralogy of Fallot • Most arrhythmias
2–3	• Individuals with these lesions may be class 2 or class 3 depending on individual factors such as symptoms, physical exam findings, and echocardiographic measurements		• Mild LV impairment • Hypertrophic cardiomyopathy • Native or tissue valvular heart disease not considered class 1 or 4 • Marfan syndrome without aortic dilation • Aorta <45 mm in aortic disease associated with bicuspid aortic valve • Repaired coarctation
3	• Maternal mortality: Significantly increased risk • Maternal morbidity: Significantly increased risk of severe morbidity	• Consider avoiding pregnancy. • If pregnancy is decided upon, intensive cardiac and obstetric monitoring are needed throughout pregnancy, birth, and the postpartum period	• Mechanical valve • Systemic right ventricle • Fontan circulation • Unrepaired cyanotic heart disease • Other complex congenital heart disease • Aortic dilation: 　• 40–45 mm in Marfan syndrome 　• 45–50 mm in aortic disease 　• Associated with bicuspid aortic valve
4	Maternal mortality: Extremely high risk Maternal morbidity: Extremely high risk of severe morbidity	Pregnancy is contraindicated. If a woman becomes pregnant, termination should be discussed. If she opts to continue the pregnancy, care for as a class 3.	• Pulmonary arterial hypertension (any cause) • Severe systemic ventricular dysfunction • LVEF <30% • NYHA class 3–4 • Previous peripartum cardiomyopathy with any residual impairment of LV dysfunction • Aortic dilation: 　• >45 mm in Marfan syndrome 　• >50 mm in aortic disease associated with bicuspid aortic valve • Native severe coarctation

ASD, Atrial septal defect; *VSD*, ventricular septal defect; *PDA*, patent ductus arteriosus; *LV*, left ventricle; *LVEF*, left ventricular ejection fraction; *NYHA*, New York Heart Association.

Adapted from Regitz-Zagrosek et al, European Heart Journal, 2011.

Case Summary

- A 28-year-old female presents for routine obstetric care.
- Her past medical history is unremarkable but she has a family history of a bicupsid aortic valve.
- An echocardiogram reveals the patient to have a bicuspid aortic valve; a fetal echocardiogram shows the same finding in the fetus.
- Her pregnancy is managed successfully with close cardiology and maternal-fetal medicine consultation.
- The patient's disease worsens after pregnancy and she eventually requires valve replacement with a mechanical valve.
- A subsequent pregnancy is managed in a similar fashion to the first, but with anticoagulation throughout pregnancy due to the high risk of thrombosis of mechanical valves during pregnancy.

References

Chan, W. S., Anand, S., & Ginsberg, J. S. (2000). Anticoagulation of pregnant women with mechanical heart valves: a systematic review of the literature. *Archives of Internal Medicine, 160*(2), 191–196.

The Criteria Committee of the New York Heart Association. (1994). *Nomenclature and criteria for diagnosis of diseases of the heart and great vessels* (9th ed.). Boston: Little, Brown & Co, 253.

Cutforth, R., & Macdonald, C. B. (1966). Heart sounds and murmurs in pregnancy. *American Heart Journal, 71*(6), 741–747.

Nishimura, R. A., Otto, C. M., Bonow, R. O., et al. (2014). 2014 AHA/ACC guideline for the management of patients with valvular heart disease: a report of the American College of Cardiology/American Heart Association task force on practice guidelines. *Circulation, 129*(23), e521–e643.

Oran, B., Lee-Parritz, A., & Ansell, J. (2004). Low molecular weight heparin for the prophylaxis of thromboembolism in women with prosthetic mechanical heart valves during pregnancy. *Thrombosis and Haemostasis, 92*(4), 747–751.

Regitz-Zagrosek, V., Blomstrom-Lundqvist, C., Borghi, C., et al. (2011). ESC guidelines on the management of cardiovascular diseases during pregnancy: the Task Force on the Management of Cardiovascular Diseases During Pregnancy of the European Society of Cardiology (ESC). *European Heart Journal, 32*(24), 3147–3197.

Warnes, C. A., Williams, R. G., Bashore, T. M., et al. (2008). ACC/AHA 2008 guidelines for the management of adults with congenital heart disease: a report of the American College of Cardiology/American Heart Association task force on practice guidelines. *Circulation, 118*(23), e714–e833.

Kathy Morris, MSSW, LCGC

A 25-Year-Old Woman Undergoes Noninvasive Aneuploidy Screening

A 25-year-old G2P1001 woman presents to establish prenatal care at about 10 weeks' gestation. She has seen advertisements about a prenatal screening test, noninvasive aneuploidy screening (NIPS), which will reveal the sex of the baby early in pregnancy. She would like to have this test done.

What is noninvasive aneuploidy screening?

NIPS utilizes DNA fragments circulating in maternal plasma to screen for certain chromosome abnormalities. These DNA fragments are primarily placental in origin, the products of apoptosis of cytotrophoblast and syncitiotrophoblast cells. NIPS became clinically available in 2011, as a screen for Down syndrome and has expanded to include screening for other common aneuploidies (trisomies 13, 18, and sex chromosome aneuploidy), triploidy, and selected microdeletions. Different molecular genetic techniques and sophisticated bioinformatic analyses are used to interpret the data. All testing techniques have high sensitivity and specificity for trisomies 21 and 18 (99% and about 96%, respectively) but are somewhat less sensitive for other chromosomal conditions (ranging from 80% to 90%). NIPS is not a karyotype or a microarray technique. As such, it remains a screening tool, not a diagnostic test. Positive NIPS results should be confirmed by karyotype or microarray, prenatally with either chorionic villus sampling (CVS) or amniocentesis, or after birth, with a newborn blood sample.

The positive predictive value of NIPS depends on the prevalence of the condition in the population. As such, the highest positive predictive value is for Down syndrome in a population at increased risk for aneuploidy. NIPS maintains high sensitivity and specificity in lower risk pregnancies, but since the prevalence of aneuploidy is lower, the positive predictive value is lower in this population. There are numerous reports of false-positive NIPS results, with various sources of discrepancy between the NIPS results and fetal karyotype.

The American College of Obstetricians and Gynecologists (ACOG) has endorsed NIPS in a population known to be at increased risk for aneuploidy, but, as of September 2015, asserts that conventional screening is the most appropriate method for the low-risk population. The American College of Medical Genetics (ACMG) recommends that all pregnant women be informed that NIPS is the most sensitive screening option for traditionally screened aneuploidies. At the same time, ACMG recommends that providers make efforts to deter patients from choosing NIPS for the sole purpose of sex identification in the absence of a clinical indication (e.g., risk of an X-linked genetic disorder) for fetal sex determination.

You are familiar with NIPS, so you counsel the patient about the pros and cons of this screening.

What facts and questions do you include in your counseling session?

NIPS is a medical test, designed to screen for certain chromosome abnormalities such as Down syndrome. NIPS is designed to identify several chromosome abnormalities which range in severity from relatively mild to life-threatening. A decision to use NIPS should be based on the parents' desire to know before birth if the baby is likely to have one of these conditions. While a secondary piece of information derived from NIPS is the fetal sex, fetal sex identification is not the purpose of the screen. NIPS is most effective in pregnancies known to be at increased risk for these chromosomal conditions. NIPS is very expensive, and insurance may not cover the screening for a low-risk patient.

This is a screening test. A positive result is concerning but does not mean that the baby definitely has a chromosome abnormality. A negative result does not rule out a fetal chromosome condition. If an abnormal result is received, follow-up testing should be done to confirm or rule out the condition. Confirmatory prenatal testing would involve an invasive procedure with a small, but real, risk to the pregnancy. Confirmatory testing could also be performed after a baby is born.

Other noninvasive screening methods exist which will identify the majority of cases of Down syndrome and trisomy 18, a very serious chromosomal condition. These "standard" screening tests are also designed to screen for open neural tube defects, serious conditions that can cause physical disability and ongoing medical concerns and that would not be detected by NIPS. Standard screening is the method recommended by ACOG for low-risk pregnancies. Fetal sex can usually be determined by ultrasound performed at 18–20 weeks.

> The patient insists on having NIPS. She is not worried about her baby having a chromosome abnormality, but she wants to have a "gender reveal" party when her parents come from out of town to visit in a few weeks. She says cost is not a factor; she will pay for the testing if insurance does not cover it. While you have discussed with the patient that sex determination is not the purpose of the screening test, you believe the patient has understood the risks, benefits, and limitations of NIPS, and, in accordance with the principle of patient autonomy, you agree to provide the NIPS.
>
> NIPS results, which return 8 days later, are read as "high risk" for trisomy 21. The lab report shows 99.9% sensitivity and 99.8 % specificity for this test for Down syndrome and indicates a "risk score" of >99/100. Fetal sex is predicted to be male. The patient is now 11 4/7 weeks pregnant.

What is the significance of these results?

While the sensitivity and specificity of NIPT are high, the risk of Down syndrome for a 25-year-old is about 1 in 1050. Taking prevalence into account, the positive predictive value is actually 32%. The "risk score" listed on the report is misleading because it suggests that there is a greater than 99% chance that the fetus truly has Down syndrome.

> The patient is very upset about these test results. She has read that NIPS is 99% accurate, and she interprets the "risk score" to mean it is a near-certainty that her baby has Down syndrome.
> How do you respond to her concerns?

What additional testing can be offered to diagnose or rule out Down syndrome?

You explain to the patient that the "risk score" on the report does not actually reflect the chance of the baby having Down syndrome. The chance of Down syndrome truly is about 1/3 or 32%, meaning a 2/3 or about 68% chance that the baby does not have Down syndrome. Expressing risk numbers in different ways often helps patients understand statistical concepts and put their specific risks in perspective.

You remind the patient that the test she has had is a screening tool. Confirmation of the suspected diagnosis is strongly recommended. Diagnostic testing for chromosome abnormalities such as Down syndrome include CVS, which is typically done between 10 and 13 weeks, and amniocentesis, which is offered after 15–16 weeks in most centers. Risks of CVS include pregnancy loss, bleeding, infection, and the small possibility of an ambiguous test result. Very recent data suggest a less than 1 in 400 risk of pregnancy loss from CVS when done by an experienced provider. The chance of an ambiguous test result is about 1%. Risks of amniocentesis include pregnancy loss, bleeding, and infection, and recent data include risk of pregnancy loss of approximately 1 in 900 (when performed by an experienced provider). The chance of an ambiguous test result from amniocentesis is about 0.25%.

> The patient is anxious to know for sure, as soon as possible, if her baby has Down syndrome or not. She opts to have CVS, which is done at 12 1/7 weeks. CVS results show mosaicism, with 5/15 cells showing a 47,XY, +21 karyotype and 10/15 cells showing a normal 46,XY karyotype. SS is now 13 2/7 weeks pregnant.

What is the significance of this test result? How do you explain the results to the patient? What additional testing do you offer?

BASIC SCIENCE PEARL   **STEPS 2/3**

A mosaic result is reported in about 1%–2% of CVS samples. In the great majority of cases (90%), the chromosome abnormality is not found in the fetus, but only in placental cells. This phenomenon is known as "confined placental mosaicism." Confined placental mosaicism can result from "trisomy rescue," in which the zygote is trisomic, but the extra chromosome is lost in an early cell division. Depending on the timing of the loss of the extra chromosome, this could result in trisomy in placental cells but a chromosomally normal fetus. Since both NIPS and CVS are performed on DNA from trophoblastic cells, a possible source of false-positive NIPS results is confined placental mosaicism.

CLINICAL PEARL   **STEPS 2/3**

About 1%–4% of infants with Down syndrome have a mosaic karyotype. While some data suggest that intellectual disability and congenital heart disease are less severe in people with mosaic versus nonmosaic trisomy 21, one cannot predict the outcome for an individual based only on their karyotype. As a result, parents of a newborn with mosaic trisomy 21 are typically given the same information about prognosis as parents of a newborn with nonmosaic trisomy 21.

You explain that the cause of Down syndrome is an extra copy of chromosome 21. The CVS showed two kinds of cells: some with the usual number of chromosomes and some with an extra copy of chromosome 21. As such, it is still not clear if the patient's baby has Down syndrome or not. If the baby has some cells with the extra chromosome, he would be expected to have features of Down syndrome, including the typical physical characteristics and intellectual disability, and he would be at risk for the medical concerns associated with Down syndrome. You tell the patient that, based on experience with this situation, it is far more likely that the cells with the extra chromosome are *only* in the placenta and *not* in the baby. Amniocentesis, which cannot be done until 15–16 weeks, should clarify whether the baby has Down syndrome or not. You review the risks of amniocentesis with the patient.

> The patient is very worried about her baby. She opts to have amniocentesis, which is done at 15 5/7 weeks. Test results show a normal 46, XY karyotype in 50/50 cells from two independent culture dishes. Fluorescence in situ hybridization analysis (FISH) for chromosome 21, run on an additional 100 cells, show two signals for chromosome 21, indicating two copies of that chromosome (Fig. 26.1).

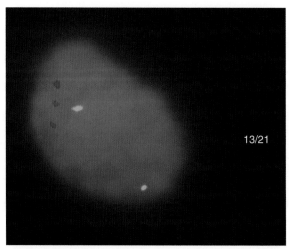

Fig. 26.1 Unlike the results of the patient in this case, this is a fluorescence in situ hybridization analysis (FISH) analysis of an interphase nucleus using locus-specific probes to chromosome 13 *(green)* and chromosome 21 *(red)*, revealing three red signals consistent with trisomy 21. *(From Kumar V, Abbas, A, Aster J et al. Genetic disorders.* Robbins and Cotran pathologic basis of disease, *9th edition. 2015: 137–83. https://www-clinicalkey-com.ezproxyhost.library.tmc.edu/#!/content/book/3-s2.0-B9781455726134000050?scroll To=%233-s2.0-B9781455726134000050-f005-019-9781455726134)*

What is the significance of these test results? What do you think caused the NIPS result? How do you counsel the patient? Do you recommend any follow-up testing? If yes, what?

BASIC SCIENCE PEARL   **STEPS 2/3**

In order to perform chromosome analysis, cytogenetics laboratories take cells from the submitted sample and grow them in separate culture flasks or dishes. Karyotype analysis includes examination of multiple cells from multiple colonies in more than one culture dish. Analysis of 30 cells in this manner rules out 15% mosaicism (i.e., 15% abnormal cells) with 99% certainty. Analysis of more cells decreases the likelihood of even lower level mosaicism. FISH analysis for aneuploidy can done on interphase cells. By applying chromosome-specific fluorescent probes, the lab is able to quickly scan large numbers of cells to look for numerical abnormalities of certain chromosomes.

The possibility of uniparental disomy (UPD, both copies of a chromosome inherited from the same parent) must be considered in cases of confined placental mosaicism. UPD could result from "trisomy rescue," explained earlier, in which a trisomic zygote loses one of the three chromosomes in early development, leaving the fetus with only two copies of the target chromosome. If the remaining two chromosomes came from the same parent, the fetus would have UPD. UPD would only be clinically important if the chromosome of interest contained imprinting regions. To date, no cases of UPD 21 as a cause of pathology have been reported, so no further testing to identify UPD would be indicated.

These test results, 150 cells in multiple colonies and independent cell cultures showing two copies of chromosome 21, suggest that the patient's baby does not have Down syndrome. While very low-level mosaicism cannot be completely ruled out, the test results are very reassuring, and the likelihood of fetal Down syndrome is very low.

You counsel your patient that there are no cells in the amniocentesis sample that show an extra chromosome 21. While one cannot test all the cells in the baby, these results essentially mean that her baby does not have Down syndrome. You recommend that she have the standard anatomy ultrasound at 20 weeks, but no further testing related to Down syndrome.

> Your patient is relieved, but also very upset about the emotional "ordeal" she has undergone. She expresses anger at what she perceives to be misleading information about the accuracy of NIPS and regrets that she decided to have this testing.

BEYOND THE PEARLS

Undergoing any prenatal testing for fetal anomalies can lead to parental anxiety when the possibility of a fetal abnormality is raised, and parental fears (and ultimate relief) can sometimes be expressed as anger. It is helpful to identify and validate patients' feelings as they go through this process and to provide perspective on the level of concern at each stage in the process. The possibility of a fetal anomaly in a patient may be challenging for providers as well, and training classes regarding communicating unexpected news to patients is helpful.

Genetic counselors, who have expertise in genetics and prenatal diagnosis, are invaluable in providing information and support to patients and providers. Genetic counselors often work in conjunction with maternal–fetal medicine specialists, in private practice, and at academic centers. Given the extensive pretest counseling recommended by the ACOG, referral to a genetic counselor should be strongly considered when a patient requests NIPS, and especially in the event of an abnormal NIPS result.

Case Summary

- A 25-year-old G2P1001 woman presents to establish prenatal care at about 10 weeks' gestation. She requests NIPS, which returns high risk for trisomy 21.
- She opts for definitive diagnosis with CVS, which demonstrates mosaicism.
- She undergoes additional genetic counseling and proceeds with amniocentesis after informed consent. The test results show a normal 46, XY karyotype.

References

American College of Obstetricians and Gynecologists. (2016). Practice Bulletin no. 162: prenatal diagnostic testing for genetic disorders. *Obstetrics and Gynecology, 127*(5), 976–978.

American College of Obstetricians and Gynecologists. (2015). Committee Opinion no. 640: cell-free DNA screening for fetal aneuploidy. *Obstetrics and Gynecology, 126*(3), e31–e37.

Bianchi, D. W., Chudova, D., Sehnert, A. J., et al. (2015). Noninvasive prenatal testing and incidental detection of occult maternal malignancies. *Journal of the American Medical Association, 14*(2), 162–169.

Goldberg, J. D., & Wohlford, M. M. (1997). Incidence and outcome of chromosomal mosaicism found at the time of chorionic villus sampling. *American Journal of Obstetrics and Gynecology, 176*(6), 1349–1352.

Grati, F. R., Malvestiti, F., Ferreira, J. C., et al. (2014). Fetoplacental mosaicism: potential implications for false-positive and false-negative noninvasive prenatal screening results. *Genetics in Medicine, 16*(8), 620–624.

Norton, M. E., & Wapner, R. J. (2015). Cell-free DNA analysis for non-invasive examination of trisomy. *The New England Journal of Medicine, 373*(26), 2582.

Papavassiliou, P., Charalsawadi, C., Rafferty, K., et al. (2015). Mosaicism for trisomy 21: a review. *American Journal of Medical Genetics. Part A, 167A*(1), 26–39.

Pergament, E., Cuckle, H., Zimmermann, B., et al. (2014). Single-nucleotide polymorphism-based noninvasive prenatal screening in a high-risk and low-risk cohort. *Obstetrics and Gynecology, 124*(2), 210–218.

Wang, J., Sahoo, T., Schonberg, S., et al. (2015). Discordant noninvasive prenatal testing and cytogenetic results: a study of 109 consecutive cases. *Genetics in Medicine, 17*(3), 234–236.

Wang, L., Meng, Q., Tang, X., et al. (2015). Maternal mosaicism of sex chromosomes causes discordant sex chromosomal aneuploidies associated with noninvasive prenatal testing. *Taiwanese Journal of Obstetrics and Gynecology, 54*(5), 527–531.

Hind N. Moussa, MD

A 27-Year-Old Woman With Vaginal Bleeding in Pregnancy

A 27-year-old G4P3003 woman presents at 26 weeks' gestation with the complaint of vaginal bleeding. This is the first time she had any bleeding during this pregnancy, and she is very concerned about it. She reports that her doctor gave her precautions about this happening especially after her last ultrasound. She is not having any pain and reports the bleeding as "similar to my period," but noted that it had stopped.

Why is it important to ask about vaginal bleeding in pregnant women?
Vaginal bleeding can occur at any time during gestation. The source in the vast majority of cases is maternal, though fetal bleeding can sometimes occur. Gestational age, amount of bleeding (light or heavy), as well as presence of associated symptoms (pain and/or contractions) is usually helpful in determining the most probable etiology. In our patient, it occurred in the second trimester, was painless and self-limited. This is most suggestive of placenta previa.

Placenta previa should be suspected in any woman beyond 20 weeks of gestation who presents with vaginal bleeding. For women who have not had a second- or third-trimester ultrasound examination, antepartum bleeding should prompt sonographic determination of placental location before digital vaginal examination is performed because palpation of the placenta can cause severe hemorrhage.

On physical exam, the patient has a temperature of 36.5°C (97.8°F), a heart rate of 95/min, and a blood pressure of 128/80 mm Hg. Her abdomen is gravid and is soft and nontender to palpation. On pelvic exam, the patient has normal external female genitalia, with no lesions and no pain on palpation. The vaginal walls are intact, with minimal blood in the vaginal vault, and the cervix is closed without any evidence of active bleeding. An ultrasound is performed. The results are shown in Fig. 27.1.

What are the risk factors for this finding? What are the conditions associated with it?
Placenta previa is defined as placental tissue that extends over the internal cervical os. Its incidence ranges from 3.5 to 4.6 per 1000 births. Etiology and risk factors are listed in Table 27.1. Our patient has a couple of these risk factors, mainly that she is multiparous and, upon asking her about her obstetric history, that she reported three previous cesarean deliveries.

Antepartum bleeding, preterm birth, as well as fetal malpresentation are the most common associated conditions. The large volume of placenta in the lower portion of the uterine cavity predisposes the fetus to assume a noncephalic presentation. Of the most serious associated conditions are velamentous umbilical cord, vasa previa, and morbidly adherent placenta.

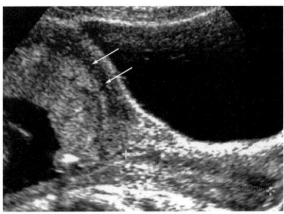

Fig. 27.1   Placenta previa. A sagittal abdominal ultrasound of the lower uterine segment shows a complete anterior placenta previa and a consistent echolucent line demarcating the placental boundary from the myometrium *(arrows)*. *(From Moore T. Placenta and umbilical cord imaging. In Creasy and Resnik's maternal–fetal medicine: principles and practice 2014;379-5. https://www.clinicalkey.com/#!/content/book/3-s2.0-B9781455711376000271?scrollTo=%233-s2.0-B9781455711376000271-f027-011-9781455711376)*

TABLE 27.1 ■ **Risk Factors for Placenta Previa**

Previous placenta previa (4%–8% of subsequent pregnancies)	Multiparity
Previous cesarean delivery (risk increases with an increasing number of cesarean deliveries)	Advanced maternal age
Multiple gestation	Previous intrauterine surgical procedure
Infertility treatment	Maternal smoking
Previous abortion	Maternal cocaine use
Male fetus	Non-white race

BASIC SCIENCE PEARL   **STEP 1**

Pathophysiology of a velamentous cord insertion and/or vasa previa:
    Thinning and expansion of the lower uterine segment as well as placental trophotropism contribute to the placental migration and possible resolution of placenta previa. Monitoring during pregnancy with ultrasound is important to identify exposed fetal vessels such as in vasa previa (Fig. 27.2).

During her subsequent clinic visit, she is at 32 weeks of gestation and undergoes a follow-up ultrasound; Fig. 27.3 shows the results.

What is your differential diagnosis?

Placenta accreta occurs when all or part of the placenta attaches abnormally to the myometrium. Three grades of abnormal placental attachment are defined according to the depth of invasion:
  1. *Accreta*: Chorionic villi attach to the myometrium, rather than being restricted within the decidua basalis.
  2. *Increta*: Chorionic villi invade into the myometrium.
  3. *Percreta*: Chorionic villi invade through the myometrium.

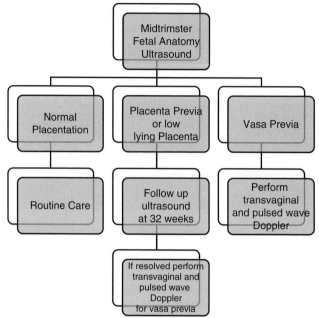

Fig. 27.2 Algorithm for diagnosis and evaluation of abnormal placentation and vasa previa; adapted from the Society for Maternal–Fetal Medicine guide for vasa previa. *(From SMFM. Diagnosis and management of vasa previa. Am J Obstet Gynecol 2015.)*

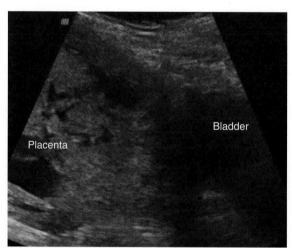

Fig. 27.3 Lower uterine segment imaging of an anterior placenta with disruption of the hyperechoic uterine serosa-bladder interface. *(From Pri-Paz S, D'Alton M. Placenta accreta. Obstetric imaging. 2012:473–7. https://www.clinicalkey.com/#!/search/placenta%2520accreta/%7B%22facetquery%22:%5B%22+contentty pe:IM%22,%22+contenttype:VD%22%5D%7D?page=2)*

CLINICAL PEARL   STEPS 2/3

Sonographic findings that have been associated with placenta accreta include:
- Loss of the normal hypoechoic retroplacental zone
- Multiple vascular lacunae (irregular vascular spaces) within the placenta, giving a "Swiss cheese" appearance
- Blood vessels or placental tissue bridging the myometrial–placental margin, myometrial–bladder interface, or crossing serosa of the myometrium
- Retroplacental myometrial thickness of less than 1 mm
- Numerous coherent vessels visualized with 3-D power Doppler

---

The patient is very concerned. She wants to understand why her placenta is behaving like this and its implications for her pregnancy. She denies any vaginal bleeding since she had this episode a few weeks back and is not having any pain or labor symptoms. What would you tell her about the etiology of placenta accreta? What complications is she at risk of having?

Placenta accreta incidence has increased from approximately 0.8 per 1000 deliveries in the 1980s to 3 per 1000 deliveries in the past decade. Of the most important risk factors for placenta accreta is placenta previa in the presence of a uterine scar (Table 27.2). Other risk factors include placenta previa, maternal age and multiparity, other prior uterine surgery, prior uterine curettage, uterine irradiation, endometrial ablation, Asherman syndrome, uterine leiomyomata, uterine anomalies, hypertensive disorders of pregnancy, and smoking. Her other risk factors are being multiparous as well as having placenta previa by itself. Because of her prior cesarean deliveries, her risk of accreta was increased from 0.1% to 40%.

CLINICAL PEARL   STEPS 2/3

Intrauterine adhesions or synechiae is a condition in which scar tissue develops within the uterine cavity. If accompanied by symptoms (infertility, amenorrhea, etc.) this is referred to as Asherman syndrome.

You explain to her that the number of prior cesarean deliveries that she had in the setting of placenta previa is the most probable contributing factor to her morbidly adherent placenta.

As for foreseen complications, you counsel her about the risk of bleeding and its consequences, including the need for blood transfusion and the need for preterm delivery as an indicated preterm birth. Additional imaging may be required or helpful. Although obstetric ultrasound is the

---

TABLE 27.2 ■ **Frequency of Placenta Accreta According to Number of Cesarean Deliveries and Presence or Absence of Placenta Previa**

Cesarean Delivery	Placenta Previa	No Placenta Previa
First (primary)	3.3	0.03
Second	11	0.2
Third	40	0.1
Fourth	61	0.8
Fifth	67	0.8
≥Sixth	67	4.7

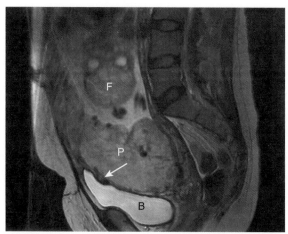

Fig. 27.4 Sagittal magnetic resonance imaging with the fetus *(F)* in vertex presentation at 25 weeks' gestation. The placenta *(P)* is anterior and low lying, with loss of the normal myometrial dark signal. Prominent vessels *(arrow)* between the uterus and bladder *(B)* are concerning for involvement of the bladder wall by placenta percreta. *(From Jauniaux E, Bhide A, Wright J. Placenta accreta.* Obstetrics: normal and problem pregnancies. *2017:456–6. https://www.clinicalkey.com/#!/content/book/3-s2.0-B9780323321082000214?scro llTo=%233-s2.0-B9780323321082000214-f021-010ab-9780323321082)*

primary tool for the diagnosis of placenta accreta, magnetic resonance imaging (MRI) can be helpful if ultrasound is inconclusive or if placenta percreta is suspected (Fig. 27.4).

Further counseling discussion includes possible:
- Damage to surrounding organs (e.g., bowel, bladder, ureters) and neurovascular structures in the retroperitoneum and lateral pelvic sidewalls from placental implantation and its removal
- Postoperative bleeding requiring repeated surgery
- Amniotic fluid embolism
- Complications (e.g., dilutional coagulopathy, consumptive coagulopathy, acute transfusion reactions, transfusion-associated lung injury, acute respiratory distress syndrome, and electrolyte abnormalities) from transfusion of large volumes of blood products, crystalloid, and other volume expanders
- Postoperative thromboembolism, infection, multisystem organ failure, and maternal death

You also discuss that maternal mortality remains a risk, with the incidence of maternal mortality related to placenta accreta and its complications being as high as 6%–7%.

> She asks about her delivery plan.

Since her diagnosis of placenta accreta is suspected antenatally, delivery should be scheduled at an institution with appropriate expertise and facilities including the ability to manage severe hemorrhage. She is given instructions that if she starts bleeding, she should present to the closest hospital with the understanding that she might need to be transferred to an accreta excellence center for further management after stabilization and that she might even be separated from her newborn.

Unless indicated earlier, scheduled late preterm delivery (34 0/7–35 6/7 weeks) is recommended with the plan/potential need for hysterectomy. Frequently postoperative intensive care unit admission is needed.

The patient elects to be hospitalized for inpatient observation close to time of delivery and understands the management plan. She is now more aware of nonimmediate risks of cesarean delivery and would like to educate women about her clinical story in the hope of reducing cesarean rates.

BEYOND THE PEARLS

- Placenta previa is defined as placental tissue that extends over the internal cervical os. Its incidence ranges from 3.5 to 4.6 per 1000 births.
- Antepartum bleeding, preterm birth, as well as fetal malpresentation are the most common associated conditions. Of the most serious associated conditions are velamentous umbilical cord, vasa previa, and morbidly adherent placenta.
- Placenta accreta occurs when all or part of the placenta attaches abnormally to the myometrium. Three grades of abnormal placental attachment are defined according to the depth of invasion: accreta, increta, and percreta.
- Multiple prior cesarean deliveries in the setting of placenta previa are associated with morbidly adherent placenta.
- Obstetric ultrasound is the primary tool for the diagnosis of placenta accreta; MRI can be helpful if ultrasound is inconclusive or if placenta percreta is suspected.
- Delivery should be scheduled at an institution with appropriate expertise and facilities with the ability to manage severe hemorrhage because the incidence of maternal mortality related to placenta accreta and its complications is as high as 7%.

Case Summary

- A 27-year-old G4P3003 woman presents at 26 weeks' gestation with the complaint of painless vaginal bleeding.
- History and physical reveals that the patient had multiple prior cesarean deliveries, and further imaging reveals a placenta previa.
- The patient's further evaluation reveals a morbidly adherent placenta consistent with accreta.
- She is hospitalized with the plan to undergo a cesarean hysterectomy at a specialized accreta center.

References

Belfort, M. A. (2010). Placenta accreta. *American Journal of Obstetrics and Gynecology, 203*(5), 430–439.

Silver, R. M., Fox, K. A., Barton, J. R., et al. (2015). Center of excellence for placenta accreta. *American Journal of Obstetrics and Gynecology, 212*(5), 561–568.

Sinkey, R. G., Odibo, A. O., Dashe, J. S., et al. (2015). Diagnosis and management of vasa previa. *American Journal of Obstetrics and Gynecology, 213*(5), 615–619.

Andrew Morado ▪ Raj Dasgupta ▪ Ahmet Baydur

A 27-Year-Old Woman With History of Asthma

A 27-year-old woman G1P0 (16 weeks of gestation) presents for outpatient evaluation of asthma management during pregnancy.

What is asthma and its clinical presentation?

Diseases of the lung can be divided in those that affect the parenchyma (interstitial lung disease), vasculature (pulmonary embolism, pulmonary hypertension), or the airways (asthma, chronic obstructive pulmonary disease) although there tends to be significant overlap in many entities. Asthma is a chronic inflammatory disorder of the airways resulting in obstruction of airflow.

Atopic reactions and immunoglobulin E cascades are the typical causes of chronic airway inflammation, of which there are many inciting factors (dust mites, animal dander, pollens, molds, etc.). Regardless of the cause, the pathologic changes that occur from this chronic inflammation are airway remodeling (smooth muscle hypertrophy/hyperplasia), goblet cell hyperplasia with excessive mucin production, and a cellular infiltration (eosinophilic and neutrophilic) of the bronchiole wall (Fig. 28.1).

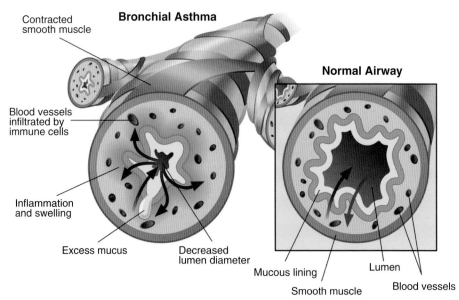

Fig. 28.1 Pathological changes from chronic airway inflammation in asthma depicting narrowed airways, bronchial wall thickening, and excessive mucin production. *(Reproduced from bioinformant.com.)*

The reduced diameter of the airway causes a reduction in airflow thereby lengthening the expiratory phase of the respiratory cycle and increasing the work of breathing, while excessive mucous plugging results in atelectasis and a derangement in ventilation/perfusion matching. This explains the commonly reported triad of wheezing, shortness of breath, and cough in poorly controlled asthmatics.

Unique to asthma are periods of relative clinical quiescence when patients report well-controlled symptoms, possibly none at all, followed by stretches of marked airflow limitation requiring increasing therapy or sometimes hospitalization. These periods of exacerbation can be linked to many triggers, including increased exposure to irritants, noncompliance with therapy, or infection.

CLINICAL PEARL STEPS 2/3

Remember, all that wheezes are not asthma. Other diseases that commonly cause wheezing include decompensated heart failure, vocal cord dysfunction, bronchiectasis, allergic bronchopulmonary aspergillosis, gastroesophageal reflux disorder, and postnasal drip.

She brings you her records from her primary care doctor and obstetrician. The records include her medical history, current medication regimen, and pulmonary function tests (PFTs) from a month ago. She has no other past medical or surgical history. Her mother was diagnosed with hypertension, and her father suffered from a myocardial infarction. She does not smoke, drink alcohol, or use illicit drugs. She has an allergy to cats and currently takes albuterol as needed for shortness of breath and inhaled low-dose budesonide daily. She asks what you think of her PFTs.

How is asthma diagnosed?

The diagnosis of asthma depends on pulmonary function testing. PFTs consist of three measurements: spirometry, lung volumes, and gas exchange. All measurements are reported as an absolute value and a percentage (%) predicted, which is derived from population-matched controls.

Spirometry is a measurement of airflow during the respiratory cycle and provides numerical values as well as flow-volumes loops. Patients are counseled to take a maximal inspiration (forced vital capacity or FVC) and exhale with peak effort. The volume of air exhaled during the first second is the FEV1. Obstructive airway disease is defined as an FEV1/FVC ratio of less than 70%. The FEV1/FVC is simply the amount of the forced vital capacity expired in 1 second and indicates airflow limitation if the ratio is less than 0.7 after maximal inspiration. In other words, in the normal population, a person should be able to exhale at least 70% of the total inspired air within the first second of expiration. The limitation in airflow in patients with obstructive airway diseases can be seen in the flow-volume loop as well, and characteristically shows the scalloped (or concave up) expiratory limb (Fig. 28.2).

Spirometry also allows for a second measurement of airflow following administration of a bronchodilator. Reversibility of airflow limitation is a key finding in asthma and is defined as an improvement in FEV1 or FVC of greater than 12% predicted or 200 mL.

Lung volumes measured using body plethysmography typically reveal increased residual volume, which is a direct byproduct of obstructive airway disease. As airflow limitation progresses, the time needed for expiration cannot be reached prior to the initiation of a second breath and leads to air trapping. This is most notable on lung volume measurements as the residual volume in the lung increases in comparison to the total lung capacity. In fact, air trapping is now considered to be a more important factor in producing dyspnea than is airflow limitation, particularly during exercise.

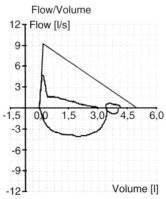

Fig. 28.2 A flow-volume loop demonstrating marked obstructive airway disease with a normal flow-volume depicted by the black line. *(From Wikimedia Commons, courtesy of Evgenios Metaxas, MD.)*

Gas exchange expressed as the DLCO typically is normal in asthmatics outside of exacerbations, though it may increase with air trapping.

CLINICAL PEARL	STEPS 2/3

Often, patients present with typical symptoms of asthma despite multiple normal PFTs. To solve this quandary, provocation testing has shown to have excellent negative predictive value and is used as the screening test of choice. Provocation testing involves administration of a bronchoconstrictor (typically methacholine) in steadily increasing concentrations until a drop in FEV1 of more than 20% is achieved. Keep in mind that all patients, including nonasthmatics, will eventually respond. Patients who require more than 16 ng/mL concentration of methacholine to induce a response indicate a negative test, and this effectively rules out asthma. This test is usually not performed during pregnancy.

Her PFTs show a flow-volume loop consistent with airflow limitation, and her FEV1/FVC is 69%. She meets criteria for bronchodilator response. Lung volumes are significant for mild air trapping, and gas exchange is normal. She tells you she uses her albuterol inhaler 2–3 times a week for shortness of breath. She is able to conduct all of her usual daily activities but does awake with shortness of breath at night 3–4 times a month. She has never been intubated for an asthma exacerbation, and her last hospitalization was several years ago. She avoids cats as this causes immediate worsening in her symptoms.

How is asthma treated?

The mainstay of asthma therapy is two-pronged: short-term control of symptoms and long-term prevention of exacerbations. As stated previously, the pathophysiology of asthma is driven by chronic inflammation of the airways. As such, the goal then is to decrease or prevent inflammation. Patients with identified triggers (cats in this case) should be instructed to avoid any undue exposure as this can be linked to acute worsening of symptoms. To control inflammation, inhaled glucocorticoids (ICS) are the therapy of choice for outpatient management and have been shown to improve lung function and decrease exacerbations.

CLINICAL PEARL	STEPS 2/3

ICS are the hallmark of asthma therapy and should never be left out of treatment regimens for persistent asthmatics. Prior studies have shown increased mortality in patients treated solely with long-acting beta agonists (LABA). The most likely explanation is due to symptom masking in the setting of continued, severe airway inflammation.

Further control of symptoms is achieved by decreasing resistance to airflow with bronchodilators. Short-acting beta agonists (SABA) like albuterol are used for acute episodes of shortness of breath. When needed, LABA can be added to provide longer lasting effects. There is also evidence for leukotriene inhibitors, although not as robust when compared to beta agonists. Theophylline, a medication with both antiinflammatory and bronchodilator properties, has lost favor recently due to a narrow therapeutic window but may be considered for refractory cases.

CLINICAL PEARL	STEPS 2/3

The majority of medications for asthma are delivered via inhalers. It is a good idea to review inhaler technique with all patients at their first visit, with reinforcement at future visits. Patients should shake and prime the inhaler on first use. The breath should be initiated from the mouth and taken slowly, beginning at the same time as dispensing of medication. Spacers allow for more effective delivery of medications and should always be used.

Vital signs are temperature 37°C (98.8°F), a heart rate of 68/min, respiratory rate of 14/min, blood pressure 112/75 mm Hg. On exam, she is a well-developed woman in no distress. She is normocephalic. The oropharynx is clear, and there is no cervical lymphadenopathy. The heart rate is regular with no murmurs, and the breath sounds are clear without evidence of wheezes. The abdomen is gravid, consistent with an early second-trimester pregnancy. The extremities are normal, with good peripheral pulses. Following the exam, she asks your opinion on her current regimen of medications and if you recommend any adjustments.

What is the significance of asthma classification and approach to management?
An approach to therapy has been established with an emphasis upon clinical findings. Patients with asthma demonstrating poor control of symptoms are more prone to exacerbations and hospitalizations. Thus, tracking the progression of symptoms during scheduled clinic visits is paramount to help guide management and decrease the chances for acute exacerbations.

The National Heart, Lung, and Blood institute in 2012 published a detailed review of asthma classification based on clinical symptoms and signs including symptoms (cough, shortness of breath, wheezing), nighttime awakenings, SABA use, physical limitation, and PFT measures of lung function. Using these five criteria, patients with asthma can be classified as intermittent, mild-persistent, moderate-persistent, and severe-persistent (Table 28.1).

These same guidelines also recommended stepwise management based on the progression or improvement in clinical presentation. Patients with intermittent asthma can be treated solely with SABA. However, once disease progresses to persistent asthma, then low-dose ICS should be started in addition to a SABA in Step 2. This is followed by a combined ICS/LABA with SABA if symptoms remain poorly controlled in Step 3 and then continued with increased doses of ICS in Steps 4 and 5. If symptoms remain poorly controlled then, Step 6 recommends systemic glucocorticoids. Alternative therapies are mentioned as well and can be tailored based on patients' characteristics (Fig. 28.3).

TABLE 28.1 ■ **Asthma Classification Based on Clinical Signs and Symptoms**

Components of Severity		Classification of Asthma Severity ≥12 Years of Age			
				Persistent	
		Intermittent	Mild	Moderate	Severe
Impairment Normal FEV$_1$/ FVC: 8–19 yr 85% 20–39 yr 80% 40–59 yr 75% 60–80 yr 70%	Symptoms	≤2 days/week	>2 days/week but not daily	Daily	Throughout the day
	Nighttime awakenings	≤2x/month	3–4×/month	>1×/week but not nightly	Often 7×/ week
	Short-acting beta$_2$- agonist use for symptom control (not prevention of EIB)	≤2 days/week	>2 days/week but not daily, and not more than 1× on any day	Daily	Several times per day
	Interference with normal activity	None	Minor limitation	Some limitation	Extremely limited
	Lung function	• Normal FEV$_1$ between exacerbations • FEV$_1$ >80% predicted • FEV$_1$/FVC normal	• FEV$_1$ >80% predicted • FEV$_1$/FVC normal	• FEV$_1$ >60% but <80% predicted • FEV$_1$/FVC reduced 5%	• FEV$_1$ <60% predicted • FEV$_1$/FVC reduced >5%
Risk	Exacerbations requiring oral systemic corticosteroids	0–1/year (see note)	2/year (see note) →		
		← Consider severity and interval since last exacerbation. → Frequency and severity may fluctuate over time for patients in any severity category. Relative annual risk of exacerbations may be related to FEV$_1$.			
Recommended Step for Initiating Treatment (See "Stepwise Approach for Managing Asthma" for treatment steps.)		Step 1	Step 2	Step 3 In 2–6 weeks, evaluate level of asthma control that is achieved and adjust therapy accordingly.	Step 4 or 5 and consider short course of oral systemic corticosteroids

NIH, National Heart, Lung and Blood Institute. Expert Panel Report 3: Guidelines for the Diagnosis and Management of Asthma (EPR-3 2007). http://www.nhlbi.nih.gov/guidelines/asthma/index.htm.

CLINICAL PEARL   **STEPS 2/3**

Studies on asthma therapy have shown increased benefit when adding a LABA to a low-dose ICS compared to doubling the dose of the ICS.

Given her current symptoms, you classify her with mild-persistent asthma and recommend continued therapy with daily low-dose budesonide and albuterol as needed. After you review inhaler technique with her, she asks what the effects are of pregnancy on her lungs.

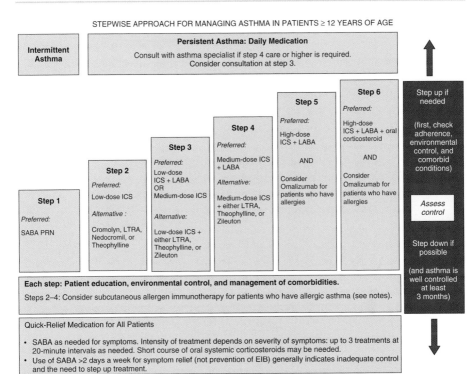

STEPWISE APPROACH FOR MANAGING ASTHMA IN PATIENTS ≥ 12 YEARS OF AGE

Intermittent Asthma

Persistent Asthma: Daily Medication
Consult with asthma specialist if step 4 care or higher is required.
Consider consultation at step 3.

Step 1
Preferred:
SABA PRN

Step 2
Preferred:
Low-dose ICS
Alternative :
Cromolyn, LTRA, Nedocromil, or Theophylline

Step 3
Preferred:
Low-dose ICS + LABA
OR
Medium-dose ICS
Alternative:
Low-dose ICS + either LTRA, Theophylline, or Zileuton

Step 4
Preferred:
Medium-dose ICS + LABA
Alternative:
Medium-dose ICS + either LTRA, Theophylline, or Zileuton

Step 5
Preferred:
High-dose ICS + LABA
AND
Consider Omalizumab for patients who have allergies

Step 6
Preferred:
High-dose ICS + LABA + oral corticosteroid
AND
Consider Omalizumab for patients who have allergies

Step up if needed

(first, check adherence, environmental control, and comorbid conditions)

Assess control

Step down if possible

(and asthma is well controlled at least 3 months)

Each step: Patient education, environmental control, and management of comorbidities.
Steps 2–4: Consider subcutaneous allergen immunotherapy for patients who have allergic asthma (see notes).

Quick-Relief Medication for All Patients

- SABA as needed for symptoms. Intensity of treatment depends on severity of symptoms: up to 3 treatments at 20-minute intervals as needed. Short course of oral systemic corticosteroids may be needed.
- Use of SABA >2 days a week for symptom relief (not prevention of EIB) generally indicates inadequate control and the need to step up treatment.

Fig. 28.3 Step-up therapy for asthma based on clinical signs and symptoms. *(From National Heart, Lung and Blood Institute. Expert Panel Report 3: Guidelines for the diagnosis and Management of Asthma. 2012.)*

What is the normal physiology of the respiratory system during pregnancy?

To better understand the dynamics of asthma and pregnancy, the normal physiologic changes of the lungs that occur with pregnancy should be reviewed. Airway mechanics do not significantly change during pregnancy and so spirometry values for FVC, FEV1, and FEV1/FVC remain normal compared to nongravid individuals. Thus, the diagnosis of asthma during pregnancy remains the same as previously stated. Lung volumes, on the other hand, have some variability. Flaring of the ribs from the enlarging uterus and unimpaired diaphragmatic excursion allows for a preserved vital capacity and total lung capacity. Due to the enlarging uterus and its impact upon the diaphragm, the residual volume and functional residual capacity are decreased compared to normal individuals.

As progesterone levels rise, minute ventilation increases beyond the metabolic demand. This has two effects: partial pressure of arterial carbon dioxide ($PaCO_2$) decreases (28–30 mm Hg) while partial pressure of arterial oxygen (PaO_2) increases (100–106 mm Hg). The chronic reduction in $PaCO_2$ causes a compensatory excretion of bicarbonate in the urine and results in a compensated respiratory alkalosis.

Fetal oxygenation is dependent upon maternal oxygenation and is typically about one-third to one-quarter the PaO_2 in the adult. It follows then that deterioration of the mother can have a substantial impact upon the developing fetus. Fetal hemoglobin (HbF) has evolved to handle such situations by having a much higher affinity for oxygen than does adult hemoglobin (HbA). This is due to difference in structure, where HbF is composed of two alpha chains and two gamma chains as opposed to the usual two alpha and beta chains seen in HbA. In addition, the placenta has higher levels of 2,3-bisphosphoglyceric acid (2,3-BPG) that causes a right shift of the HbA

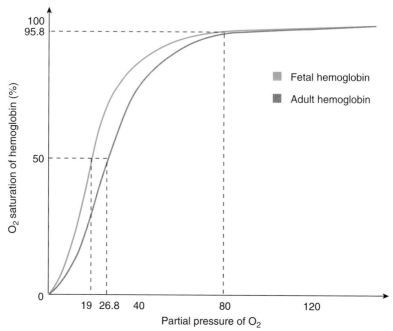

Fig. 28.4 Fetal hemoglobin dissociation curve (blue line) compared to adult hemoglobin (orange line). *(Adapted from Delivoria-Papadopoulos M, McGowan JE. Oxygen transport and delivery. In Polin RA, Fox WW, Abman SH, editors, Fetal and neonatal physiology, 3rd ed. Philadelphia: Saunders; 2004.)*

dissociation curve, coaxing oxygen release from mother's blood that is then rapidly bound by HbF in the fetal circulation. Because of the structural differences just noted, 2,3-BPG has no effect on oxygen dissociation from HbF (Fig. 28.4).

BASIC SCIENCE PEARL   **STEP 1**

Compensatory mechanisms during sustained hypoxemia in the fetus include redistribution of blood flow to vital organs, increased oxygen extraction, and slowed overall growth. This is the presumed reason for low term birth weight seen in newborns of patients with poorly controlled asthma during pregnancy.

What is the effect of pregnancy on asthma?

Most studies have demonstrated variable effects of pregnancy on asthma. Of note, a prospective study of 366 pregnancies in patients with asthma revealed worsening of symptoms in 35%, improvement of symptoms in 28%, and unchanged in the remainder. If patients did worsen, it tended to happen from weeks 29–36, and symptoms during labor were rare, occurring in only 10% of reported births.

Asthma exacerbations occur in 20%–36% of pregnancies. Peak incidence of severe exacerbation is reported to occur during weeks 14–24. The most commonly reported reason for exacerbation was ICS noncompliance following first knowledge of the pregnancy (Fig. 28.5).

What is the effect of asthma on pregnancy?

Most reported studies suggest an adverse effect of asthma upon the pregnancy. The largest study evaluated more than 281,000 pregnancies consisting of 37,000 women with asthma and 243,000

Frequency distribution of acute attacks during pregnancy

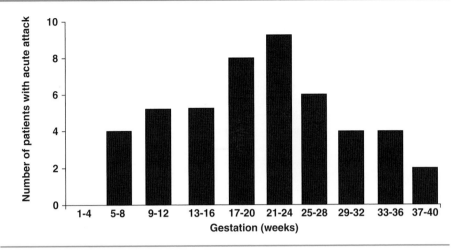

Asthma attacks during pregnancy were seen most frequently between weeks 17 and 24 of gestation.

Fig. 28.5 Incidence of acute asthma exacerbation by gestational week. *(From Stenius-Aarniala, et al. Acute asthma during pregnancy. Thorax. 1996; 51:411.)*

women without asthma. Of note, pregnancies of women with moderate to severe asthma had increased risk of miscarriage, antepartum hemorrhage, postpartum hemorrhage, anemia, depression, and cesarean delivery. Other similar studies looking at large populations of asthmatic women demonstrated increased risk for low-birth-weight infants.

How does management differ for the pregnant patient with asthma?

The strategies for controlling asthma are the same in pregnant women. The emphasis of therapy should be in avoiding triggers, decreasing inflammation, improving symptoms, and preventing exacerbations. The step-up guidelines remain pertinent but do have variation because of the pregnancy categories of current medications. To review, definitions of pregnancy categories A–X are listed.

> The patient thanks you for your time and leaves with scheduled follow-up in 2 months. Six weeks later, you are called to the ER for a stat consult. You arrive and are surprised to see your clinic patient. She was brought in by ambulance after exposure to cat dander. Shortly following the exposure, she reported increased shortness of breath, audible wheezing, and cough. She is noticeably dyspneic and in distress. Vitals reveal a respiration rate of 31/min and oxygen saturation of 91% on a 10-L face mask. On auscultation, she has tachycardia with no audible wheezing. The abdomen is gravid, consistent with 22 weeks' gestation. She has received several breathing treatments with nebulized albuterol. The ER attending asks for your opinion.

What is status asthmaticus?

Status asthmaticus is an acute asthma exacerbation not relieved with SABA. These patients present with the usual symptoms of asthma but with progressive worsening of shortness of breath and peak expiratory flow of less than 50% of their baseline. All patients with an acute asthma exacerbation not improved with initial SABA should be evaluated in an urgent care or ER setting for a higher level of care. Following the initial assessment (circulation, airway, breathing), nebulized beta-agonists should be delivered, with supplemental oxygen as needed to maintain a minimum saturation of 92%. Intravenous steroids are recommended as early treatment for a severe asthma exacerbation, although the optimal dose is unknown. Typically, 1–2 mg/kg in divided doses is a reasonable option. Though commonly administered, there is weak evidence for magnesium sulfate infusion given its potential as a bronchodilator.

As part of the initial evaluation, an arterial blood gas (ABG) should be ordered to assess for hypoxemia or hypercapnia. Additionally, a chest radiograph (CXR) should be ordered to evaluate for large areas of atelectasis or infiltrates that may suggest overwhelming mucous plugging or infection.

CLINICAL PEARL   **STEPS 2/3**

The wheeze heard in an asthma exacerbation is from the turbulent airflow moving through narrowed bronchioles. Wheezing is indicative of narrowed airways but does offer some evidence the patient is able to maintain some level of minute ventilation. The patient with a severe asthma exacerbation and no audible wheezes has deteriorated to cessation of air movement, and respiratory failure will surely follow.

Albuterol nebulized treatments are continued, and a first dose of IV Solu-Medrol is given with a 2-g magnesium sulfate infusion. The CXR reveals hyperinflation but no pulmonary infiltrates or significant atelectasis. ABG taken at the bedside results in a pH of 7.38, $PaCO_2$ 41 mm Hg, and a PaO_2 of 62 mm Hg.

What is the optimal ventilator strategy for an acute asthma exacerbation?

Knowledge of normal ABG values for pregnant women is vital to determining management in this acute scenario. As stated previously, pregnancy causes a compensated respiratory alkalosis with PCO_2 ranging from 28 to 32. This woman, now with respiratory acidosis and a "normal" PCO_2, is deteriorating to acute hypercapnic and hypoxemic respiratory failure. The decision to intubate should be made at this juncture.

The mode of ventilation for acute asthma exacerbation can be challenging. Because some patients can develop significant hypercapnia, often ventilators are set to optimize minute ventilation with high respiratory rate and/or high tidal volumes. The pathophysiology of asthma directly affects the flow of air *out* of the lungs. The narrowed airways and mucous plugging cause air trapping and increased dead space that contributes to hypercapnia. As air trapping worsens, the alveoli become overdistended, cutting off the blood supply through the capillary walls and effectively increasing dead space and further contributing to hypercapnia. Air trapping also leads to shortening of the diaphragmatic muscle fibers and reduction in diaphragmatic appositional area with respect to the abdominal wall and fatigue. Thus, the preferred ventilator strategy should be to maximize expiration and decrease minute ventilation to prevent further air trapping. This is best accomplished by setting a tidal volume of 6 mL/kg, a respiratory rate less than 20, and an inspiratory/expiratory ratio of 1:3 to 1:5. Permissive hypercapnia is allowed as long as serum pH does not drop below 7.3. This rarely happens because, as air trapping improves, the overdistention of alveoli decreases and actually improves ventilation/perfusion mismatch.

SABA therapy with IV glucocorticoids should be continued to treat the underlying asthma exacerbation and ventilator weaning should begin as soon as feasible.

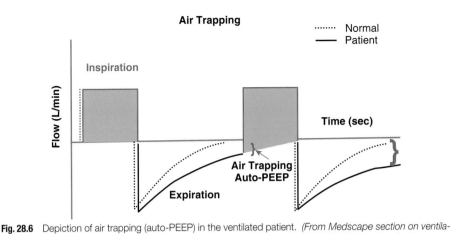

Fig. 28.6 Depiction of air trapping (auto-PEEP) in the ventilated patient. *(From Medscape section on ventilator graphics authored by Amanullah,* http://emedicine.medscape.com/article/305120-overview#a1.*)*

CLINICAL PEARL   **STEPS 2/3**

The phenomenon of air trapping (autopositive end-expiratory pressure) can be so severe that intrathoracic pressures elevate and return of blood to the right atrium is impaired. If this continues, then preload drops low enough to affect cardiac output and pulseless electrical activity arrest can ensue. Patients with severe air trapping and hemodynamic instability should first be disconnected from the ventilator to allow exhalation of excess air. Rapid improvement quickly follows (Fig. 28.6).

Your patient remains intubated for 2 days on continued SABA and IV corticosteroid therapy, following which respiratory mechanics significantly improve and spontaneous breathing trials are begun. She is extubated without complication and transferred to the floor the following day. She is discharged 2 days later, following an uncomplicated stay with follow-up with her obstetrician and your clinic in 1 week.

BEYOND THE PEARLS

- Bronchothermoplasty is a bronchoscopic technique that applies heat to the bronchiole walls, inhibiting smooth muscle hypertrophy (studies have shown an actual reduction in muscle mass in the bronchiole wall) and has been shown to decrease ER visits and hospitalization. It is reserved for severe asthmatics on maximal medical therapy.
- ER literature supports the use of ketamine as a preferred sedative agent for rapid-sequence intubation, given its potential as a bronchodilator.
- Heliox is a mixture of helium and oxygen that can be delivered through a ventilator to patients with severe asthma exacerbation. It functions by decreased resistance to airflow, thereby improving airway mechanics.
- There is no role for IV epinephrine in the treatment of an asthma exacerbation.

Case Summary
- A 27-year-old woman G1P0 (16 weeks of gestation) presents for outpatient evaluation of asthma management during pregnancy and subsequently goes to the ER for an asthma exacerbation 6 weeks later.

- In the ER, patient has shortness of breath, audible wheezing, and cough. She is noticeably dyspneic and in distress. Vitals reveal a respiration rate of 31 and oxygen saturation of 91% on a 10-L face mask.
- ABG taken at the bedside shows a pH of 7.38, $PaCO_2$ 41 mm Hg, and a PaO_2 of 62 mm Hg. The CXR reveals hyperinflation but no pulmonary infiltrates or significant atelectasis.
- The patient is diagnosed with status asthmaticus during pregnancy.
- The patient is intubated and placed on mechanical ventilation, receiving continuous bronchodilators and IV corticosteroids.

References

Källén, B., Rydhstroem, H., & Aberg, A. (2000). Asthma during pregnancy: a population based study. *European Journal of Epidemiology, 16*(2), 167–171.

Mendola, P., Laughon, S. K., Männistö, T. I., et al. (2013). Obstetric complications among US women with asthma. *American Journal of Obstetrics and Gynecology, 208*(2), 127.e1–127.e8.

National Heart, Lung and Blood Institute. (2007). *NAEPP: Expert panel report III: guidelines for the diagnosis and management of asthma.* updated 2012. https://www.nhlbi.nih.gov/.

O'Donnell DE. (2006). Hyperinflation, dyspnea, and exercise intolerance in chronic obstructive pulmonary disease. *Proceedings of the American Thoracic Society, 3*(2), 108–184.

Rodrigo, G. J., Rodrigo, C., & Hall, J. B. (2004). Acute asthma in adults: a review. *Chest, 125*(3), 1081–1102.

Schatz, M., Harden, K., Forsyth, A., et al. (1988). The course of asthma during pregnancy, post partum, and with successive pregnancies: a prospective analysis. *The Journal of Allergy and Clinical Immunology, 81*(3), 509–517.

Stenius-Aarniala, B., Hedman, J., Teramo, K. A. (1996). Acute asthma during pregnancy. *Thorax, 51*(4), 411–414.

Tata, L. J., Lewis, S. A., McKeever, T. M., et al. (2007). A Comprehensive analysis of adverse obstetric and pediatric complications in women with asthma. *American Journal of Respiratory and Critical Care Medicine, 175*(10), 991–997.

Katherine K. Green, MD MS ■ Raj Dasgupta, MD

A 34-Year-Old Woman With Sleep Disturbance During Pregnancy

A 34-year-old woman presents for a routine second-trimester prenatal visit and is feeling severely fatigued. She reports that she is able to fall asleep quickly at night and feels like she "sleeps through the night," but wakes up feeling tired in the morning. She feels tired throughout the day and is falling asleep on the couch while watching television in the evenings. Her prepregnancy body mass index (BMI) was 32 kg/m², and she has had appropriate weight gain during pregnancy.

"Fatigue" is a common and vague chief complaint, particularly common in pregnancy and often due to the increased physical and metabolic demands of pregnancy. However, as the prevalence of obesity has risen in reproductive-age women, there has also been a notable increase in obesity-related comorbid conditions, and one of the most common conditions of this type is obstructive sleep apnea (OSA). OSA is characterized by complete ("apnea") or partial ("hypopnea") obstruction in the upper airway while sleeping, despite continued respiratory effort. This results in episodes of reduction of airflow, hypoxemia, increased sympathetic discharge, and recurrent arousals from sleep. It is important that any patient with risk factors for OSA (see Clinical Pearls Box) be carefully evaluated with a thorough sleep history and review of systems to see if further testing is warranted. Traditional screening tools for OSA (e.g., the Berlin Questionnaire) have been shown to be less sensitive and specific for pregnant women.

CLINICAL PEARL   **STEPS 2/3**

Risk factors for OSA include obesity, history of OSA in primary family members, other medical conditions related to obesity (including hypertension and diabetes), history of snoring, or daytime somnolence. There are several commonly used screening tools that may be used to assess risk and can be helpful in determining which patients need further screening, including the Berlin Questionnaire and STOP-BANG, but there is evidence that these screening tools may be less sensitive and specific for pregnant women. The current recommendation is to consider further testing for anyone with symptoms and any risk factors for OSA.

The patient reports that she sleeps from 10 pm to 6 am. She denies any difficulty falling asleep or staying asleep. She denies any atypical sensations in her legs that disrupt her sleep. Prior to pregnancy, she reports that she drank three to four cups of coffee daily and sometimes would have an "energy drink" in the afternoon; however, she has cut this down to one cup of coffee per day since she became pregnant.

CLINICAL PEARL   **STEPS 2/3**

Excessive daytime sleepiness may be masked by caffeine intake or by prescription stimulants such as methylphenidate (Ritalin), dextroamphetamine/levoamphetamine (Adderall), and modafinil (Provigil). When evaluating any patient, it is always important to obtain a complete list of current medications and herbal supplements, to assess caffeine and alcohol intake, and to ask about tobacco and substance use.

She has had intermittent headaches mostly in the morning, but attributed this to "caffeine withdrawal" since cutting back on coffee. The patient denies drowsy driving, falling asleep at the wheel, and motor vehicle collisions related to sleepiness. She does not nap. Her husband has also complained that recently she has started snoring loudly every night, to the point that it is disrupting his sleep. He reports that previously she would snore only occasionally, particularly after alcohol intake or if she "had a cold," but not on a regular basis.

CLINICAL PEARL   **STEPS 2/3**

When assessing a patient who reports sleep-related difficulties, it is critical to assess safety concerns, particularly drowsy driving and if his or her occupation involves operating heavy machinery or vehicles involved in mass transit or the transportation of goods. All patients should be counseled to avoid driving and other high-risk activities when they are drowsy.

What is the most likely diagnosis for this patient's complaint of fatigue and daytime somnolence?

Although there are many reasons for fatigue and sleepiness, particularly during pregnancy, there are several "red flags" about this patient's history that should raise your suspicion for OSA.

In the general population, the prevalence of OSA in reproductive age women is significantly lower than in men, and estimates vary in the literature between 0.7% and 6.5%. The prevalence of OSA in pregnant women is not well defined in the literature, but several studies suggest that it is significantly higher than a nonpregnant cohort. One small prospective study looked at 105 women who underwent first- and third-trimester polysomnography and noted that the prevalence of OSA (as defined by an apnea-hypopnea index [AHI] of >5 events per hour) was 10.5% in the first trimester and 26.7% in the third trimester. Increased age and obesity are both known to be independent risk factors for OSA in women (both pregnant and nonpregnant), and both of these things are increasing in the population of pregnant women in the United States.

In this patient, her snoring history and obesity are risk factors for OSA, and the progression of symptoms as her pregnancy progressed is concerning for worsening OSA. Alcohol ingestion reduces upper airway tone, worsening snoring and sleep-disordered breathing in patients with OSA, and is consistent with the prepregnancy history that she provides. The worsened disruptive snoring and the development of daytime hypersomnolence are suggestive of worsening OSA, and further testing should be pursued.

Are there physiologic reasons that OSA would be worse during pregnancy?

While weight gain is a known risk factor for OSA, there are several other hormonal and physiologic changes during pregnancy that may be responsible for the increase in incidence of OSA, even during the first and second trimesters when weight gain is not yet as significant:

1. Nasal patency is reduced during pregnancy. Due to changes in estrogen and progesterone, there is an increased in blood flow and variations in the nasal mucosa, leading to increased nasal

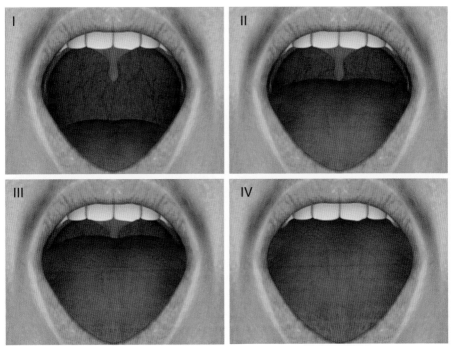

Fig. 29.1 Mallampati classification. Class I: fully visible uvula and soft palate; class II: hard and soft palate, and upper portion of uvula are visible; class III: soft and hard palate and base of uvula are visible; class IV: only hard palate visible. *(From Islam S, Selbong U, et al. Does a patient's Mallampati score predict outcome after maxillomandibular advancement for obstructive sleep apnoea? Br J Oral Maxillofacial Surg. 2015;53(1):23–7. https://www.clinicalkey.com/#!/content/journal/1-s2.0-S0266435614005877? scrollTo=%231-s2.0-S0266435614005877-gr1).*

congestion and decreased nasal airflow. This may result in increased negative intrapharyngeal pressure during inspiration and increased upper airway resistance with nasal breathing.

2. Several studies suggest that there is narrowing of the pharyngeal airway and an increase in the Mallampati grade as pregnancy progresses. The Mallampati scoring system is a visual grading scale that assesses the size of the oropharyngeal airway. It was originally developed to assess the difficulty of orotracheal intubation when undergoing general anesthesia, and the airway is graded from I to IV, depending on the space and visibility between the tongue and the roof of the mouth (see Fig. 29.1).

There is a well-established link between OSA and the size of the oropharyngeal airway in the general population. An increasing Mallampati score as pregnancy progresses may be a contributing factor to the increasing incidence of OSA in this population.

3. Finally, although no definitive studies have been performed on women during pregnancy, there are several studies that show that, in nonpregnant females, fluid displacement away from the legs and into the neck and head reduces upper airway size and increases upper airway collapsibility. Since it is well-known that maternal blood volume increases 40%–45% during pregnancy, lying down to sleep at night may result in increased fluid shifts and fluid volume in the upper airway, leading to increased collapsibility and an increased risk of OSA.

Given the preceding risk factors and this patient's clinical presentation and symptoms, you decide to proceed with further testing to confirm the diagnosis of OSA.

What are the testing options to diagnose sleep apnea?
The options for the diagnosis for OSA are the same for the pregnant and nonpregnant patient; there are no studies evaluating the efficacy of different diagnostic measures during pregnancy. The gold standard diagnostic test for OSA is an overnight, attended, in-laboratory polysomnography, which monitors and records multiple parameters including airflow, respiratory effort, oxygen saturation, limb movements, and electroencephalogram (EEG) activity, including stages of sleep and frequency of arousals. The result of the testing reports the AHI, which is a calculation of the average number of respiratory events in an hour. In adults (>age 18), an AHI of less than 5 is considered normal, AHI 5–15 is mild OSA, AHI 15–30 is moderate OSA, and an AHI of greater than 30 is severe OSA.

Unattended, in-home portable monitoring is another option for diagnostic testing for patients with a high likelihood of moderate or severe OSA, and no comorbid health conditions or concern for other sleep disorders. However, it should be noted that the American Academy of Sleep Medicine (AASM) guidelines on the use of home testing state that portable tests should be used only in patient populations with substantive data in the literature regarding sensitivity and specificity of home tests. There have been no published studies to date evaluating the reliability of portable home testing in pregnant women, and, for that reason, the recommendation for diagnosis is an in-lab study. In addition, many pregnant patients have comorbid sleep disorders, including insomnia and restless leg syndrome, and home testing would not be appropriate in these patients.

> Your patient has an overnight, in-lab polysomnography and is diagnosed with moderate OSA. Her AHI is 17.9 events per hour, with an oxygen desaturation index of 19 events per hour, and an oxygen nadir of 83%.

What are the health risks associated with untreated OSA?
In the general population, there are significant health consequences to untreated OSA, including primary hypertension, increased risk of coronary artery disease, ischemic stroke, cerebrovascular disease, and cardiac arrhythmias. In addition, the secondary consequences of daytime hypersomnolence (decreased cognitive performance, increase in motor vehicle accidents, loss of productivity) are well proven and associated with mild, moderate, and severe OSA. Several studies have also shown an increased risk of all-cause mortality with moderate or severe OSA that is untreated. The cardiac comorbidities are not strongly associated with mild OSA; however, the daytime symptoms of hypersomnolence have been associated with even very mild OSA in some patients.

Are there any additional potential risks of untreated OSA to the mother that should be considered in a patient who is pregnant?
There are several additional potential health risks to both the mother and the fetus associated with OSA during pregnancy; however, the literature is sparse and larger, controlled studies are needed. The majority of literature on the effects of apnea and snoring in pregnancy is difficult to interpret, as many of the studies are based on self-reported symptoms, and there are few studies in which standardized polysomnography was done.

In a retrospective study examining discharge codes from in-hospital stays from 1998 to 2009, OSA was found to be associated with an increased odds of several pregnancy-related morbidity events. After controlling for potential confounders, including obesity, OSA was associated with increased odds of preeclampsia (odds ratio [OR], 2.5; 95% confidence interval [CI], 2.2–2.9), eclampsia (OR, 5.4; 95% CI, 3.3–8.9), cardiomyopathy (OR, 9.0; 95% CI, 7.5–10.9), and pulmonary embolism (OR, 4.5; 95% CI, 2.3–8.9). In fact, women with OSA in this study experienced more than a fivefold increased odds of in-hospital mortality (95% CI, 2.4–11.5). The authors also note the significant increase in diagnosed OSA over the 10-year study period. In 1998, the incidence was 0.7 per 10,000 patients, which climbed to 7.3 per 10,000 in 2008, for an average increase per year of 24%. The authors speculated that this might be due to a combination of increasing rates of obesity among reproductive-aged women and an increased awareness and screening for OSA.

CLINICAL PEARLS	STEPS 2/3
The link between OSA and hypertension is thought to be a physiological response to intermittent nocturnal hypoxia. This causes an activation of the sympathetic response pathway repeatedly throughout the night. The recurrent hypoxia and reoxygenation cycles also result in oxidative stress, endothelial dysfunction, and increased oxidative vascular injury. Because this is a similar mechanism suspected to underlie the development of preeclampsia, this provides a plausible common pathway for the development of early preeclampsia among women with OSA.	

Within the general population, patients with OSA have an increased risk of type 2 diabetes and metabolic syndrome. No causal pathway has been identified, but several studies have demonstrated that glucose control improves in these patients when OSA is treated.

Several small studies have shown an increased risk of gestational diabetes in women with sleep-disordered breathing, but these results need to be extrapolated to patients with caution: the majority of the studies used patient questionnaires to evaluate symptoms and did not obtain polysomnography, so the diagnosis of OSA cannot be confirmed. In some studies, obesity was not controlled for as a confounding factor as well.

Are there any potential risks of untreated OSA to the fetus?

One relatively large population-based observational study observed an increased risk of preterm birth in patients with OSA. They also observed an increased risk of low birth weight, small for gestational age infants, and an increased risk of cesarean delivery. While there are scattered case reports and small observational studies that have found similar results, the majority of these studies did not control for preeclampsia as a potential confounding factor, so the specific effects of OSA on fetal health remain unclear.

You discuss the preceding risks of OSA with your patient, and she is interested in pursuing treatment.

What are the treatment options for OSA? Are there any specific recommendations for treatment during pregnancy?

At the time of this publication, there are no guidelines specifically for the treatment of OSA in pregnancy, but guidelines for treatment are extrapolated from the general population recommendations.

Treatment with a CPAP device is the first-line treatment for moderate to severe OSA and is the first-line treatment for mild OSA when the patient is experiencing symptoms of daytime hypersomnolence or has cardiac risk factors. A CPAP device is a mask that is worn over the nose and/or mouth and delivers positive pressure to the wearer while asleep. The goal of treatment with CPAP is to normalize the AHI and cyclic nocturnal hypoxemia. Starting CPAP would be strongly recommended in pregnant women who are newly diagnosed with moderate or severe OSA. In addition, CPAP should be recommended for patients with mild OSA who have significant daytime symptoms or nocturnal oxygen desaturations below 90%, given the potential risks of recurrent hypoxemia on the fetus. An autotitrating CPAP machine is a good choice throughout pregnancy as this provides a range of pressures to the patient, which will increase pressure as needed as OSA likely worsens throughout pregnancy.

Referral to a trained sleep medicine provider is strongly recommended as these patients will need continued follow-up for management of their treatment and monitoring for compliance. In the general population, 50%–60% of patients are adherent with their CPAP therapy, and there are no studies specifically examining compliance within a pregnant population, but it is likely similar. Nasal congestion and oral dryness are two reasons commonly cited as contributing factors for nonadherence, and, given the increased risk of rhinitis and nasal congestion during pregnancy, this may be an additional challenge.

For patients who are unable to tolerate CPAP, surgical intervention or oral appliances are considered second-line treatments for the treatment of OSA. Oral appliances often require multiple refittings and adjustments with weight gain, and therefore may not be as effective for patients throughout pregnancy. Given the increased risks of general anesthesia and difficulty with effective postoperative pain control during pregnancy, elective surgery to treat OSA is not generally indicated during pregnancy, although patients can be counseled that it may be an option in the future, if OSA persists after pregnancy.

> Your patient is referred to a sleep medicine provider and is given an autotitrating CPAP machine, which she tolerates well. At her next visit with you, she reports that she is sleeping well with it throughout the night and uses it most nights of the week. Her husband reports that she is no longer snoring since starting to use CPAP at night.

Are there specific instructions you would give to this woman regarding her delivery and postpartum recovery with regard to her OSA?

Pregnancies with associated OSA should be considered "high-risk." Among the general population, it is well documented in the literature that compliant treatment with CPAP minimizes the morbidities and secondary health risks associated with untreated OSA. While this is a likely extrapolation to the pregnant population because treatment with CPAP would normalize the nocturnal hypoxemia and likely decrease the risks to mother and fetus, few studies have been done in the literature on the effects of treatment with CPAP.

Patients using CPAP should bring their equipment with them to the hospital when they present for delivery, and patients with OSA should be monitored with continuous pulse oximetry. Any desaturations should be treated with either CPAP while asleep or with supplemental oxygen to maintain saturations of greater than 90%. There is increased risk of complications from general anesthesia in patients with untreated OSA, so early regional anesthesia placement can help to avoid the need for general anesthesia in the event of a necessary emergent cesarean delivery and can also minimize the need for narcotic pain medication.

Opioid medications can suppress respiratory drive, blunt the arousal response during sleep, and worsen nocturnal hypoxemia. There is particular concern with the use of narcotics in patients with untreated OSA as there have been reports of sudden death with the use of narcotics in patients with sleep apnea. For postpartum pain control, these patients should utilize nonsteroidal antiinflammatory medications, and narcotics should be dosed conservatively if needed.

> You see your patient for her 6-week postpartum appointment, and she asks if she will continue to require her CPAP machine now that she is no longer pregnant. You refer her back to her sleep medicine physician for follow-up.

Will OSA that was diagnosed during pregnancy "resolve" after pregnancy is over?

As discussed earlier, any patient who has OSA newly diagnosed during pregnancy should be followed by a sleep medicine provider, and this is particularly important during the postpartum period. Once the patient has had her postpartum weight stabilize, reassessment with repeat poly-somnography should be obtained to assess severity of OSA and continued CPAP needs. In this patient's case, she had risk factors for OSA prior to pregnancy (intermittent snoring, obesity), and may need continued CPAP, although often weight loss can lower CPAP pressure requirements.

BEYOND THE PEARLS

- It is common for healthcare providers and patients to think that poor sleep and excessive daytime fatigue are "normal" symptoms of pregnancy. Resulting in the under-diagnosis of sleep apnea in this population.
- Due to increased weight and swelling of tissues that occurs in pregnancy, many women have new onset of snoring in pregnancy.
- The second trimester usually has less severe disruption of sleep than earlier or later stages, but still not a normal quality sleep.
- The third trimester for most patients is associated with the most significant changes in sleep. The physical changes of pregnancy are the greatest and include general discomfort, increased nocturnal urination, heartburn, back pain and nasal congestion.
- Two main effects of untreated OSA in pregnancy include the increased risks of developing gestational diabetes and preeclampsia
- Physicians may consider screening women with OSA for diabetes early in pregnancy and repeat screening at 24 to 28 weeks in those with an initial negative screen.
- In the postpartum patient with OSA, use of analgesic that minimizes the need for systemic opioids and other drugs that suppress respiratory function and central nervous system.

Case Summary

- A 34-year-old female presents for a routine second-trimester prenatal visit and is feeling severely fatigued. Her husband has also complained that recently she has started snoring loudly every night
- Her prepregnancy BMI was 32kg/m².
- Polysomnography is performed, and she is diagnosed with moderate OSA. Her AHI is 17.9 events per hour
- She is diagnosed with moderate OSA.
- She is prescribed an autotitrating CPAP.
- Patient adherent to CPAP therapy with overall improvement in her daytime symptoms of fatigue and sleepiness.

References

Chen, Y. H., Kang, J. H., Lin, C. C., et al. (2012). Obstructive sleep apnea and the risk of adverse pregnancy outcomes. *American Journal of Obstetrics and Gynecology, 206*, 136. e1.

Izci, B., Vennelle, M., Liston, W. A., et al. (2006). Sleep-disordered breathing and upper airway size in pregnancy and post-partum. *The European Respiratory Journal, 27*, 321.

Louis, J. M., Mogos, M. F., Salemi, J. L., et al. (2014). Obstructive sleep apnea and severe maternal-infant morbidity/mortality in the United States, 1998–2009. *Sleep, 37*, 843.

Mickelson, S. A. (2007). Preoperative and postoperative management of obstructive sleep apnea patients. *Otolaryngologic Clinics of North America, 40*, 877.

Olivarez, S. A., Maheshwari, B., McCarthy, M., et al. (2010). Prospective trial on obstructive sleep apnea in pregnancy and fetal heart rate monitoring. *American Journal of Obstetrics and Gynecology, 202*, 552. e1.

Pien, G. W., Pack, A. I., Jackson, N., et al. (2014). Risk factors for sleep-disordered breathing in pregnancy. *Thorax, 69*, 371.

Pilkington, S., Carli, F., Dakin, M. J., et al. (1995). Increase in Mallampati score during pregnancy. *British Journal of Anaesthesia, 74*, 638.

Kimberly A. DeQuattro, MD, MM ■ R. Michelle Koolaee, DO

A 25-Year-Old Woman in Her Third Trimester of Pregnancy

A 25-year-old G1P0 female at 34 weeks' gestation who just moved to the area presents to your maternal–fetal medicine (MFM) clinic to establish care. She has a history of systemic lupus erythematosus (SLE), with biopsy-proven lupus nephritis (class IV), diagnosed at 23 years of age after she presented with acute renal failure and microscopic hematuria and proteinuria. Her autoantibody profile at diagnosis is shown in Table 30.1.

She was treated with intravenous (IV) cyclophosphamide for 3 months, followed by mycophenolate mofetil (MMF) for 1 year, the MMF was gradually tapered. She had quiescent disease for more than 6 months prior to this pregnancy. She has a previous history of mild inflammatory arthritis and photosensitive rash for 1 year, after which are both well controlled. Medications include hydroxychloroquine, folic acid, and a prenatal vitamin. See Table 30.2 to familiarize yourself with SLE treatments referenced in this case.

How does a prior history of SLE nephritis impact pregnancy?
Her history of SLE nephritis puts her at risk for hypertension that can lead to poor maternal and fetal outcomes if not well controlled. Factors associated with SLE flare during pregnancy include history of lupus nephritis and active lupus within 6 months of conception or cessation of hydroxychloroquine therapy. Active cytopenias (leukopenia, thrombocytopenia), serositis (pleuritis, pericarditis), and nephritis have been associated with maternal hypertension and preeclampsia, preterm (<37 weeks) delivery, and intrauterine growth restriction and fetal loss.

CLINICAL PEARL　　　　　　　　　　　　　　　　　　　　　　　　　**STEPS 2/3**

The mnemonic, "PATH to Poor Outcomes"—Proteinuria, Antiphospholipid syndrome, Thrombocytopenia, Hypertension—can help to identify SLE patients who might have difficulties in pregnancy. These signs in the first third of gestation confer a one-third risk of fetal loss in SLE patients with active disease.

From Clowse M, Siaton B. Pregnancy and rheumatic diseases. In Imboden J, Hellmann D, Stone D, editors.
  Current diagnosis and treatment in rheumatology, *3rd ed. McGraw Hill; 2013:ch 69, 533–9.*

CLINICAL PEARL　　　　　　　　　　　　　　　　　　　　　　　　　**STEPS 2/3**

The most common obstetric complication of SLE is preeclampsia/eclampsia, while common fetal complications include intrauterine growth restriction, premature delivery, premature rupture of membranes, and preterm premature rupture of membranes.

TABLE 30.1 ■ Antibody Profile History at Diagnosis

Antibody	Result
ANA	Positive at a 1:320 dilution
Anti-dsDNA	Positive at a 1:320 dilution
Anti-Sm	Positive
Anti-Ro/SSA	Positive
Anti-La/SSB	Negative
APLa	
ACL	Negative
LAC	Absent
Anti-B2GP1	Negative

ACL, Anticardiolipin; ANA, antinuclear antibody; APLa, antiphospholipid antibody; B2GP, β-2-glycoprotein-1 antibody; dsDNA, double-stranded deoxyribonucleic acid; LAC, lupus anticoagulant; Sm, smith; SSA, Sjögren's-syndrome–related antigen A; SSB, Sjögren's-syndrome–related antigen B.

TABLE 30.2 ■ Lupus Treatments Relevant to This Case

Treatment	Class/Type	Mechanism	Side Effects	Terato-genic
Glucocorticoids	Corticosteroid	Upregulates antiin-flammatory cytokines and decreases inflammatory gene transcription	Hypertension, dyslipid-emia, osteoporosis, avas-cular necrosis, adrenal insufficiency, hyperglyce-mia, obesity	In high doses, Yes
Hydroxychloro-quine	DMARD/Antimalarial	Posited to inhibit TLR activation which miti-gates inflammation	Retinopathy, myopathy, skin hyperpigmentation	No
Mycophenolate mofetil	Antimetabolite	Inhibits B- and T-lymphocyte prolif-eration and antibody production	GI (nausea, diarrhea), my-elosuppression, infection	Yes
Cyclophospha-mide	Alkylating agent	Cross-links DNA, prevents DNA replica-tion, and hastens apoptosis	Myelosuppression, acute myeloid leukemia, pulmo-nary fibrosis, hemorrhagic cystitis, transitional cell carcinoma, premature gonadal failure, infection	Yes
Rituximab	Biologic/Monoclonal antibody	Inhibits CD20 B-lymphocyte produc-tion and function	Infection	No

DMARD, Disease-modifying antirheumatic drugs; DNA, deoxyribonucleic acid; GI, gastrointestinal; TLR, Toll-like receptor.

What does the specific history of class IV nephritis mean for her pregnancy?

Table 30.3 delineates the classification of SLE nephritis. Patients like ours with proliferative class III or IV disease are at higher risk for hypertension during pregnancy. Hypertension increases the likelihood of preeclampsia and eclampsia, which in turn are associated with fetal loss and preterm delivery.

TABLE 30.3 ■ International Society of Nephrology/Renal Pathology Society Classification of Lupus Nephritis

Class I	Minimal mesangial
Class II	Mesangial proliferative
Class III	Focal (<50% glomeruli)
Class IV	Diffuse (>50% glomeruli)
Class V	Membranous (may be classified concomitantly with class III or IV)
Class VI	Advanced sclerosing (>90% globally sclerosed glomeruli without residual activity)

CLINICAL PEARL　　　　　　　　　　　　　　　　　　　　　　　　　　　　**STEPS 2/3**

Lupus nephritis is categorized histologically by class on renal biopsy and is useful for predicting clinical course and effective therapies. Class I or class II disease can be treated with angiotensin converting enzyme inhibitors or angiotensin receptor blockers alone. Classes III–V exhibit immune complex deposition and are most responsive to high-dose glucocorticoids and cytotoxic therapies. Class VI disease represents irreversible scarring that should not be treated with additional aggressive immunosuppressive regimens.

When is it safe for patients with SLE to become pregnant?

There is a direct correlation between the severity of maternal disease and pregnancy risk for the fetus and the mother; the general recommendation is for at least 6 months of quiescent, well-controlled disease prior to conception.

When should referral to a maternal–fetal medicine (MFM) specialist be considered?

The scenarios in Table 30.4 should prompt consideration for referral to MFM for preconception or prenatal counseling for potential life-threatening outcomes for both the mother and the fetus. Discussions of surrogacy, adoption, and/or multidisciplinary teams may be warranted. Table 30.5 lists contraindications to pregnancy in SLE patients.

Given this patient's past history of lupus nephritis and positive anti–Sjögren's-syndrome-related antigen-A (anti-Ro/SSA) antibodies, a referral to MFM would be appropriate.

How do you interpret her autoantibody profile as it relates to her pregnancy?

Anti-Ro/SSA antibodies alone can be present in many autoimmune disorders such as SLE, Sjögren's syndrome, dermatomyositis, polymyositis, and systemic sclerosis. In SLE, anti-Ro/SSA antibodies are associated with photosensitivity, subacute cutaneous lupus, and interstitial lung disease. Women with anti-Ro/SSA and/or anti-La/SSB antibodies have an increased fetal risk for both neonatal lupus as well as congenital heart block. Therefore, they need to undergo frequent surveillance for heart block during the second trimester of pregnancy. Early detection of heart block allows for more closer monitoring, despite lack of a treatment modality.

CLINICAL PEARL　　　　　　　　　　　　　　　　　　　　　　　　　　　　**STEPS 2/3**

Autoantibody testing alone in rheumatology is rarely diagnostic for disease. These positive laboratory tests need to be interpreted in the context of clinical history, physical examination, other laboratory testing, and any relevant imaging studies in order to determine relevance.

TABLE 30.4 ■ **Considerations for Maternal–Fetal Medicine Referral**

Clinical and/or Biochemical Status	Examples
Active or recent organ involvement	
Central nervous system	Stroke, posterior reversible encephalopathy syndrome, psychiatric
Cardiac	Coronary artery disease, myocarditis, valvular disease
Pulmonary	Pulmonary hypertension, severe interstitial lung disease
Renal	Nephritis, renal insufficiency
Cytopenia	Thrombocytopenia
Antibody profile positivity	Anti-Ro/SSA, Anti-La/SSB
	APLa (LAC, ACL, B2GP1)

SSA, Sjögren's-syndrome–related antigen A; *SSB*, Sjögren's-syndrome–related antigen B; *APLa*, antiphospholipid antibody; *ACL*, anticardiolipin; *LAC*, lupus anticoagulant; *B2GP1*, β-2-glycoprotein-1 antibody.

TABLE 30.5 ■ **Contraindications to Pregnancy in Patients With Systemic Lupus Erythematosus (SLE)**

Contraindication to Pregnancy	Recommend Deferral of Pregnancy
Severe pulmonary hypertension	Severe disease flare within the past 6 months
Severe restrictive lung disease	Stroke within the last 6 months
Advanced renal insufficiency	Active lupus nephritis
Advanced heart failure	
Prior severe preeclampsia or HELLP despite treatment	

HELLP, Hemolysis, elevated liver enzymes, low platelets.

From Lateef A, Petri M. Managing lupus patients during pregnancy. *Best Pract Res Clin Rheumatol.* 2013 June; 27(3).

In SLE, anti-Ro/SSA antibodies are associated with photosensitivity, cutaneous lupus, and interstitial lung disease. Either anti-Ro/SSA or anti-La/SSB positivity confers increased fetal risk for neonatal lupus.

What is neonatal lupus?

"Neonatal lupus" is a misnomer because the neonate does not necessarily have a full diagnosis SLE. However, anti-Ro/SSA and anti-La/SSB antibody positivity is sensitive for transient cutaneous (annular lesions (Fig. 30.1, *Panel A*), malar rash (Fig. 30.1, *Panel B*), or life-threatening irreversible cardiac disease (heart block leading to cardiomegaly (Fig. 30.2) among infants born to mothers carrying these antibodies. Neonatal lupus occurs in 1%–2% of women with autoimmune diseases like SLE and Sjögren's and can occur in asymptomatic women who unknowingly have anti-Ro/SSA or anti-La/SSB antibody positivity.

CLINICAL PEARL   **STEP 1**

Quick review of heart block:
First-degree AV (atrioventricular) block: PR interval prolongation
Second-degree AV block:
   Type 1 second-degree AV block (Mobitz I aka Wenckebach): PR prolongation then dropped beat
   Type 2 second-degree AV block (Mobitz II): No prolongation prior to dropped beat, usually due to a block in or below the bundle of His
Third-degree AV block (complete heart block): AV dissociation; consider permanent pacemaker

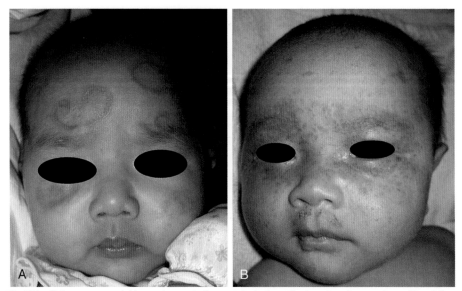

Fig. 30.1 Cutaneous neonatal lupus demonstrating annular lesions of subacute cutaneous lupus (*Panel A*) as well as malar rash sparing nasolabial folds (*Panel B*). *(From Chantorn R, Lim HW, Shwayder TA. Photosensitivity disorders in children: part II.* J Am Acad Dermatol. *2012 Dec;67(6):1113.e1–15; quiz 1128, 1127.)*

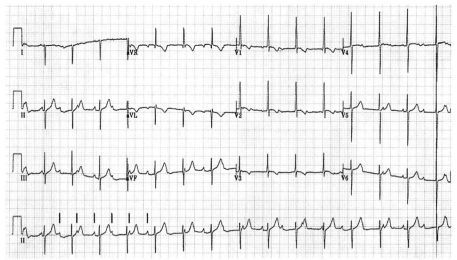

Fig. 30.2 Example of neonatal heart block on electrocardiogram. *(From Skinner JR, et al. Detection and management of life threatening arrhythmias in the perinatal period.* Early Hum Dev. *2008;84(3):161–72.)*

What causes congenital heart block to occur?

During weeks 18–30 of gestation, maternal anti-Ro/SSA and anti-La/SSB antibodies cross the placenta and affect fetal cardiac growth via irreversible remodeling of the sinoatrial and atrioventricular nodes. The pathophysiology is thought to be driven by antibody binding to fetal cardiomyocytes and failure of apoptosis (Fig. 30.3). Together, these processes lead to cytokine release, triggering inflammation in and damage to the myocardium and resulting in heart block.

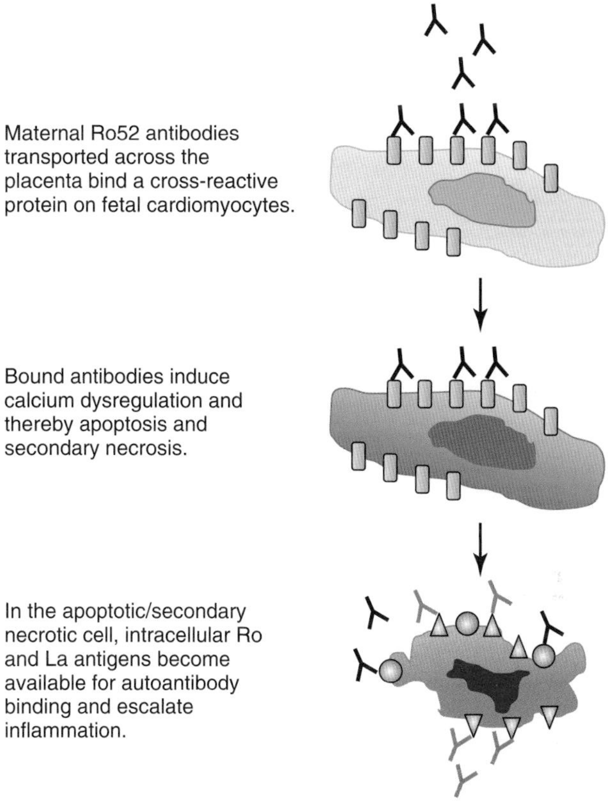

Maternal Ro52 antibodies transported across the placenta bind a cross-reactive protein on fetal cardiomyocytes.

Bound antibodies induce calcium dysregulation and thereby apoptosis and secondary necrosis.

In the apoptotic/secondary necrotic cell, intracellular Ro and La antigens become available for autoantibody binding and escalate inflammation.

Fig. 30.3 Purported pathogenesis of anti-Ro/SSA and anti-La/SSB antibodies and neonatal lupus. *(From Wahren-Herlenius M, Sonesson SE, Clowse MEG. Chapter 37 - Neonatal lupus erythematosus. In D J Wallace, BH Hanh, editors. Dubois' lupus erythematosus and related syndromes. 8th ed. Philadelphia: WB Saunders; 2013:464–72.)*

CLINICAL PEARL   **STEPS 2/3**

Neonatal lupus accounts for 80%–95% of congenital complete heart block in the antepartum or neonatal periods and is most often diagnosed within the first 3 months of life.

What is the risk of her child developing cardiac neonatal lupus?

Table 30.6 indicates risks for developing neonatal lupus. In this case, since the patient is only anti-Ro/SSA antibody positive and has not previously had a child with cutaneous neonatal lupus or congenital heart block, the risk of her child developing cardiac neonatal lupus is 2%.

How does her historical treatment course impact her current pregnancy?

At her diagnosis of class IV lupus nephritis, cyclophosphamide was appropriately given. Like some cancer regimens, immunosuppressive therapy in SLE for class III or IV nephritis occurs in two phases: induction and maintenance. Induction is an aggressive, high-dose regimen of glucocorticoids and cyclophosphamide or MMF. Once there is a renal response, maintenance follows with lower dose MMF to prevent disease progression.

TABLE 30.6 ■ Risks for Development of Neonatal Lupus (NL)

History	Risk of cardiac-NL in offspring
Women who are anti-Ro/SSA antibody positive	2%
Women who are anti-La/SSB antibody positive	
Women who have previously given birth to a child with cutaneous	15%
NL with or without cardiac NL	

SSA, Sjögren's-syndrome–related antigen A; SSB, Sjögren's-syndrome–related antigen B; NL, neonatal lupus

---

CLINICAL PEARL   **STEPS 2/3**

A complete response to renal immunosuppression is defined by improvement in clinical manifestations and resolution of biochemical measures such as serum creatinine, proteinuria, hematuria, pyuria, and cellular casts or dysmorphic red blood cells.

What are the side effects of cyclophosphamide, and how could they impact this woman of childbearing age?

Cyclophosphamide has numerous risks (see Table 30.2), both immediate and chronic. Of note, treatment with cyclophosphamide before 25 years confers a lower risk of infertility than after 30 years. The total cumulative dose of cyclophosphamide increases ovarian toxicity risk.

Are her current medications safe?

Yes. Cyclophosphamide was stopped over a year ago, and MMF was stopped more than 6 weeks prior to conception (according to American College of Rheumatology guidelines on SLE nephritis; refer to Case 31 for more information regarding immunosuppressive medications in pregnancy). Hydroxychloroquine is safe during pregnancy and breastfeeding.

CLINICAL PEARL   **STEPS 2/3**

Hydroxychloroquine decreases the risk for developing SLE flares and neonatal lupus when continued during pregnancy.

As you are gathering history, prior records demonstrate no fetal bradycardia and no heart block on second-trimester evaluation. Your patient has been adherent to her medication regimen of hydroxychloroquine and asks whether her recent increased leg swelling is an expected finding of her pregnancy or something more concerning. On physical examination, her temperature is 36.4°C (97.6°F), blood pressure is 150/92 mm Hg (baseline 128/82 mm Hg), heart rate is 72 beats/min, and respirations are 20 breaths/min. S1/S2 heart sounds are auscultated without a prominent S2 heart sound. A third-trimester gravid uterus is palpated with good fetal Doppler tones. 2+ symmetric pretibial edema is present.

In a patient with a history of lupus nephritis, what specific physical exam findings should you look for?

Assess vital signs in the context of the case and keep in mind that there are expected physiologic changes due to pregnancy, such as fixed split systolic flow murmurs, prominent pulses, or increased jugular venous pressure. Think about your patient's history and what you expect to find. There is a past history of SLE nephritis, arthritis, and photosensitive rash, but she was treated and had quiescent disease with a normal blood pressure for more than 12 months prior to this evaluation. Her elevated blood pressure from baseline raises the suspicion for a flare of her nephritis or preeclampsia.

CLINICAL PEARL   **STEPS 2/3**

Indicators of SLE flare on physical exam include pallor or petechiae (suggestive of cytopenias), malar or photosensitive skin rash (see Fig. 30.4), oral lesions (mucocutaneous involvement), pericardial or pleural friction rub with dyspnea (serositis), a loud S2 (suggestive of pulmonary hypertension), crackles on lung exam with abdominal distention and lower extremity pitting edema (overload from active renal disease), and/or arthritis with synovitis.

Routine laboratory testing is performed; results are shown in Table 30.7.

TABLE 30.7 ■ **Routine Laboratory Testing**

Hematocrit	28%
Leukocyte count	8800/uL (8.8 ×10⁹/L)
Platelet count	100,000/uL (130 × 10⁹/L)
Mean corpuscular volume	77 fL
Blood urea nitrogen	20 mg/dL (mmol/L)
Serum creatinine	1.9 mg/dL (baseline 0.9 mg/dL)
AST	30 units/L
ALT	28 units/L

ALT, Alanine transaminase; *AST*, aspartate transaminase.

What is your differential diagnosis based on the laboratory testing?

Our patient has new elevated blood pressure in her third trimester, pretibial edema, and laboratory findings demonstrating microcytic anemia, thrombocytopenia, and an elevated creatinine more than doubled from baseline. Taken together, this clinical picture is most concerning for lupus flare versus preeclampsia/eclampsia. There is also consideration for diseases associated with microangiopathic hemolytic anemia (MAHA) such as HELLP syndrome (hemolysis, elevated liver enzymes, low platelet count), and thrombotic microangiopathies, thrombotic thrombocytopenia (TTP), and hemolytic uremic syndrome (HUS). Since HELLP, TTP, and HUS are associated with MAHA, a lack of evidence of hemolysis would be reassuring and decrease the likelihood of these processes. More information will help narrow the diagnosis. She will need inpatient admission for further monitoring, workup, and management.

On inpatient admission, the primary team asks whether additional labs are warranted. What labs should be recommended and why?

You recommend peripheral smear, lactate dehydrogenase, total and direct bilirubin, haptoglobin, uric acid, urinalysis with microscopy, urine protein to creatinine ratio, anti–double-stranded deoxyribonucleic acid (anti-dsDNA) antibodies, and C3/C4 complement levels.

- A peripheral smear with schistocytes as well as elevated lactate dehydrogenase, elevated indirect bilirubin, and low haptoglobin together are evidence of hemolysis.
- Uric acid and aspartate aminotransferase/alanine aminotransferase (AST/ALT) are elevated in preeclampsia more so than in a SLE flare.
- Active urinary sediment (presence of erythrocytes or leukocytes in urine microscopy) is typically more consistent with SLE nephritis flare than preeclampsia, which has bland sediment.
- Elevated dsDNA can indicate significant disease in some SLE patients, although this is not always reliable.
- Low serum complement level compared to baseline suggests increased immune-complex deposition in the tissues and disease activity flare.

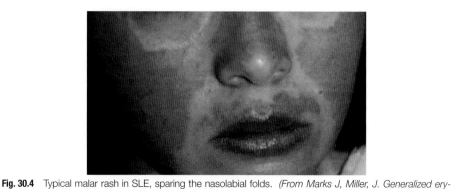

Fig. 30.4   Typical malar rash in SLE, sparing the nasolabial folds. *(From Marks J, Miller, J. Generalized erythema. In Lookingbill and Marks' principles of dermatology. Amsterdam: Elsevier; 2013:14, 183–95.)*

CLINICAL PEARL   **STEPS 2/3**

Because estrogens increase hepatic synthesis of complement, in pregnancy, complement may be normal or elevated. Closely monitor the trend and not the absolute value; falsely normal complement may still represent SLE flare.

CLINICAL PEARL   **STEPS 2/3**

Do not repeatedly order an ANA test. Only order anti-Ro/SSA and anti-La/SSB if the results have never been checked or are unknown because of associations with neonatal lupus. Once SLE is diagnosed, repeating these tests is not advised and will not change management. Furthermore, absolute changes in ANA titers are not relevant clinically and do not predict disease activity or outcome.

What other antibodies would be useful to evaluate this patient?
Obtain antiphospholipid antibodies (lupus anticoagulant (LAC), anticardiolipin (ACL), and β2-glycoprotein-1) if they have not been checked prior. During pregnancy, the antiphospholipid syndrome (APLS), which requires antibody positivity and history of thrombus and/or miscarriages, confers increased risks for uteroplacental insufficiency (preeclampsia, HELLP, intrauterine growth restriction) and thrombosis. Some women with APLS may need aspirin and/or heparin prophylaxis antepartum, and some will require postpartum anticoagulation as well.

Additional labs results are in. She has developed a faint rash on her cheeks, sparing her nasolabial folds (Fig. 30.4). Her wrists are painful, and there is synovitis on exam.

How do you interpret this new information and additional labs from Table 30.8 and Figs. 30.5 and 30.6?
Her clinical and biochemical picture is consistent with active SLE and demonstrates a severe exacerbation. She exhibits her typical clinical manifestations of malar rash and inflammatory arthritis. For this patient whose dsDNA is 1:1280, her serologies appear to parallel her disease activity. In addition to cytopenias, our suspicion for renal involvement is supported. Her

TABLE 30.8 ■ **Additional Laboratory Information**

Peripheral smear	Microcytic anemia, schistocytes absent
Lactate dehydrogenase, total and direct bilirubin, haptoglobin	Normal
Urinalysis	2+ protein, 2+ blood with 10–15 dysmorphic erythrocytes/hpf; 5–10 leukocytes/hpf
Spot urine protein to creatinine ratio	2
Uric acid	Normal
dsDNA	1:1280 (baseline 1:320)
C3	Low from baseline
C4	Low from baseline

C3, Complement 3; *C4*, complement 4; *dsDNA*, double-stranded deoxyribonucleic acid.

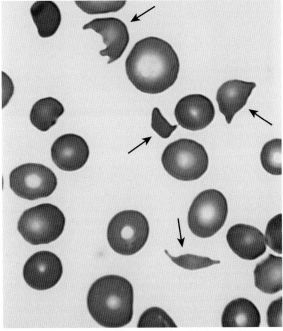

Fig. 30.5 Our patient lacks schistocytes typical in microangiopathic hemolytic anemia. Arrows depict fragmented red blood cells, known as "helmet cells." *(From Kumar V, Fausto N, Abbas A. Robbins and Cotran's pathologic basis of disease. 7th ed. Philadelphia: WB Saunders; 2004, fig. 13-17.)*

creatinine is twice her baseline, with substantial proteinuria and an active sediment with dysmorphic erythrocytes and low complement from baseline. Taken together, our patient has a severe flare of lupus nephritis. For the remaining findings, normal transaminases without abdominal pain make HELLP less likely. A normal smear and hemolysis labs further eliminate HELLP, HUS, and TTP. Low uric acid is less concerning for preeclampsia. Table 30.9 reviews the differential diagnosis for a patient with new hypertension and proteinuria in the third trimester. Table 30.10 distinguishes causes of new hypertension in the third trimester by clinical features and laboratory findings.

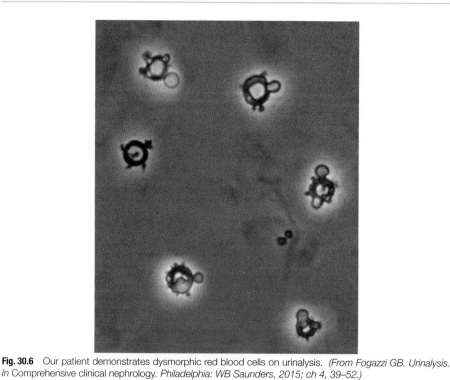

Fig. 30.6 Our patient demonstrates dysmorphic red blood cells on urinalysis. *(From Fogazzi GB. Urinalysis. In* Comprehensive clinical nephrology. *Philadelphia: WB Saunders, 2015; ch 4, 39–52.)*

CLINICAL PEARL   **STEPS 2/3**

Serum complements (C3/C4) and anti-dsDNA antibodies are not perfect markers of disease activity in SLE. It is helpful to trend them to see if there is reliability in each lupus patient. Some patients can have low serum complements and high anti-dsDNA antibodies and do not have other features of active disease; use your clinical judgment in the context of each individual case.

Fetal heart tones are reassuring. Lower extremity Doppler ultrasonography are negative for deep vein thrombosis. Renal biopsy is not pursued at this time.

When would a repeat renal biopsy be indicated?

It is safe to perform renal biopsies during pregnancy, particularly for definitive diagnosis and if results will change management. The decision to rebiopsy is made on an individual basis. In general, if there is reason to suspect a different class of lupus nephritis (based on urinalysis findings), or if there is uncertainty regarding the degree of active renal disease (versus irreversible damage as noted by sclerotic features on biopsy), a biopsy is helpful. If the biopsy reveals irreversible damage, there would be less of a role for aggressive immunosuppression. In this case, her biopsy was only performed 2 years ago, and her clinical presentation of acute renal failure, proteinuria, and hematuria mimic her initial lupus nephritis manifestation (class III and IV disease are treated similarly, and both classes present with hematuria/proteinuria). Therefore, a biopsy would not likely change management.

TABLE 30.9 ■ Differential Diagnosis for New Hypertension and Proteinuria in Third Trimester

HELLP	Typically occurs in the third trimester; often co-occurs in 10%–20% of those with preeclampsia/eclampsia. Features include abdominal pain, emesis, malaise, hypertension, and proteinuria. Platelets are <100,000 cells/mL, total bilirubin is >1.2 mg/kL, and serum aspartate aminotransferase is greater than twice the upper limit of normal.
Hemolytic uremic syndrome	Characterized by thrombocytopenia, MAHA, and marked renal injury. Commonly associated with Shiga toxin–producing *Escherichia coli*.
Thrombotic thrombocytopenia	Known for the pentad of fever, thrombocytopenia, MAHA, and central nervous system and renal involvement. Pathogenesis is from acquired or inherited deficiency of ADAMTS13, which normally degrades large von Willebrand multimers. Persistence of large multimers increases platelet aggregation and thrombus formation.
Preeclampsia	New onset hypertension (SBP >140 mm Hg, DBP >90 mm Hg) and proteinuria or kidney injury at >20 weeks' gestation. In absence of proteinuria, can be diagnosed as severe in presence of CNS symptoms (AMS, severe headache, visual disturbance), platelet count <100,000/uL, pulmonary edema, 2× normal transaminases, serum creatinine >1.1 mg/dL, or 2× creatinine in absence of other renal disease. Patients with SLE have 3–5 times the risk for preeclampsia, which can occur in 15%–30% of SLE pregnancies.
Eclampsia	New generalized tonic-clonic seizures or coma in a woman with preeclampsia without other CNS conditions. Uric acid may be elevated.

ADAMTS13, A disintegrin and metalloproteinase with a thrombospondin type 1 motif, member 13; *AMS*, altered mental status; *CNS*, central nervous system; *SBP*, systolic blood pressure; *DBP*, diastolic blood pressure; *MAHA*, microangiopathic hemolytic anemia; *HELLP*, hemolysis, elevated liver enzymes, low platelets.

TABLE 30.10 ■ Distinguishing Causes of New Hypertension in Third Trimester

Frequency of Clinical and Laboratory Features Among Imitators of Preeclampsia/Eclampsia

	HELLP	TTP	HUS	Preeclampsia	SLE exacerbation
Clinical Features					
Hypertension	85%	20%–75%	80%–90%	100%	80% w APLa/nephritis
Proteinuria	90%–95%	With hematuria	80%–90%	Present	100% with nephritis
Fever	Absent	20%–50%	?	Absent	Common during flare
Jaundice	5%–10%	Rare	Rare	Rare	Absent
Central nervous system	40%–60%	60–70%	?	Eclampsia if present	50% with APLa
Laboratory findings					
Hemolysis	50%–100%	100%	100%	—	14%–23% with APLa
Thrombocytopenia	>20,000	<20,000	>20,000	>100,000	>20,000
Elevated transaminases	100%	Usually mild	Usually mild	2× normal levels	With APLa
Renal dysfunction	50%	30%	100%	Present	40%–80%

[a]Common, reported as the most common presentation.

APLa, Antiphospholipid antibodies; *HELLP*, hemolytic anemia, elevated liver enzymes, low platelets; *HUS*, hemolytic uremic syndrome; *TTP*, thrombotic thrombocytopenic purpura; *SLE*, systemic lupus erythematosus.

Adapted from Sibai BM. Imitators of severe pre-eclampsia. *Semin Perinatol*. 2009;33(3):196–205.

Your diagnosis is lupus nephritis flare in a pregnant patient in her third trimester. She is given 3 days of intravenous (IV) pulse dose glucocorticoids (Solu-Medrol 1 g IV daily), followed by reduction to high-dose glucocorticoids (prednisone 60 mg daily) because both MMF and cyclophosphamide are teratogenic agents. She is induced, and the fetus is late preterm, delivered at 35 weeks.

What are some other management considerations in patients with lupus nephritis in pregnancy?

Please see Case 31 for more details on medications safe to use in pregnant SLE patients with active disease, as well as details on the use of glucocorticoids in third-trimester pregnancy.

If this clinical scenario of severe SLE nephritis had occurred in the first or second trimesters and necessitated high-dose pulse glucocorticoids or cyclophosphamide, it would likely have prompted a discussion regarding pregnancy termination in order to save the patient. These circumstances are ethically challenging, and risks and benefits to mother and fetus must be addressed on a case-by-case basis.

On follow-up, the patient's rash, arthritis, blood pressure, hematuria, and proteinuria improve. She continues hydroxychloroquine. Although she does desire to breastfeed, she understands that her active lupus nephritis can be life-threatening, so she defers breastfeeding in order to be able to restart MMF to treat her SLE nephritis. To prevent pregnancy while on a teratogenic medication, she elects placement of a long-acting reversible subdermal implant for safe contraception given her complex history.

BEYOND THE PEARLS

- Congenital heart block develops in the second trimester of gestation and can be fatal. There are no formal guidelines for the type or frequency of testing for fetal heart block, but weekly pulsed Doppler fetal echocardiography from weeks 18–26 of pregnancy and every other week until 32 weeks should be strongly considered.
- There may be some role for glucocorticoids in first- or second-degree fetal heart block; however, complete heart block is irreversible even with glucocorticoid therapy.
- Having SLE confers increased risk for lymphoma, lung, and cervical malignancy. There are no consensus guidelines for Pap tests in immunocompromised patients due to autoimmune disease. Regular human papilloma virus (HPV) testing is important to evaluate for cervical neoplasia.
- Treatment with cyclophosphamide (in patients with severe lupus) before 25 years of age confers a lower risk of infertility than after 30 years of age. The total cumulative dose of cyclophosphamide increases ovarian toxicity risk. Giving Lupron (leuprolide) as a means of preserving ovarian function is not necessary with certain protocols, but fertility should be addressed prior to initiating cyclophosphamide therapy in any woman of childbearing age.
- Nephrotic syndrome, pregnancy, and SLE are independently associated with prothrombotic states. In a pregnant SLE patient with nephritis, be wary of new venous thromboembolism. Ensure that antiphospholipid antibodies are checked with new pregnancies in SLE patients. If antiphospholipid antibodies are positive, low-dose aspirin throughout the pregnancy can be considered.

Case Summary

- A 25-year-old G1P0 woman in her third trimester with a history of quiescent SLE nephritis develops new hypertension and leg swelling.
- Exam reveals malar rash, inflammatory arthritis, and pitting edema.
- Testing demonstrates elevated anti-dsDNA antibodies from baseline, bone marrow suppression, and hypocomplementemia. Hemolysis labs are negative. She develops acute renal failure, microscopic hematuria, dysmorphic erythrocytes on urinalysis, and proteinuria.

- A diagnosis is made of lupus nephritis flare in a pregnant patient in her third trimester.
- Hydroxychloroquine is continued. High-dose glucocorticoids are administered, the fetus is delivered, and postpartum MMF is initiated, with improvement of disease.

References

Dall'era, M. (2013). Systemic lupus erythematosus. In J. Imboden, D. Hellmann, & D. Stone (Eds.), *Current diagnosis and treatment in rheumatology* (3rd ed.) (pp. 187–197). McGraw Hill. ch. 21.

D'Cruz, D., Khamashta, M., & Hughes, G. (2007 Feb 17). Systemic lupus erythematosus. *Lancet, 369*(9561), 587–596.

Doria, A., Tincani, A., & Lockshin, M. (2008). Challenges of lupus pregnancies. *Rheumatology (Oxford), 47*(Suppl. 3), iii9–12.

Ben-Chetrit, E. (1993). Lucky lady. *The New England Journal of Medicine, 328*, 636–639.

Gladman, D. D., Tandon, A., Ibañez, D., & Urowitz, M. B. (2010). The effect of lupus nephritis on pregnancy outcome and fetal and maternal complications. *The Journal of Rheumatology, 37*(4), 754–758.

Hahn, B., McMahon, M., Wilkinson, A., et al. (2012). American College of Rheumatology. American College of Rheumatology guidelines for screening, treatment, and management of lupus nephritis. *Arthritis Care and Resuscitation (Hoboken), 64*(6), 797–808.

Lateef, A., & Petri, M. (2013). Managing lupus patients during pregnancy. *Best Practice & Research. Clinical Rheumatology* (3), 27.

Sibai, B. M. (2009). Imitators of severe pre-eclampsia. *Seminars in Perinatology, 33*(3), 196–205.

Tedeschi, S. K., Guan, H., Fine, A., Costenbader, K. H., & Bermas, B. (2016 Jul). Organ-specific systemic lupus erythematosus activity during pregnancy is associated with adverse pregnancy outcomes. *Clinical Rheumatology, 35*(7), 1725–1732.

Beatrice Kenol, MD ■ R. Michelle Koolaee, DO

A 29-Year-Old Woman With Systemic Lupus Erythematosus Planning Pregnancy

A 29-year-old nulligravid (G0P0) woman is evaluated in the office for preconception planning. She has a history of systemic lupus erythematosus (SLE) diagnosed 5 years ago, with manifestations of polyarthritis, malar rash, and biopsy-proven class V nephritis. At diagnosis she had positive antinuclear (ANA), anti–double-stranded DNA (anti-dsDNA) and anti-smith (anti-Sm) antibodies. Table 31.1A shows laboratory data at diagnosis. She is recently married and expresses to you that she would like to become pregnant as soon as possible but is concerned due to her underlying lupus.

What questions should you ask any patient with SLE who is interested in becoming pregnant?

The most important consideration is evaluation of the patient's current disease severity; disease should be well-controlled prior to the onset of pregnancy. The probability of flare during pregnancy depends on the severity and activity of disease; if conception occurs after remission of SLE, the risk of flare falls below 10%. It is recommended that maternal disease should be controlled for at least 6 months prior to planning a pregnancy, especially in patients with known renal disease.

In addition, the patient's medications should be reviewed because some of the medications used in the treatment of SLE may affect maternal and/or fetal health, infant development and survival, and/or length of gestation and labor.

TABLE 31.1A ■ Initial Laboratory Testing

Leukocyte count	8000/μL (8.0 × 10⁹/L)
Hemoglobin	11.8 g/dL (118 g/L)
Platelet count	200,000/μL (200 × 10⁹/L)
Leukocyte differential	Normal
Erythrocyte sedimentation rate	86 mm/h
Serum creatinine	0.6 mg/dL
Urinalysis	3+ protein; 0–2 erythrocytes/hpf
Chest radiograph	No acute cardiopulmonary disease
Anti–double-stranded DNA antibody	Negative
Anti-smith antibody	Positive
Anti-SS-A/Anti-SS-B antibodies	Negative
Complement C3	Normal
Complement C4	Normal
Rheumatoid factor	Negative

It is also important to inquire about obstetric history, particularly any history of miscarriages or complicated pregnancy. Usual family planning factors, such as emotional motivation, available support system, and socioeconomic situation, should also be evaluated.

How does SLE affect fertility and pregnancy?

There is no evidence that SLE affects fertility. The patient and her partner should be informed that the chances of becoming pregnant are the same as if the patient did not have SLE. However, there is an increased rate of high-risk pregnancy in patients with SLE. For example, hypertension and preeclampsia are more common in patients with lupus nephritis or with positive antiphospholipid antibodies. In addition, if the disease activity is uncontrolled at the time of pregnancy, there are increased risks of maternal lupus flare (active renal or central nervous system disease in pregnancy can be potentially life threatening), fetal loss, or prematurity and intrauterine growth restriction (IUGR).

Prematurity has been reported as high as 80% in patients with active SLE and IUGR in 30% of these cases.

CLINICAL PEARL   **STEPS 2/3**

Patients with SLE are considered as fertile as women in the general population, unless they have received medications that are known to decrease fertility (i.e., cyclophosphamide).

At diagnosis 5 years ago, she was treated with intravenous (IV) methylprednisolone and mycophenolate mofetil (MMF) induction treatment with improvement of disease activity. Since then, she has been on maintenance therapy with mycophenolate mofetil 1000 mg orally twice daily and hydroxychloroquine 200 mg orally twice daily. She reports mild intermittent hand and wrist pain, which is improved with ibuprofen. She has no chest pain, dyspnea, or rashes for the past 3 years. She has no history of thrombosis or miscarriage.

On physical examination, her temperature is 37.2°C (99°F), blood pressure is 115/80 mm Hg, heart rate is 90 beats/min, and respiration rate is 20 breaths/min. Cardiac exam reveals no murmurs, and pulmonary exam is without any wheezing, rales, or rhonchi. There is moderate tenderness and swelling of the wrists and metacarpophalangeal and proximal interphalangeal joints bilaterally, as well as small bilateral knee effusions.

Laboratory results from this visit are provided in Table 31.1B.

Does this patient have active lupus? If so, how can you tell?

Detailed information obtained through history, physical examination, and laboratory testing helps to determine whether or not lupus is active. Some clinical features of active disease may include fatigue, fevers, oral ulcers, photosensitive rashes (particularly the classic malar rash of SLE), alopecia, new hypertension (which can sometimes indicate a flare of lupus nephritis), and arthritis. During a flare manifesting with arthritis, the joint examination may reveal synovitis, which is characterized classically by boggy, tender, and swollen joints.

Laboratory testing suggestive of lupus flare may include:
- *Elevated sedimentation rate or C-reactive protein*: These are nonspecific markers of inflammation in the blood, but in some patients may correlate with disease flare
- *Elevated anti-dsDNA antibody levels and hypocomplementemia*: In select patients, these strongly correlate with disease flare.

In this patient, the presence of synovitis on exam, along with elevated sedimentation rate, elevated anti-dsDNA antibodies, and hypocomplementemia are suggestive of an arthritic flare of

TABLE 31.1B ■ Follow-Up Laboratory Testing

Antinuclear antibody	1:1280 dilution
Anti–double-stranded DNA antibody	Positive
Anti-smith antibody	Positive
Anti–SS-A/Anti-SS-B antibodies	Negative
Complement C3	Low
Complement C4	Low
Erythrocyte sedimentation rate	52 mm/h
Serum creatinine	0.6 mg/dL
Urinalysis	No proteinuria, no hematuria

her underlying SLE. A normal blood pressure, lack of signs of fluid overload (no rales on exam, no pedal edema), along with normal renal function and lack of proteinuria or hematuria, are reassuring that this is not a flare of her underlying lupus nephritis.

CLINICAL PEARL   **STEPS 2/3**

It is important to distinguish between synovitis (which is suggestive of an inflammatory arthritis, such as rheumatoid arthritis) and bony hypertrophy (which is more typical of osteoarthritis). In patients with synovitis, the joints have features including tenderness, swelling, "bogginess," and warmth indicating active inflammation. In contrast, in patients with osteoarthritis, the affected joints have bony hypertrophy, and while they may be tender, the joints are typically firm to touch, without any warmth or bogginess.

What is the role of mycophenolate mofetil in SLE treatment? What is the associated maternal or fetal risk?

The patient is currently on MMF, an inosine monophosphate dehydrogenase inhibitor that interferes with purine synthesis and has been well described as effective in the treatment of lupus nephritis.

MMF has been associated with first-trimester pregnancy loss. In addition, there are reports of various fetal malformations including cleft lip and palate and anomalies of the distal limbs, heart, esophagus, and kidneys. Therefore, it is contraindicated in pregnancy. Contraception is imperative while on MMF. Furthermore, MMF is excreted in breast milk and therefore contraindicated in lactation.

What immunosuppressive medications are safe to be given during pregnancy?

Table 31.2 details the immunosuppressive medications used in patients with autoimmune illnesses and their risks in pregnancy. There is limited evidence regarding toxicity and teratogenicity of many medications used for treatment of autoimmune disease.

Nonsteroidal antiinflammatory drugs (NSAIDs) and low-dose aspirin are thought to present very low fetal or maternal risk during the first two trimesters of pregnancy. Use in the third trimester may be associated with premature closure of the ductus arteriosus. Of the immunosuppressive medications, hydroxychloroquine, sulfasalazine, and azathioprine are considered safe to use during pregnancy.

Tumor necrosis factor (TNF) inhibitors are a class of biologic medications used in the treatment of various autoimmune conditions such as rheumatoid arthritis or inflammatory bowel disease, but these have a limited role in SLE treatment. Examples of TNF inhibitors include infliximab (a chimeric mouse/human monoclonal antibody to TNF), adalimumab

TABLE 31.2 ■ Risk of Immunosuppressives for Rheumatology Patients in Pregnancy

Minimal Fetal or Maternal Risk	Selective Use Allowed During Pregnancy	Moderate to High Fetal Risk	Unknown Fetal Risk
Hydroxychloroquine	NSAIDs (in 1st–2nd trimesters) and aspirin	Cyclophosphamide	Anakinra
Sulfasalazine	Glucocorticoids	Methotrexate	Rituximab
	Azathioprine	Mycophenolate mofetil	Abatacept
	TNF-inhibitors	Leflunomide	Tocilizumab
	Intravenous immune globulin	Third-trimester use of NSAIDs and aspirin	
	Cyclosporine		
	Tacrolimus		

TNF, Tumor necrosis factor; *NSAIDs*, nonsteroidal antiinflammatory drugs.

(a humanized monoclonal antibody to TNF-α), and etanercept (a soluble fusion protein combining a TNF receptor moiety to the constant Fc portion of the immunoglobulin G1 antibody). There is no known increased risk during pregnancy and breastfeeding with TNF inhibitors when analyzed in observational studies and case reports. Although they are probably safe to use, there are no randomized controlled studies that can show this conclusively. As such, if TNF inhibitors are needed to control disease activity and prevent flares, they can be used, but, in general, most rheumatologists try to use them only if absolutely necessary during pregnancy.

CLINICAL PEARL   **STEPS 2/3**

The use of TNF inhibitors has been associated with numerous case reports of drug-induced lupus, so they are generally avoided in patients with existing SLE (so as not to exacerbate underlying disease).

What is the role of hydroxychloroquine in SLE treatment? What is the associated maternal or fetal risk?

Hydroxychloroquine has not only been shown to decrease frequency of lupus flares, but it also has antithrombotic properties. It is widely used as an antimalarial agent, and anyone with any degree of SLE should be taking hydroxychloroquine. There are no known associated fetal malformations, and expert opinion deems it appropriate during pregnancy. In addition, discontinuation has been associated with a threefold increased incidence of flare in a randomized double-blind controlled trial. This patient should therefore continue hydroxychloroquine throughout pregnancy.

BASIC SCIENCE PEARL   **STEP 1**

The exact mechanism of action of hydroxychloroquine in SLE is unknown. One hypothesis is that it may impair complement-dependent antigen–antibody interactions. It may also impair chemotaxis and neutrophil migration.

Your patient is treated for a mild arthritic flare of lupus with a 2-week glucocorticoid taper, starting with prednisone 20 mg daily for 1 week, followed by 10 mg daily for 1 week. She returns for follow-up 1 month later with resolution of her synovitis, improvement of inflammatory markers, improvement of hypocomplementemia, and decrease in anti-dsDNA antibody levels.

What medication recommendations should you make for the maintenance treatment of nephritis in this patient who desires pregnancy?

Azathioprine is a purine metabolite and is considered a generally milder immunosuppressive. Some examples of its use include in patients with organ transplantation, systemic vasculitis (as part of a maintenance regimen), and SLE.

Although not first-line for lupus nephritis, it is much safer in pregnancy than either cyclophosphamide or MMF. Furthermore, while it carries the label of pregnancy category D, it is actually considered relatively safe for use in pregnancy and is widely used. The data on the use of azathioprine come primarily from studies of patients with organ transplantation or with Crohn's disease.

BASIC SCIENCE PEARL   **STEP 1**

Azathioprine is a purine metabolite, converted by the enzyme inosinate phosphorylase to 6-mercaptopurine (6-MP), which inhibits synthesis of nucleic acids and thereby interferes with cellular metabolism and mitosis.

Her MMF is discontinued and she is started on azathioprine 50 mg daily, gradually increased to a dose of 2 mg/kg per day. She returns 5 months later and is 8 weeks pregnant. There is some mild swelling noted in the metacarpophalangeal joints, which are not limiting her function significantly. Laboratory data show no significant change, and there is no evidence of nephritis flare at this time.

Diagnosis: Mild flare of lupus arthritis in pregnancy

How should her mild arthritic flare be treated now that she is pregnant?

Since she is early on in her pregnancy and her flare is mild, NSAIDs are a reasonable option. These can either be taking on an as-needed basis or can be taken on a standing basis for 1–3 weeks, or until symptoms improve.

In moderate to severe arthritic flares, glucocorticoids may be considered. Studies in rodents suggest possible risk of cleft palate, which has also been reported in humans exposed to glucocorticoids in utero. It is therefore recommended to avoid high-dose glucocorticoids in the first trimester during palate formation unless absolutely necessary.

In addition, there are other adverse effects of glucocorticoid therapy including increased risk of impaired glucose tolerance and gestational diabetes.

What medications should be avoided at this time for treatment of her arthritis?

Unless disease is life threatening, known embryotoxic medications should be avoided.

Methotrexate has been associated with various fetal malformations, such as cleft palate, hydrocephalus, anencephaly, and meningoencephalocele, as well as skeletal deformities (including congenital stenosis of tubular long bones and abnormal facial features of low-set ears, micrognathia, and delayed ossification).

Leflunomide, a pyrimidine synthesis inhibitor, has a role in treatment of rheumatoid arthritis and is also occasionally used in SLE. It is a known embryotoxic drug and has been associated with many fetal malformations in animal studies, so its use in pregnancy is contraindicated.

BASIC SCIENCE PEARL	STEP 1

There are several proposed mechanisms of action of methotrexate. One hypothesis is that it increases serum adenosine release (adenosine has potent anti-inflammatory properties), which contributes to decreases in leukocyte migration to tissues, thereby decreasing systemic inflammation.

The patient is started on naproxen 500 mg, which she takes twice daily for a week and on an as-needed basis thereafter prior to the third trimester. This regimen is helpful for her pain. The remainder of the gestation period is unremarkable. She undergoes spontaneous vaginal delivery of a healthy baby at 39 weeks and now wants to breastfeed.

Is it advisable for this patient to breastfeed?

Many immunosuppressive medications are excreted in breast milk in varying doses. Multiple factors need to be considered. The American Academy of Pediatrics (AAP) and the Drugs and Lactation Database (LactMed) database via the National Institute of Health (NIH) and the Toxicology Data Network are resources with information on drugs to which breastfeeding mothers may be exposed.

Hydroxychloroquine is considered safe to use in lactation. It is recommended that hydroxychloroquine be continued during pregnancy and lactation in patients with SLE to prevent disease flares.

As for glucocorticoids, while they are also excreted in breast milk, the benefits to the mother sometimes justify their use, per the AAP. If there is concern about prednisone exposure in breast milk, it can be advised to discard breast mild for the first 4 hours after ingestion. In this patient who desires to breastfeed, she should continue hydroxychloroquine, with judicious use of glucocorticoids only if indicated and at the lowest dose possible. There are some instances where postpartum lupus patients have more active disease and require potent immunosuppression in order to preserve organ function, in which case breastfeeding cannot be recommended.

Methotrexate and leflunomide are generally contraindicated in lactation. Although there are limited data suggesting that only low levels of methotrexate are excreted in breast milk, expert opinion is that methotrexate is contraindicated in pregnancy as well as lactation. No data are available on the use of MMF during lactation and use is therefore not recommended per the AAP.

Since she has a history of lupus nephritis, the azathioprine is cautiously withheld when she is breastfeeding. She has close monitoring of her laboratory and urine tests in order to ensure stable renal function. She is maintained on hydroxychloroquine while breastfeeding. She finishes breastfeeding after 6 months and is then restarted on her MMF while maintaining hydroxychloroquine. Her joint pain is very mild and is improved with periodic naproxen.

BEYOND THE PEARLS

- The FDA no longer endorses the labeling of medications with the widely known "Letter Categories." Per the current FDA website (http://www.fda.gov/), "FDA has decided to eliminate the pregnancy categories because they are often viewed as confusing and overly simplistic and don't effectively communicate the risk a drug may have during pregnancy and lactation and in females and males of reproductive potential."
- Teriflunomide is the major metabolite of leflunomide, and it has a half-life of years. In case of unplanned pregnancy and inadvertent exposure to leflunomide, cholestyramine may be used to accelerate the decrease in levels after leflunomide is discontinued.
- Belimumab is human monoclonal antibody that inhibits B-cell activating factor (BAFF, also known as B-lymphocyte stimulator, BLyS); it is the newest agent available for the treatment of SLE. Its use is contraindicated in pregnancy due to unknown risk.
- Studies of the use of combined oral contraceptives in SLE patients have shown no increased risk of flares as compared to placebo. However, there is limited evidence indicating a possible increased risk of thrombosis in women with positive antiphospholipid antibodies and history of oral contraceptive use.
- Sometimes, even with a trained eye, it can be difficult to determine the presence of synovitis on joint exam. In these cases, there is a role for imaging modalities such as musculoskeletal ultrasound (MSK US) or magnetic resonance imaging (MRI) to best evaluate the soft tissue and joints.
- Remember to always ask any patients with SLE about history of miscarriages or thrombosis and to evaluate for the presence of anticardiolipin IgG or IgM antibodies, anti-β-2-glycoprotein IgG or IgM antibodies, and lupus anticoagulant.
- The classification criteria for antiphospholipid syndrome requires both a clinical manifestation (documented arterial or venous thrombus; or one or more miscarriages beyond 10 weeks' gestation; or 3 or more first-trimester miscarriages) as well as persistent laboratory abnormalities as noted in the previous bullet point item (repeatedly positive, at least 12 weeks apart).

Case Summary

- A 29-year-old woman with a history of class V lupus nephritis, which is now well controlled, wishes to become pregnant and comes to you for evaluation. She has mild intermittent joint pains in the hands.
- She is normotensive, without any pedal edema. There is synovitis in the metacarpophalangeal joints, with limited pain and preserved range of motion.
- Labs reveal hypocomplementemia, elevated anti-dsDNA antibody levels, and an elevated sedimentation rate. Serum creatinine is normal, and there is no hematuria or proteinuria.
- After becoming pregnant, you diagnosis a mild flare of lupus in early pregnancy.
- Since she is in her first trimester, she started on NSAIDs and the symptoms improve. Her MMF is transitioned to azathioprine during pregnancy. She has a healthy delivery. Since she is interested in breastfeeding, the azathioprine is temporarily held (with frequent laboratory and urine monitoring to ensure stable renal disease), with the continuation of only hydroxychloroquine while breastfeeding. She finishes breastfeeding after 6 months and is then restarted on MMF while maintaining hydroxychloroquine.

References

Clowse, M. E., Magder, L., Witter, F., & Petri, M. (2006). Hydroxychloroquine in lupus pregnancy. *Arthritis and Rheumatism, 54*, 3640.

Culwell, K., et al. (2009). Safety of contraceptive method use among women with systemic lupus erythematosus: a systematic review. *Obstetrics and Gynecology, 114*(2 Pt 1), 341–353.

Johns, D. G., et al. (1972). Secretion of methotrexate in human milk. *American Journal of Obstetrics and Gynecology*, *112*, 978–980.

Kitridou, R. C. (1997). The mother in systemic lupus erythematosus. In D. J. Wallace, & B. H. Hahn (Eds.), *Dubois' lupus erythematosus* (5th ed.) (pp. 967–1028). Baltimore: Williams & Wilkins.

LactMed Drugs and Lactation Database. https://toxnet.nlm.nih.gov.

Parke, A., & West, B. (1996). Hydroxychloroquine in pregnant patients with systemic lupus erythematosus. *The Journal of Rheumatology*, *23*, 1715.

Petri, M., et al. (2005 Dec 15). Combined oral contraceptives in women with systemic lupus erythematosus. *The New England Journal of Medicine*, *353*(24), 2550–2558.

Petri, M. (2003). Immunosuppressive drug use in pregnancy. *Autoimmunity*, *36*, 51.

Pistilli, B., et al. (2013). Chemotherapy, targeted agents, antiemetics and growth-factors in human milk: how should we counsel cancer patients about breastfeeding? *Cancer Treatment Reviews*, *39*, 207–211.

Temprano, K. K., Bandlamudi, R., & Moore, T. L. (2005). Antirheumatic drugs in pregnancy and lactation. *Seminars in Arthritis and Rheumatism*, *35*(2), 112–121.

Andrew Morado ■ Raj Dasgupta ■ Ruth Minkin

A 29-Year-Old Woman With Shortness of Breath

A 29-year-old healthy G1P0 woman (32 weeks of gestation) presents to the emergency room complaining of shortness of breath (SOB).

What is the differential diagnosis of SOB in pregnancy?

SOB in pregnancy can manifest for numerous reasons and involve multiple organ systems. Generally speaking, common etiologies include cardiovascular (systolic heart failure, myocardial infarction), pulmonary (asthma, pneumonia, pulmonary embolism), and hematopoietic systems (anemia). The differential diagnosis can be narrowed based on ancillary history as well as demographics. In a young, previously healthy woman in her third trimester, a few disorders should come to mind.

Pregnancy, due to increased estrogen, is a pro-coagulopathic state. Pregnant women have increased risk of both deep venous thrombosis (DVT) and pulmonary embolism. Overall, DVT occurs in all trimesters antepartum, while pulmonary embolism occurs most often peripartum. The length of hypercoagulability can extend beyond delivery (venous thromboembolism [VTE] is 2–5 times more common postpartum) with highest risk in the first 6 weeks postpartum. Although the risk persists until 12 weeks, the absolute risk beyond 6 weeks appears to be low. Patients may complain of unilateral lower extremity edema as well as acute chest pain with hypoxia, all suggesting the possibility of VTE.

Anemia can occur in pregnancy for several reasons. The increased plasma volume tends to dilute hemoglobin, with the nadir typically occurring in the early portion of the third trimester. This effect dampens as the pregnancy reaches term due to minimal further expansion of the plasma volume relative to the increase in red blood cells. Additionally, the placenta and developing fetus utilize large amounts of dietary iron and can further exacerbate anemia. Iron supplementation is paramount in prenatal care and should exceed 1 g/day to ensure adequate stores.

Peripartum cardiomyopathy is a rare disorder resulting in impairment of left ventricular ejection fraction (LVEF of <45%) with or without left ventricular dilatation. These patients without previously known cardiovascular disease present near term (after 36 weeks of gestation) and up to 6 months after delivery. The typical clinical presentation mirrors systolic heart failure with signs of volume overload including pulmonary and lower extremity edema. Management aims at restoring left ventricular function, but, in some instances, the condition is irreversible and heart transplant may be required.

CLINICAL PEARL   **STEPS 2/3**

Progesterone in pregnancy stimulates the respiratory center to increase minute ventilation (respiratory rate × tidal volume). This is primarily achieved through increase in tidal volume. Tachypnea is not an expected finding during pregnancy and should always be investigated for an underlying cause.

The patient reports an insidious onset of her SOB that has progressed over the 4 weeks since her last visit. She admits to decreased exercise tolerance as well as new-onset bilateral lower extremity edema. She has severe SOB with ambulation around her home. She has no past medical or surgical history. Both her mother and father have hypertension. She is taking her prenatal vitamins as instructed and takes no other medications at this time. Five years prior, she did take herbal supplements for weight loss, which she bought online from Europe. She has no drug allergies. Review of systems is otherwise negative.

How does heart failure present on physical exam?

Heart failure is a ubiquitous term meant to describe a wide array of clinical diseases. The left ventricle, responsible for systemic tissue perfusion, can be subject to both systolic and diastolic dysfunction. Systolic dysfunction (low ejection fraction) is most commonly caused by coronary disease and/or myocardial infarction, while diastolic dysfunction (heart failure with preserved ejection fraction) is strongly associated with long standing, poorly controlled HTN. Regardless of the type, the common physical exam findings when in heart failure exacerbation are jugular venous distention, orthopnea, peripheral edema, accessory heart sounds, and inspiratory crackles.

Commonly overlooked is the right ventricular function, which plays just as important a role as the left ventricle. The right ventricle delivers blood to the pulmonary arteries for subsequent offloading of carbon dioxide and uptake of oxygen from the ambient air. The pulmonary circulation is a low-pressure, high-flow system with a great capacity for recruitment of normally unperfused vessels. As a consequence, the walls of pulmonary arteries are thin, in keeping with their low transmural pressure. This explains the discrepancy in myocardial thickness between the right and left ventricles. Failure of the right ventricle can occur as a consequence of left ventricular disease, but isolated right ventricular dysfunction is most commonly caused by a myocardial infarction involving the right coronary artery or pulmonary hypertension. Physical exam findings associated with right ventricular dysfunction are increased intensity of the pulmonic component of the second heart sound with accentuated splitting, precordial heave, holosystolic murmur signifying tricuspid regurgitation, and peripheral edema. Typically, the lung sounds are clear (Fig. 32.1).

CLINICAL PEARL   **STEPS 2/3**

The most specific exam finding for heart failure is the presence of an S3. It occurs in the middle third of diastole after the S2 heart sound due to turbulent blood flow from the atrium to a dilated left ventricle. An S4 occurs after the atrial kick and just before the S1 heart sound. It results from the forceful ejection of blood from the atria into a stiffened left ventricle.

On exam, she is afebrile with blood pressure 103/54 mm Hg, a heart rate of 107/min, respiratory rate of 22/min, and oxygen saturation of 97% on room air. She appears to be in mild respiratory distress. She has obvious jugular venous distention up to the angle of the mandible. Her lungs are clear, and she has a loud P2 with a 3/6 holosystolic murmur best heard at the 5th intercostal space, parasternal border. She has 2+ peripheral, pitting edema. The remainder of the physical exam is normal. Her chest radiograph (CXR) is shown in Fig. 32.2. She is admitted to the obstetrics floor for further evaluation. Pulmonology is consulted from the emergency room.

What is pulmonary hypertension?

Pulmonary hypertension classification was recently restructured to include five classes of disease, all characterized by elevated pressure within the pulmonary vasculature. Just as systemic hypertension has a pressure criteria, pulmonary hypertension is defined as a mean pulmonary arterial pressure (mPAP) greater than 25 mm Hg. From there, the classes of pulmonary hypertension are

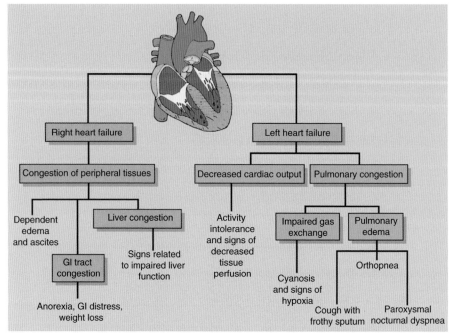

Fig. 32.1 Comparison of physical exam findings resulting from right and left heart failure.

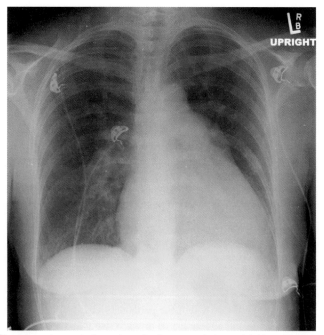

Fig. 32.2 Chest x-ray demonstrating enlarged pulmonary arteries and right ventricular enlargement.

further delineated based on history and hemodynamic measurements. It is extremely important to correctly identify the type of pulmonary hypertension because management can vary significantly between the classes. The most important distinction to make is between classifying the disease into precapillary (mPAP >25 mm Hg, pulmonary capillary wedge pressure [PCWP] <15 mm Hg) or postcapillary (mPAP >25 mm Hg, PCWP >15 mm Hg) pulmonary hypertension as the approach to these conditions varies considerably.

Group 1 pulmonary arterial hypertension (PAH), "true" precapillary disease, is defined as mPAP greater than 25 mm Hg, PCWP less than 15 mm Hg, and a pulmonary vascular resistance (PVR) greater than 3 Woods Units (WUs). It includes idiopathic PAH, heritable PAH, drug- and toxin-associated PAH, and PAH with associated conditions (i.e., collagen vascular disease, human immunodeficiency virus [HIV] infection, portal hypertension, congenital heart diseases, and schistosomiasis). The pathogenesis and treatment of Group 1 PAH will be discussed shortly.

Group 2 pulmonary venous hypertension (PVH), postcapillary disease, is due to left ven- tricular heart disease and is differentiated based on a PCWP greater than 15 mm Hg. As the left ventricle fails, increased pressure is transmitted back through the pulmonary veins to the pulmonary arteries. Over time, the elevated pressure from the left side of the heart will result in failure of the afterload-intolerant right ventricle. This is by far the most common cause of pulmonary hypertension, and the mainstay of treatment is optimization of cardiac function and blood pressure control.

Group 3 pulmonary hypertension is due to chronic hypoxia and usually has a PCWP of less than 15 mm Hg and a history of underlying lung disease or sleep apnea. Chronic hypoxia leads to physiologic pulmonary arterial vasoconstriction, and, if subjected to long periods of hypoxia, permanent remodeling at the vascular level occurs resulting in identifiable pulmonary hyperten- sion. As with Group 2, the mainstay of therapy for Group 3 disease is optimizing lung function and addition of supplemental oxygen to maintain adequate oxygen saturation.

Group 4 pulmonary hypertension includes chronic thromboembolic pulmonary hyperten- sion (CTEPH). Up to 4% of patients diagnosed with acute pulmonary embolism will develop CTEPH, and this is a direct result of an unresolved thrombus that becomes coalescent and organized, resulting in obstructive blood flow and increased vascular resistance. With time, this increased pulmonary vascular resistance results in right heart failure. A ventilation/perfusion scan is the test of choice to make this diagnosis as it is more sensitive in detecting organized clots than computed tomography (CT) pulmonary angiogram.

Group 5 is a miscellaneous category of different causes of pulmonary hypertension. Manage- ment depends on the underlying etiology (Fig. 32.3).

CLINICAL PEARL   **STEP 2/3**

CTEPH is the one class of pulmonary hypertension that is primarily treated with surgery. When there is a significant amount of proximal clot burden noted on V/Q scan, referral should be made to a center specializing in pulmonary arterial endarterectomy. In centers with experience, the mortality rate following this surgery is less than 2%.

What is the best screening test for pulmonary hypertension?

The best screening test for pulmonary hypertension is a transthoracic echocardiogram (TTE). Now readily available in most hospitals, ultrasonography at the bedside allows for a rapid non- invasive evaluation of the heart function and anatomy. While specificity is lacking, the high sensitivity and excellent negative predictive value make TTE a great test to rule out pulmonary hypertension.

Findings indicative of pulmonary hypertension are right ventricular dilation and a reduced func- tion. Most importantly, TTE can estimate pulmonary artery systolic pressure using the simplified

TABLE 2. Clinical classification of pulmonary hypertension	
GROUP 1	Primary pulmonary hypertension: idiopathic, familial, drug and toxin induced (appetite suppressant drugs), rare medical conditions
GROUP 2	Secondary to left ventricular disease: mitral valve disease, left ventricular systolic or diastolic failure.
GROUP 3	Secondary to pulmonary disease or hypoxia: COPD, sleep disordered breathing, obesity hypoventilation
GROUP 4	Secondary to chronic thromboembolism
GROUP 5	Unclear and multifactorial etiologies
Abbrevations: COPD: chronic obstructive pulmonary disease	

Fig. 32.3 World Health Organization group classification system for pulmonary hypertension.

Simplified Bernouli Equation

$$\Delta P = 4\ (V^2)$$

Fig. 32.4 Simplified Bernoulli equation, where delta P is the difference in pressure of the right ventricle and right atrium, and V is the velocity of regurgitated blood through the tricuspid valve.

Bernoulli's equation, a property of fluid dynamics stating that an increase in speed of fluid occurs simultaneously with a decrease in pressure. In other words, the pressure gradient between the right atrium and right ventricle is equal to four times the square of the velocity of blood flow through the tricuspid valve. With normal anatomy, the right ventricle systolic pressure is equal to the pulmonary artery pressure and inferences regarding pulmonary hypertension can be made (Fig. 32.4).

CLINICAL PEARLS   **STEP 1**

Sensitive tests have low false negative rates while specific tests have low false positive rates. The negative predictive value is the proportion of patients who, with a negative test, do not in fact have disease. The positive predictive value is the proportion of patients with a positive test who do in fact have disease.

A screening TTE reveals severe right ventricular dilation and a markedly reduced right ventricular function. The pulmonary artery systolic pressure is estimated at 65 mm Hg. The left ventricle is normal in size and function.

What is the most specific test for pulmonary hypertension?
Once TTE suggests the presence of pulmonary hypertension, the results must be further explored and diagnosis confirmed with a right heart catheterization. Invasive measurement of hemodynamics is the gold standard for the evaluation of pulmonary hypertension as it further defines the etiological group as well as guides therapy and can contribute to prognosis. Using a small inflatable balloon, the catheter is inserted through a large vein; it naturally follows the flow of blood through the right atrium and ventricle until it wedges in the pulmonary artery. Once appropriately positioned, the pulmonary artery pressure, right atrial and ventricular pressures, cardiac output, and PCWP can be measured. The cardiac index (cardiac output divided by body surface area) as well as pulmonary and systemic vascular resistance can be then calculated (Fig. 32.5).

If the measurements fit with Group 1 PAH (PAP >25 mm Hg, PCWP <15 mm Hg, and PVR >3 WU) then a vasodilator challenge is performed next. This is done most commonly with inhaled nitric oxide, a potent vasodilator. If a patient is deemed a vasodilator responder, then her prognosis tends to be more favorable than if she is a nonresponder.

CLINICAL PEARL   **STEPS 2/3**

A positive vasoreactive study is defined as a decrease of the mPAP by more than 10 mm Hg and below 40 mm Hg overall without a decrease in cardiac output. Unique to those patients who respond is the option to treat with a calcium channel blocker.

CLINICAL PEARL   **STEPS 2/3**

The decision to place a PAC in a pregnant patient should be made on a case-by-case basis after carefully weighing the potential benefits against the risks for the individual patient and the fetus. Common complications of PAC insertion include the occurrence of atrial and/or ventricular arrhythmias. Perforation of a cardiac chamber and rupture of a cardiac valve or the pulmonary artery are rare complications that can be catastrophic. Complications of catheter use include pulmonary artery rupture, pulmonary infarction, thromboembolic events, infection, and data misinterpretation.

CLINICAL PEARL   **STEP 1**

The PCWP is measured when the balloon is inflated and occludes the distal pulmonary artery. Assuming normal anatomy, the static column of blood exerts a pressure from the balloon to the left ventricle and thus estimates left ventricular end diastolic pressure. This can be used as a surrogate for left ventricular end diastolic volume or preload of the left ventricle.

The patient undergoes right heart catheterization which reveals a mPAP 45 mm Hg, PCWP 12 mm Hg, cardiac output 3.5 L/min, cardiac index 2.1, SVR 1300 dynes, and a PVR of 9.5 WU. She is not responsive to a vasodilator challenge. Based on these findings, she is diagnosed with Group 1 PAH, likely as an effect of the dietary supplements she took several years prior.

What is the pathogenesis of PAH?
Idiopathic PAH as well as PAH with associated conditions have similar pathophysiology. The latter involves three main pathways occurring at the level of the pulmonary artery: endothelial cell proliferation, nitric oxide (NO) dysregulation, and dysregulated prostacyclin synthesis. Understanding the pathophysiology behind PAH will elucidate targeted therapies used to treat this disease.

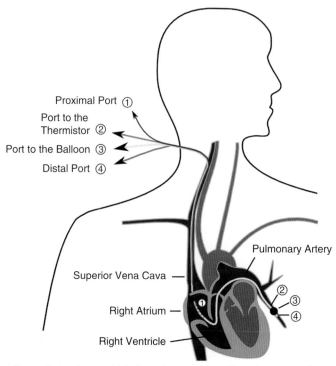

Proximal Port ①
Port to the
Thermistor ②
Port to the Balloon ③
Distal Port ④

Pulmonary Artery

Superior Vena Cava —

Right Atrium —

Right Ventricle —

Fig. 32.5 Swan-Ganz catheter placement into the pulmonary artery. The pulmonary capillary wedge pressure estimates left atrial pressure, an indirect measurement of volume status.

Patients with PAH have increased endothelial cell growth regulated through the endothelin receptor-1. This results in thickening of the arterial wall, vasoconstriction, and smooth muscle proliferation. The plexiform lesion, hallmark of the disease, is commonly found on lung biopsy specimens of patients with PAH and is formed mainly through the endothelin pathway. In most cases, plexiform lesions are located near the origin of small pulmonary arteries.

NO is a potent vasodilator operating primarily through a cyclic-guanosine monophosphate (GMP) pathway to relax smooth muscle. Arginine is a required substrate for NO and is profoundly reduced in patients with PAH, leading to unopposed vasoconstriction through the endothelin pathway.

Prostacyclin promotes vasodilation through cyclic-adenosine monophosphate (AMP), inhibits smooth muscle proliferation, and has antithrombotic properties. Similar to NO, synthesis of prostacyclin is disproportionately reduced in the pulmonary artery of patients with PAH leading to unregulated effects of endothelin and increased thrombosis within small arteries, further contributing to increased vascular resistance (Fig. 32.6).

CLINICAL PEARL   **STEPS 2/3**

There is evidence for anticoagulation in patients with either Group 1 PAH or Group 4 CTEPH suggesting improved mortality. The choice of anticoagulant remains warfarin for this indication though its use in pregnancy is absolutely contraindicated. If impossible to avoid, warfarin should not be given in the first trimester due to teratogenicity nor in the weeks leading up to delivery to decrease the risk of bleeding.

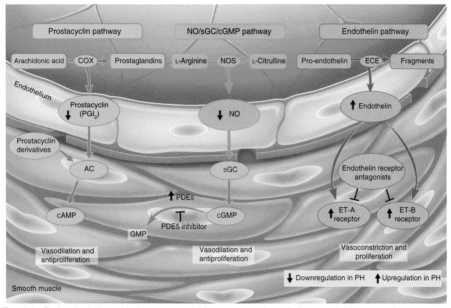

Fig. 32.6 Pathophysiology of pulmonary arterial hypertension through the endothelin, nitric oxide, and prostacyclin pathways.

What are targeted therapies for PAH?

The current therapies for PAH are targeted at the individual pathways just outlined. Endothelin receptor antagonists block the proliferative effects of endothelin and have been shown to improve quality of life and cardiopulmonary function. In the acute setting, NO can be delivered continuously mixed with oxygen via different devices (nasal cannula, mask, mechanical ventilator) to promote vasodilation but is not available as an outpatient therapy. Fortunately, phosphodiesterase-5 (PDE-5) inhibitors demonstrate similar effects by increasing endogenous levels of cyclic-GMP.

Prostacyclin and its analogues have intravenous (IV), subcutaneous, inhaled, and oral routes of administration. IV and subcutaneous prostacyclin and its analogues must be given by continuous infusions due to their very short half-life and potential for rebound worsening of the disease with abrupt termination of the medication. IV prostacyclin analogs have been manufactured and can be given through long-term indwelling catheters.

The timing of implementation of these therapies as well as choice of therapy is based on the patient's New York Heart Association (NYHA) functional class scale. Numerous studies are published and currently are ongoing on whether a monotherapeutic or upfront multitherapeutic approach should be the initial offering. The response to therapy is typically followed mainly by frequent functional assessment rather than repeated hemodynamic measurements (Figs. 32.7 and 32.8).

In addition to the PAH-specific therapy, all patients should be evaluated for home oxygen therapy, diuretics with the goal to keep net even, and pulmonary rehabilitation. All female patients of childbearing potential should be advised on contraception and the potential risk of pregnancy for a PAH-affected person. Supervised gradual exercise is being advised and is demonstrated to be a safe option for stable patients with PAH.

Table 2 – World Health Organization functional classification for pulmonary hypertension

Functional class	Symptoms
Class I	*Symptoms do not limit physical activity.* Ordinary physical activity does not cause undue discomfort.
Class II	Slight limitation of physical activity. The patient is comfortable at rest, yet experiences *symptoms with ordinary physical activity.*
Class III	Marked limitation of activity. Patient is comfortable at rest, yet experiences *symptoms with minimal physical activity.*
Class IV	Inability to carry out any physical activity. The patient may experience *symptoms even at rest.* Discomfort is increased by any physical activity. Manifest signs of right-sided heart failure.

Fig. 32.7 World Health Organization functional classification for pulmonary hypertension.

INITIAL THERAPY WITH PAH APPROVED DRUGS				
YELLOW: Morbidity and mortality as primary end-point in randomized controlled study or reduction in all-cause mortality (prospectively defined) *Level of evidence is based on the WHO-FC of the majority of the patients of the studies. †Approved only: by the FDA (macitentan, riociguat, treprostinil inhaled); in New Zealand (iloprost i.v); in Japan and S.Korea(beraprost). ‡Positive opinion for approval of the CHMP of EMA				
Recommendation	Evidence*	WHO-FC II	WHO-FC III	WHO-FC IV
I	A or B	Ambrisentan Bosentan Macitentan†‡ Riociguat† Sildenafil Tadalafil	Ambrisentan Bosentan Epoprostenol i.v. Iloprost inhaled Macitentan†‡ Riociguat† Sildenafil Tadalafil Treprostinil s.c., inhaled†	Epoprostenol i.v.
IIa	C		Iloprost i.v. † Treprostinil i.v.	Ambrisentan, Bosentan Iloprost inhaled and i.v† Macitentan†‡ Riociguat† Sildenafil, Tadalafil Treprostinil s.c., i.v., Inhaled†
IIb	B		Beraprost†	
IIb	C		Initial Combination Therapy	Initial Combination Therapy

Fig. 32.8 Targeted therapies and timing of use based on New York Heart Association functional class. *(Adapted from 2015 ESC/ERS Guidelines for the diagnosis and treatment of pulmonary hypertension. Eur Heart J. 2015.)*

CLINICAL PEARL   **STEPS 2/3**

Of the available therapies for PAH, endothelin receptor antagonists (bosentan, macitentan, ambrisentan) are category X for pregnancy, as is riociguat, a recently approved medication for Group 1 and Group 4 disease. PDE5 inhibitors (sildenafil, tadalafil) and prostacyclin and its analogues are category B.

The patient is categorized as NYHA functional class 3 based on symptoms with minimal activity, and the choice is made to begin IV epoprostenol. Fetal monitors show no abnormalities. She is anxious to know the management plan for her pregnancy.

How does pregnancy impact PAH?

To understand how pregnancy affects a patient with PAH, normal cardiovascular changes that occur with pregnancy must be reviewed. Total body volume increases by as much as 8 L while plasma volume can increase by 1.5 L when at term. Cardiac output increases by as much as 50% and occurs as a function of metabolic demand needed for the mother and developing fetus. Cardiac output is augmented by the change in plasma volume, which increases preload; reduced afterload through the vasodilatory effects of estrogen; and increased maternal heart rate.

These changes place higher stress on the heart and cardiovascular system but proceed normally in the healthy individual. In a woman with PAH, the right ventricle is compromised by the increased effort of working against high pressures. Once the system is taxed further by increasing the overall volume of blood and the need for higher cardiac output, the right heart inevitably fails and cardiovascular collapse ensues.

Given this, women with known PAH are recommended against pregnancy, and dual contraception should be employed in all reproductive-age women. In those who do become pregnant, a multidisciplinary discussion involving the obstetrician and pulmonary hypertension specialist regarding the risks and benefits of elective abortion and continuation of the pregnancy must occur.

Women who chose to proceed with pregnancy in the setting of PAH should be referred to a tertiary care center with high-risk obstetrics as well as a pulmonary hypertension team available. There is no consensus to the time of delivery, and either an elective cesarean with concurrent right catheterization can be performed as early as 34 weeks or a vaginal delivery can be pursued between 34 and 37 weeks if the mother and fetus are stable.

CLINICAL PEARL   **STEPS 2/3**

For patients with decompensated right heart failure, management goals focus on right ventricular support. This can be done with IV inotropes like norepinephrine, dobutamine, or milrinone. Inhaled NO can also be given for added pulmonary vascular dilation, effectively offloading strain from the right ventricle.

The patient shows good initial response to IV epoprostenol, and, after multidisciplinary discussion between obstetrics and pulmonology, she is discharged home for weekly follow-up in the outpatient clinic. She chooses to proceed to 34 weeks of pregnancy and then undergo an elective cesarean delivery. She undergoes an uncomplicated delivery and is monitored in the medical intensive care unit. After an uncomplicated hospital course, she and her child are discharged home with follow-up in the pulmonary hypertension clinic in 1 week.

BEYOND THE PEARLS

- Large shifts in volume status are poorly tolerated in PAH. Volume management should be conservative, with small boluses given for resuscitation if needed and low-dose drips for diuresis.
- Patients without contraindications should be referred for lung transplantation if still having NYHA 4 disease despite maximal medical therapy.
- IV epoprostenol, while very effective, has significant side effects including diarrhea, nausea, jaw pain, flushing, and headache. These symptoms tend to minimize over time with continued use of the medication.
- Inhaled (iloprost, treprostinil) and oral (treprostinil) prostacyclin analogues as well as prostacyclin receptor agonist(Selexipag) are available, thus negating the need for indwelling IV catheters while still achieving therapeutic effects comparable to IV epoprostenol in patients with NYHA 3 disease. However, for more advanced patients with class 4 disease, systemic prostacyclin still remains the drug of choice for this therapeutic class.

Case Summary

- A 29-year-old woman at 32 weeks of gestation presents with worsening SOB.
- Physical exam reveals jugular venous distension, a loud P2 with 3/6 holosystolic murmur, lungs clear to auscultation, and bilateral pitting lower extremity edema.
- TTE shows severe right ventricular dilation with a pulmonary artery systolic pressure estimated at 65 mm Hg.
- The diagnosis is WHO Group 1 PAH.
- Based on symptoms and NYHA functional class, the patient is started on IV epoprostenol and has an elective cesarean delivery.

References

Beghetti, M., & Galie, N. (2009). Eisenmenger syndrome: a clinical perspective in a new therapeutic era of pulmonary arterial hypertension. *Journal of the American College of Cardiology, 53*(9), 733–740.

Berg, C. J., Chang, J., Callaghan, W. M., et al. (2003). Pregnancy-related mortality in the United States 1991–1997. *Obstetrics and Gynecology, 101*(2), 289–296.

Davie, A. P., Francis, C. M., Caruana, L., et al. (1997). Assessing diagnosis in heart failure: which features are any use? *Quarterly Journal of Medicine, 90*(5), 335–339.

Galie, N., Corris, P. A., Frost, A., et al. (2013). Updated treatment algorithm of pulmonary arterial hypertension. *Journal of the American College of Cardiology, 62*(Suppl 25), D60–D72.

Heit, J. A., Kobbervig, C. E., James, A. H., et al. (2005). Trends in the incidence of venous thromboembolism during pregnancy or postpartum: a 30-year population-based study. *Annals of Internal Medicine, 143*(10), 697–706.

Kiely, D. G., Condliffe, R., Webster, V., et al. (2010). Improved survival in pregnancy and pulmonary hypertension using a multiprofessional approach. *British Journal of Obstetrics and Gynaecology, 117*(5), 565–574.

Pengo, V., Lensing, A. W. A., Prins, M. H., et al. (2004). Incidence of chronic thromboembolic pulmonary hypertension after pulmonary embolism. *The New England Journal of Medicine, 350*(22), 2257–2264.

Pereira, A., & Krieger, B. P. (2004). Pulmonary complications of pregnancy. *Clinics in Chest Medicine, 25*(2), 299–310.

Sandham, J. D., Hull, R. D., Brant, R. F., et al. (2003). Canadian Critical Care Clinical Trials Group. A randomized, controlled trial of the use of pulmonary artery catheters in high-risk surgical patients. *The New England Journal of Medicine, 348*(1), 5–14.

Simonneau, G., Gatzoulis, M. A., Adatia, I., et al. (2013). Updated clinical classification of pulmonary hypertension. *Journal of the American College of Cardiology, 62*(Suppl 25), D34–D41.

Sliwa, K., Hilfiker-Kleiner, D., Petrie, M. C., et al. (2010). Heart failure association of the European Society of Cardiology Working Group on Peripartum Cardiomyopathy. Current state of knowledge on aetiology, diagnosis, management, and therapy of peripartum cardiomyopathy: a position statement from the Heart Failure Association of the European Society of Cardiology Working Group on peripartum cardiomyopathy. *European Journal of Heart Failure, 12*(8), 767–778.

Van Oppen, A. C., Stigter, R. H., Bruinse, H. W., et al. (1996). Cardiac output in normal pregnancy: a critical review. *Obstetrics and Gynecology, 87*(2), 310–318.

Young, P., & Johanson, R. (2001). Haemodynamic, invasive and echocardiographic monitoring in the hypertensive parturient. *Best Practice & Research Clinical Obstetrics & Gynecology, 15*(4), 605–622.

Linda Shiber, MD

A 42-Year-Old With Heavy Vaginal Bleeding

A 42-year-old woman presents to the emergency department with a 2-week history of heavy vaginal bleeding, pelvic pressure, and fatigue. She denies any new medications. She has had to miss work as a nurse's assistant due to weakness and multiple episodes of soiling her clothing with blood. Her past medical history is significant for obesity (body mass index of 39 kg/m²) as well as hypertension, for which she takes hydrochlorothiazide daily. On physical examination, her blood pressure is 138/78 mm Hg, heart rate is 102/min, respiration rate is 22/min, and oxygen saturation is 86% on room air. Hemoglobin is 7.2 mg/dL. Abdominal exam is significant for mild suprapubic tenderness, particularly on the left. Speculum exam reveals a large amount of dark red clotting and 200 mL of blood in vaginal vault. No cervical lesions are noted. Bimanual exam finds an 8 cm mass anterolaterally on the left aspect of the uterus and tenderness with uterine palpation.

What are the next steps in evaluating this patient?
A thorough history including menstrual history, family history of bleeding problems, family history of cancer, a review of medications and contraception, and a cervical screening history is imperative in the evaluation of a patient with abnormal vaginal bleeding. Next, an assessment for possible coagulation problems should be done by asking screening questions about the onset of the heavy bleeding, excessive bleeding after childbirth or surgery, and a history of hemorrhagic nose bleeds, gum bleeds, or easy bruising. If the patient gives a positive answer to these questions, consider coagulation testing, such as testing of von Willebrand factor. Basic laboratory evaluation for this patient would include a pregnancy test with β-chorionic gonadotropin (β-hCG), coagulation factors, thyroid stimulating hormone (TSH), and a complete blood count (CBC). An endometrial biopsy should be performed in any woman older than 45 years with abnormal bleeding or in younger women with risk factors for endometrial cancer such as obesity or nulliparity.

CLINICAL PEARL   **STEPS 2/3**

When taking a history and physical on a female patient, it is very important to obtain a thorough gynecologic and obstetric history. This includes questions about menstrual pattern, sexual activity, gynecologic surgeries and infections, contraceptive method, and pregnancy outcomes. It is equally important not to ignore the patient's general medical, surgical, and family histories as these factors can impact treatment options even for gynecologic conditions.

    The patient reports a history of normal menstrual periods until approximately 4 years ago when she underwent tubal ligation. Menarche was age 11 years. Menses used to last 3–5 days with 1 day of heavy flow until 1 year ago; it now lasts 7–10 days with heavy, painful flow and passage of "golfball-sized" clots. She uses up to nine overnight pads per day. She denies a family history of gynecologic cancer but reports that her mother and both older sisters had hysterectomies in their 30s. She denies a family or personal history of easy bruising or bleeding. She has a history of three term cesarean sections, a tubal ligation, and one spontaneous miscarriage. She has never required a blood transfusion. Her last Pap smear was normal 2 years ago. A urine β-hCG in the emergency room is negative.

What is the definition of abnormal menstrual bleeding, and what are the causes?
A normal menstrual period lasts approximately 5 days with a cycle length (time between menses) ranging from 21 to 35 days. Assessment of "normal" menstrual blood loss is difficult and highly subjective. Heavy menstrual bleeding has been defined as greater than 80 mL, but this research definition is not clinically helpful and a woman's perception of blood loss is most useful in assessing excessive blood loss.

What is the best imaging test to evaluate this patient's abnormal physical exam?
Transvaginal ultrasonography is the most cost-effective and useful initial imaging modality for evaluation of pelvic masses suspected to be gynecologic in origin. If the endometrial lining appears to contain a lesion or a better assessment of the endometrial cavity is needed, either a saline infusion sonogram or an office hysteroscopy can be performed. If a pelvic mass is not clearly evaluated on ultrasound, in some cases magnetic resonance imaging (MRI) can be used to better characterize the mass.

A pelvic ultrasound is ordered and shows a uterus measuring 12 × 7.5 × 9 cm. The endometrial thickness is 5 mm. The myometrium contains multiple hypoechoic lesions, the largest of which is in the left anterior uterine body and measures 7.2 × 6.8 × 6.5 cm. Both ovaries are small (2 × 4 cm) and normal in appearance, and no adnexal masses are noted.

What is the diagnosis? How do you counsel the patient about the ultrasound?
This patient has uterine leiomyoma, otherwise known as uterine fibroids. The large left anterior fibroid just described accounts for the mass that was palpated on exam.

What are fibroids, and how are they related to bleeding and symptoms?
Fibroids (leiomyomas) are benign masses and can occur in many sizes and in different locations within the uterus; they are the leading indication for hysterectomy in the United States. The most common type are intramural, located within the myometrium of the uterus. These may or may not impact bleeding and fertility. Submucosal fibroids, located closest to the endometrium, are the least common but most likely to cause abnormal bleeding. Subserosal fibroids distort the external contour of the uterus and can cause bulk symptoms such as pain or pelvic pressure but have less impact on bleeding. Pedunculated fibroids extend off the serosa of the uterus on a stalk and can be mistaken for an adnexal mass (Fig. 33.1).

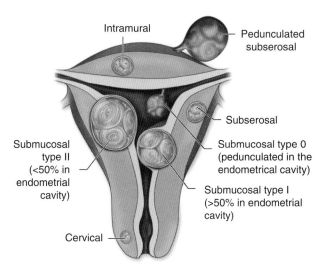

Fig. 33.1 Uterine fibroid types as demonstrated by location, including intramural, pedunculated, subserosal, and submucosal (type I, II, and III) fibroid locations. *(From Fielding JR et al.* Gynecologic Imaging. *Philadelphia: WB Saunders; 2011.)*

How are fibroids related to hormones?

Fibroids are comprised of hormonally responsive tissues and contain progesterone receptors. In premenopausal women, fibroids can grow in response to endogenous hormones and become very large. In postmenopausal women who no longer have significant hormone production by the ovaries, fibroid-related symptoms tend to resolve.

What are the next steps in managing this patient's bleeding and acute anemia?

In a patient who is hemodynamically unstable, uterine curettage is the first-line treatment for heavy, ongoing uterine bleeding as it will generally result in a rapid cessation of blood loss, usually in less than an hour. Medical management can be combined with curettage in the hemodynamically unstable patient or can be used alone in women who are hemodynamically stable. In patients presenting with hemorrhage and symptomatic anemia or a hemoglobin less than 7 mg/dL, blood transfusion may be necessary. Medical management most commonly involves the use of high-dose intravenous (IV) estrogen, oral estrogen, oral combined contraceptive pill tapers, or high-dose oral progestins. IV estrogen promotes endometrial stabilization and regrowth and usually stops bleeding within 5 hours of initial administration. The most common side effect is nausea and vomiting; antiemetics can be given to patients during this therapy.

CLINICAL PEARL   **STEPS 2/3**

A personal history of venous thromboembolism, myocardial infarction, cerebrovascular accident or stroke, active cancer, or thrombophilia is an absolute contraindication to estrogen therapy. Other conditions such as hypertension, diabetes mellitus, smoking over the age of 35, or lupus are relative contraindications, meaning that acute therapy with estrogen may be safe in the short term, and risks and benefits must be weighed.

An oral contraceptive pill taper using a pill containing 35 μg ethinyl estradiol can be used in women with moderate bleeding. Generally, five pills are given on day 1, four pills on day 2, three pills on day 3, two pills on day 4, and one pill a day to complete the pack. This method usually stops bleeding within 48 hours. For women who have contraindications to estrogen-containing therapy, progestin therapy can be used. Progestins manage bleeding by preventing further proliferation of the endometrium. Medroxyprogesterone acetate (Provera) 10–20 mg twice daily or megestrol acetate (Megace) 20–60 mg twice daily can be continued for 1–2 months to stop bleeding and improve anemia. Side effects of these medications include bloating, weight gain, acne, and mood changes.

The patient receives IV fluid resuscitation in the emergency room. The decision is made to administer a high-dose oral conjugated equine estrogen 2.5 mg four times daily to stop her acute bleeding episode. Oral iron three times daily and antiemetics are ordered. She is admitted for observation to the gynecology service.

What treatment options can the patient be offered once her acute bleeding episode is resolved and her anemia is stabilized?

The treatments for uterine leiomyoma include medical, procedural, and surgical options. Treatment is tailored to the patient's symptoms and her future pregnancy plans. Medical management for heavy bleeding as discussed earlier may be less effective in women with fibroids, so treatment to remove or interrupt blood flow to fibroids may be needed. However, for women who desire to avoid surgery or want to preserve fertility, medications can provide short-term symptom relief. For women considering surgery who have anemia and bulk symptoms related to very large uterine leiomyoma, gonadotropin-releasing hormone (GnRH) agonists such as leuprolide acetate can improve hemoglobin and reduce fibroid size preoperatively.

BASIC SCIENCE PEARL   **STEP 1**

GnRH agonists work by binding pituitary GnRH receptors, creating an initial surge in luteinizing hormone (LH) and follicle-stimulating hormone (FSH). With time, as these receptors become saturated, LH and FSH secretion decreases, leading to suppression of ovarian function and decreased production of estrogen and progesterone from the ovaries. This creates an artificial, menopause-like state, so side effects include hot flashes, night sweats, and vaginal dryness.

For women who desire to retain their uterus for future pregnancy, a surgical procedure called *myomectomy* can be offered to remove the fibroids. Depending on fibroid burden and symptoms, this fertility-preserving surgery may or may not improve bleeding and bulk symptoms. Young patients with multiple fibroids must be counseled that new fibroids may occur later in life, potentially requiring future surgery. Myomectomy can be done through an open incision or laparoscopically through the abdomen or hysteroscopically through the endometrium, based on the location and number of fibroids. For women who have completed childbearing, two procedural options exist: uterine artery embolization and hysterectomy. Uterine artery embolization is an interventional radiology procedure in which the vessels feeding the uterine fibroids are catheterized and occluded using polyvinyl alcohol particles or trisacryl gelatin microspheres. This procedure is intended to improve heavy bleeding and will generally decrease uterine size by only a small amount. Hysterectomy definitively treats heavy menstrual bleeding as well as the pelvic pain and pressure many women experience with large fibroids, but it is the most aggressive treatment, so typically is not considered before alternative management has been considered or attempted.

The patient's bleeding stops within 6 hours of beginning estrogen therapy. Her hemoglobin remains stable on hospital day 2, and she is discharged with oral iron therapy and a continuous oral contraceptive pill. She is strongly considering hysterectomy and plans to follow up in the office in 1 week to discuss this option.

BEYOND THE PEARLS

- Alternate treatment options for fibroids have been innovated in recent years, including the newest offering of radiofrequency fibroid ablation. This is administered via laparoscopy, with ultrasound used to localize each fibroid. A needle tip is inserted into the fibroid and radiofrequency energy is applied to heat and ablate the leiomyoma. Successful pregnancy has been attained in women who have undergone this procedure.
- The impact of fibroids on infertility is not entirely clear. In general, fibroids that are completely or partially submucosal are believed to negatively impact pregnancy since they distort the endometrial cavity, preventing implantation and increasing the likelihood of miscarriage and/or preterm birth. Subserosal and pedunculated fibroids are generally not thought to affect the ability to become pregnant, and the effect of intramural fibroids is unclear.
- After menopause, fibroids generally do not grow because hormone stimulation is lacking. If rapid growth of a fibroid is seen in a postmenopausal woman, one's index of suspicion for a malignant process should be high.

Case Summary

- A 42-year-old woman presents with vaginal bleeding, a pelvic mass, and acute anemia.
- A transabdominal and transvaginal ultrasound is performed to better assess the mass palpated on her pelvic exam; this is consistent with uterine leiomyoma.
- She is assessed to be hemodynamically stable. Her acute bleeding is treated with oral ethinyl estradiol and she receives fluid resuscitation.
- The patient's bleeding stops over the next few hours. She is counseled about her management options for fibroids and plans to follow up in an outpatient clinic. She is discharged with medication to prevent further bleeding and iron for her anemia.

References

American College of Obstetricians and Gynecologists (2008). Alternatives to hysterectomy in the management of leiomyomas. ACOG Practice Bulletin No. 96. *Obstet Gynecol, 112*, 201–207.

American College of Obstetricians and Gynecologists (2012). Diagnosis of abnormal uterine bleeding in reproductive-aged women. ACOG Practice Bulletin No. 128. *Obstet Gynecol, 120*, 197–206.

Galen, D., et al. (2014). Laparoscopic radiofrequency fibroid ablation: phase II and phase III results. *J Soc Laparoendoscop Surg, 18*, 182–190.

Marjoribanks, J., Lethaby, A., & Farquhar, C. (2006). Surgery versus medical therapy for heavy menstrual bleeding. *Cochrane Database Syst Rev* (2), CD003855.

Valerie Valant, BA ▪ Christy Williams, BS ▪ Jessica Shepherd, MD, MBA

A 38-Year-Old Woman With Acute Pelvic Pain

A 38-year-old G0 woman presents to your outpatient clinic complaining of pelvic pain for the past 2 days. The pain is localized to the left side, intermittent throughout the day, and mild (3/10) in severity but causes her to wake up at night. She has no past medical or surgical history, does not take any medications, and her menses are regular. She denies fevers, nausea, vomiting, or vaginal discharge, but reports intermittent constipation over the past few months. Vitals signs include a temperature of 37°C (98.7°F), blood pressure of 128/78 mm Hg, heart rate of 64/min, respiratory rate of 14/min, and an oxygen saturation of 99% on room air.

What is your initial differential diagnosis?
When formulating a differential diagnosis for pain, it is important to think about the structures surrounding the location of the pain. Systems relevant to the patient's left pelvic pain and constipation include gastrointestinal, musculoskeletal, urinary, and reproductive. Diagnoses to consider would include appendicitis, urinary tract infection (UTI), kidney stones, ectopic pregnancy, ovarian cysts, and pelvic inflammatory disease (PID).

CLINICAL PEARL   **STEPS 2/3**

Always start off with a broad differential diagnosis. As you collect the patient's history and physical, begin to rank each diagnosis as either (1) most likely, (2) least likely, or (3) most dangerous or potentially fatal. These categories will help you determine the most important tests you should order and prevent you from missing the diagnoses that are most dangerous to the patient.

Why is it important to consider the age of the patient?
The patient's history includes symptoms suspicious for an adnexal mass, such as unilateral pelvic pain and constipation. The adnexa are the spaces between the pelvic sidewalls and the uterus and contain the ovaries, fallopian tubes, and support ligaments. When an adnexal mass is suspected, the age and reproductive status of the patient narrows the differential diagnosis. In women of reproductive age, masses are most likely gynecologic and related to the menstrual cycle. In women of peri- or postmenopausal age, masses are most commonly benign tumors, but the incidence of malignancy is higher in this population. Since the patient is perimenopausal, our differential should include both benign and malignant etiologies. A family history of gynecologic malignancy and family members' ages at diagnosis could be helpful in raising suspicion for malignancy as well.

CLINICAL PEARL STEPS 2/3

A pregnancy test should be ordered for every woman of reproductive age who is reporting abdominal pain, nausea, vomiting, or vaginal bleeding. Ectopic pregnancies are the most common cause of pregnancy-related deaths in the first trimester and should not be missed.

BASIC SCIENCE PEARL STEP 1

Family history should always be taken in the setting of an adnexal mass, specifically about breast, ovarian, or colon cancer, since a family history of these increases a patient's lifetime risk of ovarian cancer. Inherited mutations in the breast cancer (BRCA) genes 1 and 2 increase the lifetime risk of developing breast or ovarian cancer, as do Lynch syndrome or hereditary nonpolyposis colorectal cancer (HNPCC).

During your history, the patient shares that her sister was diagnosed and successfully treated for breast cancer at the age of 38. Her maternal grandmother also died of an unknown cancer type at the age of 67.

What other risk factors should you ask about in the history?

In addition to age and family history, other risk factors that increase the risk of ovarian cancer include nulliparity (having never given birth), early menarche, late menopause, and history of primary infertility and endometriosis. The use of combined oral contraceptives decreases the risk of certain ovarian cancers.

On the patient's physical exam, the abdomen is negative for tenderness, guarding, or peritoneal signs. During the bimanual pelvic exam, you palpate a mass in the left lower pelvis. The mass is motile and feels soft, but size is difficult to assess, and she is tender to palpation in that region. No other masses were appreciated on rectovaginal exam.

What negative physical exam findings are important in this case?

Pertinent negatives are as important to report as pertinent positives in helping make the diagnosis. In this patient, the rectovaginal exam is important to help rule out gastrointestinal-related diagnoses, to locate a mass in the posterior pelvis, or to assess for certain manifestations of malignancy, such as nodularity in the posterior cul-de-sac associated with metastatic ovarian cancer. The abdominal exam is also important to evaluate for more life-threatening presentations, such as ovarian torsion, ruptured ovarian cysts, or a ruptured ectopic pregnancy, which present with more severe pain, or signs of peritonitis (such as abdominal rebound or guarding). Because this patient has intermittent pain, the possibility of intermittent ovarian torsion (the ovary twisting and untwisting on its vascular axis, causing intermittent ischemia) is also still a possibility.

CLINICAL PEARL STEPS 2/3

The absence of a palpable mass on pelvic exam cannot completely exclude an adnexal cyst or tumor. The mass may be too small to palpate, may have decompressed if it has ruptured, or may have shifted into a different location within the pelvis or abdomen.

Which laboratory test should be ordered for this patient?

Because our patient is of reproductive age, she should first receive a pregnancy test by measuring the urine or serum β-human chorionic gonadotropin (β-hCG). A complete blood count (CBC) can detect possible anemia from bleeding caused by an ectopic pregnancy or a ruptured cyst and assess for leukocytosis (white blood cell elevation) caused by PID or another infectious process. Last, if you are suspicious of malignancy, a number of serum biomarkers can be obtained. The most common type of ovarian cancer, epithelial ovarian cancer (EOC), is associated with an elevated cancer antigen 125 (CA 125) in 80% of patients. This biomarker is useful for establishing a baseline CA 125 level and for monitoring patients during and after treatment. It is not useful as a screening test, because fewer than 50% of patients with stage 1 EOC have abnormal CA 125 and many noncancerous conditions, such as menstruation, pregnancy, uterine fibroids, PID, and endometriosis, can have elevated CA 125 levels. Other tests for the evaluation of EOC risk include the human epididymis protein (HE4), OVA1 biomarker panel (Vermillion, Inc.), and the Risk of Malignancy Algorithm (ROMA). Non-EOC types of ovarian tumors, such as germ cell tumors or stromal tumors, are associated with distinct serum biomarkers such as α-fetoprotein (AFP), human chorionic gonadotrophin (hCG), lactate dehydrogenase (LDH), estradiol (E2), inhibin A or B, dehydroepiandrostenedione (DHEA), or antimullerian hormone (AMH). Additionally, while not useful in identifying malignant adnexal masses, carcinoembryonic antigen (CEA) can be helpful in identifying metastatic ovarian malignancy, and cancer antigen 19-9 (CA 19-9) is associated with certain germ cell tumors.

Her pregnancy test is negative. CBC is within normal range. The patient's CA 125 is 22 U/mL (normal <35 U/mL), which is equivocal for our diagnostics.

What type of imaging test should be ordered for this patient's evaluation?

A transvaginal ultrasound (TVUS) is the imaging study of choice for the evaluation of an adnexal mass. It is inexpensive and is highly sensitive and specific in determining whether the mass is benign or malignant. The "Simple Rules" are TVUS criteria used to determine risk of malignancy. The benign characteristics include the following: unilocular cyst, solid components present (<7 mm), acoustic shadows, smooth multilocular tumor with largest diameter (<100 mm), and no blood flow (color score 1). Malignant features include an irregular, solid tumor; ascites; at least four papillary structures; irregular multilocular-solid tumor with largest diameter (≥100 mm); and very strong flow (color score 4). If the TVUS result is indeterminate, or if further imaging is needed, magnetic resonance imaging (MRI) can be used for diagnostic evaluation. (Fig. 34.1)

A transvaginal ultrasound identifies an 11.3 cm cyst in the left ovary. The cyst is multilocular, with sonographically detectable septations. The wall appears to have a regular surface with no nodularity or projections noted.

CLINICAL PEARL   **STEPS 2/3**

When following up on imaging studies for your patients, first examine the image yourself without looking at the radiologist's impression. Frequent practice will help you to learn radiologic appearance and better understand the pathophysiology of your patients.

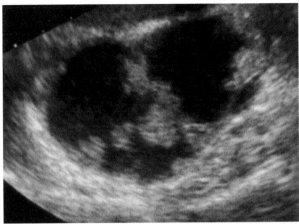

Fig. 34.1 Transvaginal ultrasound of a complex ovarian mass that proved to be cancerous. Note the appearance of solid component (echogenic vs. fluid-filled), septations, and the irregularities in wall thickness.

What is our next step in management?

Management depends on the patient's age, clinical presentation, and cyst characteristics. In reproductive-aged women, conservative management may be considered for asymptomatic simple cysts with no suspicious features on initial ultrasound. Current guidelines state that simple cysts of 5 cm or less do not need follow-up, whereas simple cysts of 5–7 cm should have yearly TVUS because cyst size increase is associated with risk of ovarian torsion. Surgical evaluation and removal of the cyst becomes the standard of care when the cyst exceeds 7 cm, or is persistent, complex, or associated with pain or signs of malignancy. In postmenopausal women, annual follow-up can be considered for cysts in the size range of 1–7 cm, but it is important to note that surgery is the only means of definitively ruling out malignancy. In our patient, her age, presentation of intermittent pain, and constipation make torsion or mass effect more likely, and the presence of a multiloculated cyst with septations on TVUS makes surgical evaluation the best choice.

CLINICAL PEARL   **STEPS 2/3**

During your preoperative interview for a woman of reproductive age, it is important to ask about her interest in future fertility. Certain types of ovarian cysts can have high risk of recurrence or malignant potential. If a woman desires children in the future, it is appropriate to remove only the cystic ovary (or in certain cases only the cyst itself, leaving the ovary in place). However, if a woman is not planning future pregnancies, risk of a contralateral mass or cyst is weighed against the risks of menopause.

The patient undergoes a laparoscopic surgery to evaluate her cyst. On entry into the abdomen, she is found to have a large left ovarian cyst with one twist of torsion seen in the ovary, but the ovary on untwisting appears perfused and viable. Before the surgery, the patient shared that she is considering having children in the next few years, and a unilateral left oophorectomy is performed in order to preserve her fertility. She recovers from surgery without any complications. Pathology demonstrates a benign, multilocular cyst with clear watery fluid and small papillary projections along the inner lining.

Based upon this information, what is the most likely diagnosis in this patient?
Ovarian serous cystadenoma is the most likely diagnosis, because this is the most common epithelial ovarian neoplasm. Of serous cystadenomas, 70% are benign, 10% have malignant potential, and 20% are malignant. The optimal treatment is surgical due to the risk of future ovarian torsion and malignant transformation.

How are adnexal masses categorized?
The classification of adnexal masses is quite broad but can be organized into three groups: functional ovarian cysts, benign ovarian neoplasms, and malignant ovarian neoplasms.

1. *Functional ovarian cysts*: Arising from normal ovarian function, these include follicular cysts, corpus luteum cysts, and theca lutein cysts. These cysts are benign and are the most common reason for a mass in reproductive-aged women. Most will resolve spontaneously in 1–3 months and can be managed expectantly.

2. *Benign ovarian neoplasms*: Masses are categorized based on the cell type of origin and include germ cell tumors (benign cystic teratoma/dermoid cyst), epithelial cell tumors (serous cystadenoma, mucinous cystadenoma, endometrioid tumor, Brenner cell), and stromal cell tumors (granulosa cells, Sertoli-Leydig, ovarian fibroma). Benign neoplasms are the most common cause of masses in postmenopausal women, but malignancy should be thoroughly ruled out for this age group because the rate of ovarian cancer increases with age.

3. *Malignant ovarian neoplasms*: Ovarian cancer is the fifth leading cause of cancer-related death among women in the United States, with presentation most commonly occurring in the fifth to sixth decades of life. Classification is by cell type of origin: malignant germ cell tumors, malignant epithelial cell tumors, and malignant stromal cells. Of the gynecologic malignancies, ovarian cancers have the highest rate of mortality because they are difficult to detect before metastasis occurs. Therefore, risk assessment is key to early diagnosis.

Two weeks later, the patient is doing well, and her pelvic pain and constipation have resolved. It is recommended that she returns to her primary care physician for annual gynecologic care. However, considering her family history, you advise the patient to consider genetic counseling.

CLINICAL PEARL   **STEPS 2/3**

When considering sending a patient for genetic counseling, it is important to know factors that will increase her risk. For ovarian cancer, this includes a known BRCA gene mutation identified on testing, a family history of gynecologic cancer, a family history of HNPCC, or another history suggestive of a hereditary cancer syndrome. Genetic counseling allows patients to have their personal and family cancer risk assessed. The American College of Obstetricians and Gynecologists (ACOG) recommends that risk-reducing salpingo-oophorectomy, complete removal of the ovaries and fallopian tubes, be offered by age 40 years for women with BRCA mutations because these patients have a 12%–46% lifetime risk of ovarian cancer.

BEYOND THE PEARLS

- Pregnancy distorts abdominal and pelvic anatomy as the uterus grows during fetal gestation. If a woman presents with upper abdominal pain or vague back pain, it is important to include ovarian cyst/torsion/rupture and appendicitis on your differential even though this is not the usual location of these structures.

BEYOND THE PEARLS—cont'd

- While both ovarian arteries come directly off the abdominal aorta, the right ovarian vein connects directly to the inferior vena cava while the left ovarian vein joins the left renal vein before connecting to the inferior vena cava. Both the artery and vein bilaterally are located within the suspensory or infundibulopelvic (IP) ligament of the ovary.
- As noted earlier, risk factors for development of ovarian cancer include nulliparity, early menarche, and late menopause. It is hypothesized that uninterrupted ovarian cycles during the reproductive years or periods of repeated ovarian stimulation lead to malignant transformation. Conversely, combined oral contraceptive use and breast-feeding, which prevent ovulation, are demonstrated to have protective effects by the same mechanism.
- There are currently no effective or recommended methods to screen for ovarian cancer. Although various tools have been assessed, such as serial CA 125 levels or pelvic ultrasounds, neither have shown to improve morbidity or mortality outcomes in women with ovarian cancer. The U.S. Preventative Services Task Force (USPSTF) currently states that for women with no symptoms, screening for ovarian cancer is not helpful and may actually lead to harm.
- Recent evidence suggests that many primary peritoneal, primary tubal, and some ovarian cancers actually originate in the fallopian tube. This is why the ACOG recommends bilateral salpingo-oophorectomies for women at an increased risk for ovarian cancer, such as those with BRCA mutations.

Case Summary

- A 38-year-old woman presents with acute pelvic pain, and her pelvic exam reveals a palpable mass and tenderness in the left adnexa. A transvaginal pelvic ultrasound displays an 11.3 cm complex left ovarian cyst.
- Based on her age, a family history of breast cancer, and appearance of the cyst, the decision is made for surgical exploration. A laparoscopic left oophorectomy is performed to allow the patient to preserve her fertility, and pathologic evaluation reveals a benign ovarian serous cystadenoma.
- Two weeks after surgery, the patient's pain resolves, and she is referred for genetic counseling due to her family history of gynecologic malignancy.

References

American College of Obstetricians and Gynecologists (ACOG) (2009). ACOG Practice Bulletin No. 103: hereditary breast and ovarian cancer syndrome. *Obstetrics and Gynecology, 113,* 957–966.

American College of Obstetricians and Gynecologists (ACOG) (2007). ACOG Practice bulletin No. 83: management of adnexal masses. *Obstetrics and Gynecology, 110*(1), 201–214.

Bozkurt, M., Yumru, A. E., & Aral, I. (2013). Evaluation of the importance of the serum levels of CA-125, CA15-3, CA-19-9, carcinoembryonic antigen and alpha fetoprotein for distinguishing benign and malignant adnexal masses and contribution of different test combinations to diagnostic accuracy. *European Journal of Gynaecological Oncology, 34*(6), 540–544.

Erickson, B. K., Conner, M. G., & Landen, C. N., Jr. (2013). The role of the fallopian tube in the origin of ovarian cancer. *American Journal of Obstetrics and Gynecology, 209*(5), 409–414.

Epithelial ovarian cancer. (2016). In B. L. Hoffman, J. O. Schorge, & K. D. Bradshaw, (Eds.), *Williams gynecology* (3rd ed.) (p. 735). New York: McGraw-Hill Education.

Lacey, J. V., & Sherman, M. E. (2009). Ovarian neoplasia. In S. L. Robboy, G. L. Mutter, & J. Prat (Eds.), *Robboy's Pathology of the female reproductive tract* (2nd ed.) (p. 601). Oxford: Churchill Livingstone Elsevier.

Levine, D., Brown, D. L., Andreotti, R. F., et al. (2010). Management of asymptomatic ovarian and other adnexal cysts imaged at US: society of radiologists in ultrasound consensus conference statement. *Radiology, 256*(3),943–954.

Lyons, Y. A., Soliman, P. T., & Frumovitz, M. M. (2014). The pelvic mass workup. *Contemporary Ob/Gyn, 59*(4).

Sagi-Dain, L., Lavie, O., Auslander, R., & Sagi, S. (2015). CA 19-9 in evaluation of adnexal mass: retrospective cohort analysis and review of the literature. *The International Journal of Biological Markers, 30*(3), 333–340.

Sagi-Dain, L., Lavie, O., Auslander, R., & Sagi, S. (2015). CEA in evaluation of adnexal mass: retrospective cohort analysis and review of the literature. *The International Journal of Biological Markers, 30*(4), 394–400.

Wei, S., Li, H., & Zhang, B. (July 2016). The diagnostic value of serum HE4 and CA-125 and ROMA index in ovarian cancer. *Biomedicine Report, 5*(1), 41–44.

Zimmerman, D., Van Calster, B., Testa, A., et al. (2016). Predicting the risk of malignancy in adnexal masses based on the simple rules from the international ovarian tumor analysis group. *American Journal of Obstetrics and Gynecology, 214*(4), 424–437.

Mark Dassel, MD

A 17-Year-Old Girl With Recent Onset of Pelvic Pain

A 17-year-old G0 girl presents to the emergency department with her mother reporting a dull, pelvic "ache" for 3 weeks. She has intermittent chills without fevers. She denies sexual activity and has an active lifestyle playing for the school basketball team. She has regular monthly periods that are "a little bit crampy," and her last period was 3 weeks ago. She denies any vaginal discharge or itching. Her vital signs show a temperature of 37.6°C (99.7°F) and a heart rate of 100/min with normal blood pressure, respiratory rate, and oxygen saturation. On physical exam, her lower abdomen is tender without guarding or rebound. A pelvic exam shows bilateral adnexal tenderness and discomfort on motion of the cervix, and the cervix is friable.

What are common causes of pelvic pain in a young female?

It is common to consider pelvic pain in a female as being of genital origin, but it is important to consider an expanded differential. For example, the gastrointestinal system ends in the pelvis, so inflammatory bowel disease, intestinal diseases, and irritable bowel syndrome can cause pelvic pain, as can urinary disorders such as interstitial cystitis or calculi. Pelvic pain may also be neuromuscular, such as pelvic floor tension myalgia or myofascial abdominal pain. Psychological stressors such as anxiety disorders, posttraumatic stress disorder, and physical or sexual abuse are also linked to abdominal pain. Pregnancy complications, such as an ectopic pregnancy, must always be considered. In a young and possibly sexually active female, common etiologies include endometriosis, sexual assault, ectopic or intrauterine pregnancy, urinary tract infection (UTI), appendicitis, pelvic inflammatory disease (PID), and tubo-ovarian abscess (TOA). In this patient with a recent onset and some signs of a pelvic infection, PID and TOA must be kept high on the differential.

What should be done to evaluate this patient?

First, in this young woman of reproductive age, regardless of reported sexual activity, a pregnancy test must be performed. Ultrasound or computed tomography (CT) imaging can evaluate for TOA. Laboratory tests to evaluate for infection include C-reactive protein (CRP), a complete blood count (CBC), and gonorrhea/*Chlamydia* testing. However, it is important to know that the diagnosis of PID is clinical, made primarily on physical exam, and no one test is diagnostic or can rule it out.

CLINICAL PEARL STEPS 2/3

When fluid can be seen in the fallopian tubes or uterine cavity, suspicion increases for PID as the diagnosis. However, this finding is neither sensitive nor specific.

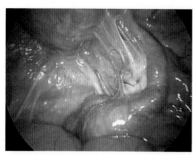
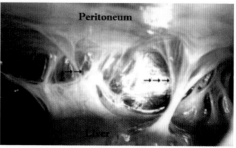

Fig. 35.1 Laparoscopic view of pelvic inflammatory disease (PID), with purulent swelling of the right fallopian tube and pelvic adhesions *(left)* and a laparoscopic view of perihepatic adhesions *(arrows)* caused by PID, otherwise known as Fitz-Hugh-Curtis syndrome *(right)*. Left image https://www.clinicalkey.com/#!/content/book/3-s2.0-B9780702031205000242?scrollTo=%233-s2.0-B9780702031205000242-f10. Right image https://www.clini-calkey.com/#!/content/journal/1-s2.0-S2213307013001032?scrollTo=%231-s2.0-S2213307013001032-gr2.

What is pelvic inflammatory disease?

PID is an infection of the lower female genital tract caused by ascension of microorganisms from the vagina or cervix into the uterus, fallopian tubes/ovaries, or peritoneal cavity. It occurs in 750,000 women per year in the United States. Most PID is polymicrobial, but the majority of cases result from sexually transmitted infections (STIs), with 15% of untreated *Chlamydia trachomatis* and *Neisseria gonorrhea* cervical infections progressing to PID. *N. gonorrhoeae* is present in 30%–80% of PID; *C. trachomatis* is present in 20%–40% of PID and higher in women with perihepatic adhesions (Fitz-Hugh-Curtis syndrome). However, 15% of PID results from respiratory or enteric sources, such as *Escherichia coli* or *Enterococcus* species. Chronic PID (symptoms >30 days) is more commonly caused by *Mycobacterium tuberculosis* or *Actinomyces* species (Fig. 35.1).

BASIC SCIENCE PEARL   **STEP 1**

Bacterial vaginosis produces enzymes that degrade cervical mucus, which impairs the barrier to ascending infection and facilitates bacterial spread to the upper genital tract.

How does PID present? What are the risks of not recognizing PID?

The diagnosis of PID is difficult to confirm, and the symptoms can mimic other conditions. The typical clinical scenario is subacute pelvic or abdominal pain following a menstrual period in a woman with risk factors for STI, and pain is often severe enough to seek medical care. Physical exam often reveals cervical motion, uterine, or adnexal tenderness, and there may be signs of pelvic inflammation such as mucopurulent discharge from the cervix, copious white blood cells on a wet prep (often with coexistent bacterial vaginosis [BV]), and a friable cervix. The diagnostic criteria for PID require cervical motion tenderness and/or pelvic organ tenderness not be explained by other causes. Other diagnostic criteria, such as a temperature of greater than 38.3°C (101°F), white blood cells in vaginal secretion microscopy, or elevated inflammatory markers like CRP are more specific but have decreased sensitivity. It is important to note that approximately 60% of PID is subclinical, stressing the importance of screening asymptomatic patients at risk: women aged 16–25 who are sexually active or women of any age with multiple or new sexual partners. Failure to recognize and treat PID can result in tubal factor infertility, ectopic pregnancy, and chronic pelvic pain.

What history is needed when PID is suspected, and what are risk factors for PID?

Because of the nonspecific diagnostic criteria of PID, a history detailing the patient's risk factors for PID is very important in identifying candidates for empiric antibiotic therapy. Risk factors for

PID include adolescence, a prior diagnosis of PID or gonorrhea/*Chlamydia* infection, male partners with gonorrhea/*Chlamydia*, multiple sex partners, douching, BV, oral contraceptive use, lower socioeconomic status, and insertion of an intrauterine device (IUD) in the past 21 days. The risk associated with IUD placement is decreased with negative prescreening for gonorrhea/*Chlamydia*.

BASIC SCIENCE PEARL	STEP 1

Genetic factors play a role in susceptibility to PID, including toll-like receptor (TLRs) variants that allow increased progression of *C. trachomatis* into PID infection.

CLINICAL SCIENCE PEARL	STEPS 2/3

Gynecologic procedures such as endometrial sampling and hysteroscopy break the cervical infection barrier, increasing the risk for women to develop ascending infections including endometritis and PID.

The patient has a CT scan that finds no diagnostic abnormalities. Her CBC demonstrates a white blood cell count of 9.5×10^9 cells/L. During your discussion with the patient and her mother, the patient denies sexual activity in the past, but you think you see some relief in her face when you mention her pregnancy test is negative.

How should the physician address sensitive issues with a patient when family members are present?

Because 85% of cases of PID are related to genital tract infections, sexual activity is related to the development of PID. Often parents and adolescent patients may have different religious and cultural views regarding sexual activity, making an adolescent presenting for evaluation of a pelvic infection a potentially volatile situation. For this reason, and to screen for a history of abuse, it is vital to speak to all patients, particularly adolescents, without other family members or accompanying parties in the room. It is essential that the practitioner is aware of the regional legality of providing medical care to minors, because laws significantly differ among states. Some states allow the treatment of a minor without the consent of a legal guardian only if the minor is pregnant, while others also allow the treatment of STIs, including PID, and provision of contraception without guardian involvement. The first step is to politely explain to the patient and the accompanying person that it is important that you speak to the patient alone and assure them that it is best for patient safety and compliance with laws. Any questions about sexual activity or abuse (mental, physical, or sexual) should then be addressed. Questions about other sensitive issues, such as alcohol or drug use and contraception needs, can be asked at this time as well. It is also a good idea to obtain a safe contact number so the results of sensitive tests or certain conversations can be discussed with the patient without violating her privacy. Patients should be informed of the Health Insurance Portability and Accountability Act (HIPAA) privacy laws—as well as the exceptions, such as if a patient shares information that will put her or another in danger if not disclosed to a third party.

Once the patient's family leaves the room, she tells you that she has had unprotected sex with two partners in the last 6 months. She reports that all encounters were consensual and denies any physical, mental, or sexual abuse. She also requests information on contraception. You explain to her that, based on her findings, she may have PID. You explain her treatment options.

What makes a patient a candidate for empiric treatment of PID?

When the diagnosis of PID is suspected and other etiologies reasonably ruled out, the practitioner should feel comfortable empirically treating PID. Error should be on the side of overtreatment, and treatment should be initiated per the Centers for Disease Control and Prevention (CDC) published guidelines. Most PID can be treated in an outpatient setting, and this has similar results to inpatient parenteral antibiotic regimens in low-risk populations. Regardless of treatment setting, success should be reevaluated within 72 hours, and if substantial clinical improvement is not seen, the diagnosis should be reevaluated. If the diagnosis is confirmed, a parenteral regimen should be initiated with the addition of metronidazole (if not already used). Inpatient admission is indicated when a patient is nonresponsive to oral therapy, is pregnant, a surgical emergency cannot be excluded (appendicitis, ectopic pregnancy), the patient is severely ill (vomiting, high fever, evidence of septic shock) or has a TOA, or the patient is unable follow-up or tolerate her oral antibiotics. Surgical intervention is indicated when a diagnosis cannot be distinguished from an emergent cause or when a TOA is nonresponsive to antibiotic therapy and unable to be drained percutaneously (Box 35.1).

> After discussion with the patient, and given her lack of TOA and stability, you opt to treat her as an outpatient. You practice in a state where you can treat STIs without consent of a guardian, and the patient asks you not to tell her mother the specifics of her diagnosis. She gives you a private cell phone number to call her in follow-up. Prior to the patient leaving, you discuss ways to reduce her risk of recurrence of PID, including condom use and treating her current partner. You also discuss contraceptive options with her, and she is interested in oral contraceptive pills (OCPs). She receives intramuscular (IM) ceftriaxone in the emergency room and a 2-week prescription for doxycycline and metronidazole.

How can the patient reduce her risk for recurrent PID? How does this affect her future fertility?

A single episode of PID increases the risk of tubal factor infertility to 8%, while recurrence increases the risk to 20%. A second recurrence increases tubal factor infertility to 50%. Abstinence, monogamy, reduced number of sex partners, cessation of douching (if relevant), and the use of latex condoms can decrease the risk of PID recurrence. Furthermore, a patient with PID should be instructed to abstain from sex until she and her sex partner have been treated. Some states permit that therapy be prescribed to a known partner without seeing the partner in clinic (expedited partner therapy), while other states require sexual partners to be evaluated by medical personnel prior to receiving treatment.

What contraception is safe for a woman with PID?

There are no contraindicated contraceptive methods for women with a history of PID. An IUD should not be placed in a woman with active PID until resolution of symptoms and completion of antibiotics, but it can be placed safely after treatment. If an IUD is present when PID is diagnosed, it can be left in place unless symptoms persist despite treatment. There is conflicting data on the use of OCPs and PID because sexual activity is a risk factor for both OCP use and PID, but there are no contraindications to OCP use after treatment.

> The patient is contacted by phone 48 hours after leaving the emergency room. She states that she is tolerating the antibiotics, has no fevers, and notes resolution of her abdominal pain. She has started using her OCPs and is abstaining from sex with her male partner until he is treated.

CENTERS FOR DISEASE CONTROL AND PREVENTION (CDC) RECOMMENDED TREATMENT REGIMENS FOR EMPIRIC TREATMENT OF PELVIC INFLAMMATORY DISEASE (PID)	BOX 35.1

Oral Treatment Regimens

Oral Regimen A

Ceftriaxone 250 mg intramuscularly in a single dose *plus*
Doxycycline 100 mg orally twice daily for 14 days
With or without metronidazole 500 mg orally twice daily for 14 days

Oral Regimen B

Cefoxitin 2 g intramuscularly in a single dose *plus*
Probenecid 1 g orally administered concurrently in a single dose *plus*
Doxycycline 100 mg orally twice daily for 14 days
With or without metronidazole 500 mg orally twice daily for 14 days

Oral Regimen C

Other parenteral third-generation cephalosporin *plus*
Doxycycline 100 mg orally twice daily for 14 days
With or without metronidazole 500 mg orally twice daily for 14 days

Parenteral Treatment Regimens (Continue for 24 Hours after Clinical Improvement)

Parenteral Regimen A

Cefotetan 2 g intravenously (IV) every 12 hours *or*
Cefoxitin 2 g IV every 6 hours *plus*
Doxycycline 100 mg orally or IV every 12 hours

Parenteral Regimen B

Clindamycin 900 mg IV every 8 hours *plus*
Gentamicin loading dose IV or intramuscularly 2 mg/kg *followed by*
Gentamicin maintenance dose 1.5 mg/kg IV every 8 hours *or*
Gentamicin IV 3–5 mg/kg once daily

Alternative Parenteral Regimen

Ampicillin/Sulbactam 3 g intravenously every 6 hours *plus*
Doxycycline 100 mg orally or intravenously every 12 hours

Oral Therapy after Parenteral Therapy (14 Days after Parenteral Completed)

Doxycycline 100 mg orally twice a day *or*
Clindamycin 450 mg orally four times a day

BEYOND THE PEARLS

- Historical treatment of PID was total abdominal hysterectomy, bilateral salpingo-oophorectomy, and pelvic washout, but with modern antibiotics and interventional radiologic techniques, such as percutaneous placement of drains into abscesses, these less invasive approaches typically cure PID.
- Genital tuberculosis, present in 1% of tuberculosis-positive cases, is almost always secondary to hematogenous spread, but can be spread primarily by sexual contact.
- One of the definitive trials that identified treatment efficacy in PID is the Pelvic Inflammatory Disease Evaluation and Clinical Health (PEACH) trial. It demonstrated that cefoxitin-doxycycline therapy was equally effective among mild to moderate cases of PID whether it is given in an inpatient or outpatient setting.
- Fitz-Hugh-Curtis syndrome is caused by an inflammation on Glisson's capsule, a thin layer of connective tissue surrounding the liver. This results in right upper quadrant pain and characteristic "violin string" adhesions anterior to the liver.

Case Summary

- A 17-year-old sexually active girl presents with abdominal-pelvic pain of 3 weeks' duration. Laboratory testing indicates that she is not pregnant and has a normal white blood cell count. CT scan yields no abnormal findings.
- The patient is diagnosed with PID based on clinical symptoms and exclusion of other etiologies for her pain. An outpatient regimen of intramuscular ceftriaxone followed by oral doxycycline and metronidazole is initiated, and the patient is improved within 48 hours.
- The patient also receives counseling on prevention of recurrent PID and STIs and initiates contraception with OCPs.

References

Brunham, R. C., Gottlieb, S. L., & Paavonen, J. (2015). Pelvic inflammatory disease. *The New England Journal of Medicine*, *372*(21), 2039–2048.

Centers for Disease Control and Prevention (CDC) (1991). Pelvic inflammatory disease: guidelines for prevention and management. *Morbidity and Mortality Weekly Report*, *40*(RR-5), 1–21.

Centers for Disease Control and Prevention (CDC). (2015). *Pelvic inflammatory disease (PID); Sexually Transmitted Diseases; Treatment, STD Treatment Guidelines*. http://www.cdc.gov/std/tg2015/pid.htm.

Ness, R. B., et al. (2002). Effectiveness of inpatient and outpatient treatment strategies for women with pelvic inflammatory disease: results from the Pelvic Inflammatory Disease Evaluation and Clinical Health (PEACH) randomized trial. *American Journal of Obstetrics and Gynecology*, *186*, 929–937.

Traci Ito, MD ■ Shan Biscette, MD, MSc

A 28-Year-Old Woman With Abdominal Pain and Vaginal Bleeding

A 28-year-old G3P0020 woman presents to the emergency department with intermittent vaginal bleeding and mild, colicky right lower abdominal pain for 2 days. Her last menses was approximately 6 weeks ago, although her menses are typically "irregular." She has no significant medical or surgical history except a history of *Chlamydia* diagnosed and treated 4 years ago. Her past pregnancies resulted in firsttrimester miscarriages, but she had a positive home pregnancy test yesterday.

What are your differential diagnoses for this patient?
Abdominal pain and vaginal bleeding are often nonspecific symptoms that can be seen in cases of spontaneous abortion, appendicitis, pelvic inflammatory disease, (PID) ovarian torsion, ruptured ovarian cyst, or a normal or abnormal pregnancy. The finding of a positive urine pregnancy test suggests that the most likely diagnosis is pregnancy, and further evaluation is needed to rule out serious complications of pregnancy.

CLINICAL PEARL	**STEPS 2/3**

Evaluation of any reproductive-age woman with symptoms of abdominal pain and vaginal bleeding should include a thorough history and physical exam as well as a prompt pregnancy test. The history should review menstrual pattern, previous sexually transmitted infections (STIs), contraceptive use, and obstetric history, including any ectopic pregnancies or assisted reproductive technology (ART) use. The physical exam should include vital signs and circulatory exam to assess hemodynamic stability and abdominal and pelvic exams to assess for location of pain, evaluate the source and volume of bleeding, and obtain any pertinent vaginal tests such as cervical cultures.

What is your next step in the evaluation of this patient?
A transvaginal ultrasound (TVUS) and blood tests are performed, including a complete blood count (CBC) to evaluate for anemia that could result from intra-abdominal bleeding, such as from a bleeding ovarian cyst like a corpus luteum or an ectopic pregnancy. The patient should also have a blood type and screen done to ensure, as she is pregnant, that she is not rhesus D (RhD) antigen negative and at risk for Rh isoimmunization disease.

The patient's abdominal exam shows a soft abdomen with tenderness in the left lower quadrant without guarding or rebound. Her pelvic exam shows a mobile, nontender uterus without palpable adnexal masses, and she has 10 mL of dark red blood in the vaginal vault and a normal cervix. Her blood type is A Rh negative, β-human chorionic gonadotropin (β-hCG) is 1000 mIU/mL, white blood cell count is 11 × 10⁹ cells/L, hemoglobin is 11 g/dL, hematocrit is 33%, and platelets are 210,000 /mcL. The TVUS shows an irregular fluid collection in the uterine cavity, no fetal pole or yolk sac, and normal adnexal structures.

Based on these findings, what diagnoses are possible or likely?

The triad of amenorrhea, irregular vaginal bleeding, and abdominal pain can occur in normal pregnancy, but also in abnormal pregnancies such as spontaneous abortion or ectopic pregnancy. TVUS and β-hCG may not be diagnostic on initial testing, so it is important to be complete, repeat testing, and look for trends. For example, an ectopic pregnancy usually cannot be diagnosed by TVUS alone on initial evaluation unless a gestational sac with a yolk sac and an embryo is clearly seen outside the uterus, so ultrasound findings should be correlated with physical exam findings and β-hCG levels.

CLINICAL PEARL   **STEPS 2/3**

Risk factors for ectopic pregnancy include prior ectopic pregnancy, previous gonorrheal or chlamydial cervical infection or pelvic inflammatory disease, previous tubal surgery, current use of intrauterine device, ART, and cigarette smoking.

What findings are suggestive of a normal intrauterine pregnancy (IUP) or an ectopic pregnancy on ultrasound?

An IUP develops between the endometrial layers and creates a "double sac sign" seen as early as 4–5 weeks' gestation, where double echogenic rings surround a hypoechoic center. By contrast, a pseudo-sac, seen within the uterus in some ectopic pregnancies, has irregular borders and no "double sac." Other TVUS signs that are suggestive of ectopic pregnancy include an extrauterine gestational sac with or without a yolk sac or an embryo, fetal cardiac activity outside the uterus, the presence of an adnexal mass with a hyperechoic ring that illuminates on Doppler flow studies ("ring of fire"), and free fluid that would suggest ectopic bleeding (Fig. 36.1).

What physical exam findings would be concerning for an ectopic pregnancy?

In a patient with a stable ectopic pregnancy, abdominal pain can be generalized, unilateral, or bilateral. Additional signs such as cervical motion tenderness (CMT), a palpable adnexal mass, or rebound tenderness may or may not be present. Ruptured ectopic pregnancies may demonstrate peritoneal signs of intraabdominal hemorrhage such as rebound and guarding on abdominal exam and signs of shock such as hypotension and tachycardia. This patient has a lower β-hCG level, and her physical exam and TVUS findings are not consistent with an acute emergency, so it would be appropriate for the patient to follow-up in 48 hours for a repeat β-hCG level and TVUS. If her pregnancy is normal, her β-hCG should double in 48 hours, whereas a β-hCG increase of less than 53% in 48 hours is diagnostic of an abnormal pregnancy.

Before the patient leaves the emergency room, you administer Rho(D) immune globulin due to her RhD negative status and first-trimester bleeding. The patient returns to the office for a follow-up β-hCG and TVUS 2 days later, and her β-hCG is now 1800 mIU/mL. Repeat ultrasound reveals an empty uterus and a 1.4 cm adnexal, cystic structure without a gestational sac. Her pain is unchanged since her last visit, and her vaginal bleeding has lessened to intermittent spotting.

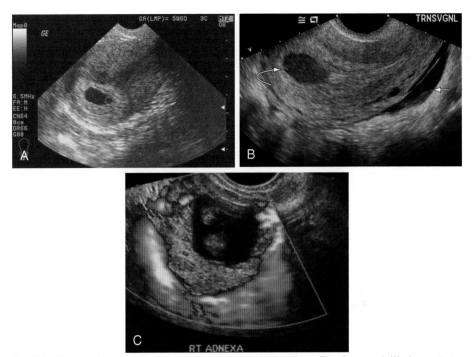

Fig. 36.1 Sonographic appearances of different pregnancy locations. The first panel (A) demonstrates a round, "double-ring" intrauterine gestational sac, consistent with an intrauterine pregnancy (IUP). The second panel (B) shows a pseudo-sac of heterogeneous material in the uterus consistent with an abnormal pregnancy or a pregnancy that is outside the uterus. The last panel (C) demonstrates the "ring of fire" sign of a mass in the adnexa with surrounding vasculature demonstrated by Doppler imaging. This mass in the adnexa is suspicious for an ectopic pregnancy. A image: *https://www.clinicalkey.com/#!/content/ journal/1-s2.0-S0733862712000338?scrollTo=%231-s2.0-S0733862712000338-gr2* B image: *https://www. clinicalkey.com/#!/content/book/3-s2.0-B9781437715750100210?scrollTo=%233-s2.0- B9781437715750100210-f21-03-9781437715750* C image: *https://www.clinicalkey.com/#!/content/journal/1- s2.0-S088721710800005X?scrollTo=%231-s2.0-S088721710800005X-gr15*

BASIC SCIENCE/CLINICAL PEARL	**STEPS 1/2/3**

RhD antigens on blood cells are an autosomal recessive trait, so women who are RhD negative have no genetic copies for RhD antigens, have serum antibodies to RhD, and are at risk of developing antibodies when exposed to RhD-positive fetal red blood cells (a process called isoimmunization). Fetal cells may have Rh antigens if the father of the baby is RhD positive. Future pregnancies with RhD-positive fetuses of isoimmunized women may result in those fetuses having their erythrocytes lysed by maternal antibodies to RhD, causing hemolytic disease of the fetus and newborn. Rho(D) immune globulin, RhD antibodies that can bind fetal blood cell antigens in maternal blood and prevent isoimmunization, is given in any circumstance where the mother may be exposed to fetal genetic material, including ectopic pregnancy.

Why are these findings concerning for a pregnancy of abnormal location?

The discriminatory zone for β-hCG between 1500 and 2000 mIU/mL is a reliable marker for when an intrauterine gestational sac should be visualized in the uterus in the case of a normal IUP. Therefore, when a β-hCG exceeds these levels and an IUP is not visualized, this is highly suggestive of an ectopic pregnancy.

You discuss your concerns that the pregnancy is ectopic and discuss treatment options for the patient. However, she states that this is a desired pregnancy and prefers to "wait and see" as her bleeding has improved.

What would be your concerns about observing this patient further?
Any patient in whom you suspect a pregnancy of abnormal location should be counseled on the risks of ectopic rupture and intraabdominal bleeding. She should be counseled that ectopic pregnancies cause severe blood loss, shock, and death that can occur minutes to hours after onset of bleeding, making it imperative that she is close to emergent care.

CLINICAL PEARL   **STEPS 2/3**

Ectopic pregnancies may be located in the cervix, ovary, abdominal cavity, cornua of the uterus, or a previous cesarean section scar, but 97% of ectopic pregnancies implant in the fallopian tube, making it the most common site.

The patient is scheduled for a follow-up visit in 48 hours, and you strongly advise her to return urgently to the emergency room for any symptoms such as worsening pain, syncope, or weakness.

Is medical management an option for this patient?
There are several questions that need to be answered prior to considering methotrexate (MTX) as an option for treatment of a suspected ectopic pregnancy. MTX is a folic acid antagonist. Specifically, it inactivates dihydrofolate reductase thereby preventing production of tetrahydrofolate from the precursor dihydrofolic acid. The patient in this scenario is hemodynamically stable and there is no evidence of an IUP. Both factors allow the use of MTX. In addition to the β-hCG, type and screen, and CBC this patient had earlier, a complete metabolic panel is needed for evaluation of hepatic and renal function. If there is no evidence of hepatic or renal dysfunction, history of sensitivity to MTX, pulmonary disease, peptic ulcer disease, immunodeficiency, or residual concern that a normal pregnancy may be present, MTX use can be considered. There are features about the pregnancy based on size and appearance on TVUS that may diminish the success of MTX and are therefore relative contraindications. MTX would be a good option for this patient if she was willing and had normal laboratory findings (Table 36.1).

TABLE 36.1 ■ Relative and Absolute Contraindications to the Use of Methotrexate (MTX) in the Medical Treatment of Ectopic Pregnancy

Absolute Contraindications	Relative Contraindications
• Intrauterine pregnancy	• Embryonic cardiac activity on TVUS
• Hemodynamically unstable patient	• β-hCG >5000 mIU/mL
• Hepatic or renal deficiency	• Ectopic pregnancy >3.5 cm in size on TVUS
• Sensitivity to MTX	
• Immunodeficiency	
• Pulmonary disease	
• Peptic ulcer disease	
• Breast feeding	

Based on history and physical exam, laboratory evaluation, and transvaginal ultrasound (TVUS) criteria.

The patient returns to the emergency department 5 days later with sudden-onset severe abdominal pain, a constant urge to defecate, and dizziness with ambulation. Her blood pressure is 105/78, heart rate is 112/min, respiratory rate is 19/min, and oxygen saturation is 98% on room air. Her physical exam is significant for tenderness of the lower right side of her abdomen accompanied by rebound and guarding. Her labs reveal a β-hCG of 2400 mIU/ml, hemoglobin of 8.0 g/dL, and hematocrit of 24%. TVUS shows an empty uterus, a complex right adnexal mass measuring 3.0 cm, and moderate free fluid in the pelvis.

What is the patient's diagnosis?

This patient has a ruptured ectopic pregnancy, which is a surgical emergency. Given the risk for hemorrhagic shock and death, prompt surgical evaluation and control of bleeding is indicated, along with readiness for fluid resuscitation and blood transfusion. Laparoscopy or laparotomy may be performed as the surgical approach. Laparoscopy is preferred if the ectopic pregnancy is unruptured, and it is sometimes feasible even in ruptured pregnancies. Laparotomy should only be used if the surgeon is not comfortable with the laparoscopic approach, the patient is hemodynamically unstable, or if good visualization is not possible during laparoscopy. Surgery may include a salpingectomy (removal of the fallopian tube) or a salpingostomy (opening of the tube with removal of the pregnancy tissue inside, which allows for tubal preservation) if the ectopic is tubal in location.

The patient undergoes an emergent laparoscopic procedure with a right salpingectomy and evacuation of hemoperitoneum. She receives 2 units of packed red blood cells due to symptomatic anemia and a postoperative hemoglobin of 6 g/dL. She is discharged on postoperative day 1. At her follow-up visit 10 days later, the patient has no complaints.

How would you counsel a patient with one former ectopic pregnancy and unilateral salpingectomy about future pregnancy?

The patient should not have any negative effect on her ability to become pregnant in the future, provided that her ovaries and remaining tube are normal in function. However, the rate of ectopic pregnancy after a single ectopic pregnancy is 20% (range 8%–72%). Therefore, women with a history of ectopic pregnancies should have early monitoring with pelvic ultrasound in subsequent pregnancies.

BEYOND THE PEARLS

- Interstitial pregnancy (commonly referred to as cornual pregnancy) accounts for up to 2.5% of ectopic pregnancies. These pregnancies occur in the proximal segment of the fallopian tube within the wall of the uterus. They present as ruptured ectopic pregnancies in 20%–50% of cases due to delays in diagnosis associated with the eccentric location of the pregnancy.
- Ovarian pregnancies account for 0.5%–3% of ectopic pregnancies. For a pregnancy to be characterized as a true ovarian pregnancy, four Spiegelburg's criteria must be met: (1) the gestational sac is in the region of the ovary, (2) the pregnancy is attached to the uterus by the ovarian ligament, (3) ovarian tissue is histologically demonstrated in the walls of the gestational sac, and (4) the tube on the involved side is intact.
- A heterotopic pregnancy is defined as a combined intrauterine and extrauterine pregnancy and has an incidence of 1 in 4000 pregnancies in the general population. The incidence is increased to 1% in women who have undergone in vitro fertilization.
- In women who desire future fertility, salpingostomy is the preferred surgical method in unruptured tubal ectopic pregnancies. However, studies have shown similar intrauterine pregnancy rates following salpingostomy versus salpingectomy and the preserved fallopian tube is at increased risk of forming a future ectopic pregnancy, so this should be discussed with a woman prior to a surgery if possible .

Case Summary

- A 28-year-old woman presents with abdominal pain and vaginal bleeding. Initial serum β-hCG is 1000 mIU/mL and pelvic ultrasound indicates a pregnancy of unknown location. Rho(D) immune globulin is given for prophylaxis due to RhD-negative status.
- Follow-up evaluation 2 days later shows a β-hCG of 1800 mIU/mL and TVUS shows an empty uterus with an adnexal mass, suspicious for ectopic pregnancy. The patient declines treatment.
- The patient presents to the emergency room 5 days later with a ruptured ectopic pregnancy. An emergent laparoscopic right salpingectomy is performed, the patient is given blood products, and she recovers well.

References

Alkatout, I., Honemeyer, U., Strauss, A., et al. (2013). Clinical diagnosis and treatment of ectopic pregnancy. *Obstetrical & Gynecological Survey*, *68*, 571.

Farquhar, C. M. (2005). Ectopic pregnancy. *Lancet*, *366*, 583.

Lipscomb, G. H., Bran, D., McCord, M. L., et al. (1999). Predictors of success of methotrexate treatment in women with tubal ectopic pregnancies. *The New England Journal of Medicine*, *341*, 1974.

Ashley Bergin, MD, MPH

A 19-Year-Old With Postoperative Fever and Lower Abdominal Pain

A 19-year-old woman, G1P0, presents for an induced abortion at 11 weeks' gestation by dilation and curettage (D&C). Four days after the D&C, she presents to the emergency room with fevers, abdominal pain and cramping, and light vaginal bleeding (using three to four incompletely soaked pads/day). On physical examination, her temperature is 38.1°C (100.6°F), blood pressure is 100/58 mm Hg, heart rate is 105/min, respiration rate is 24/min, and oxygen saturation is 98% on room air. Her lower abdomen is diffusely tender to palpation, and speculum exam demonstrates 10 mL of blood in the vaginal vault. A urine pregnancy test is positive. Complete blood count (CBC) results show that the patient's white blood cell count is 15,000/uL, and her hemoglobin is 9.6 g/dL.

What is the differential diagnosis for this patient?

Following induced abortion, it is not uncommon for patients to experience pelvic cramping and unpredictable uterine bleeding. The β-human chorionic gonadotropin (β-hCG) hormone can remain detectable in serum for around 30 days and sometimes as long as 60 days after an induced abortion. Fevers, nausea, vomiting, and diarrhea can occur following administration of misoprostol, a medication used in medical abortion. As this patient had a surgical abortion (D&C), the findings of fever, leukocytosis, and abdominal pain point to an infectious process. Infection following induced abortion is most commonly due to endometritis, abscess, or retained products of conception (RPOC). Persistent "cramping," lower abdominal pain, or continued bleeding after an induced abortion is characteristic of RPOC, while any of the above with the addition of fever or leukocytosis is more characteristic of postabortion endometritis. If pain, fever, or leukocytosis is severe, a pelvic abscess should be considered.

CLINICAL PEARL	STEPS 2/3

When evaluating a patient postoperatively following an induced abortion, a complete obstetric and gynecologic history should be obtained, specifically in regards to risk for sexually transmitted infections such as gonorrhea or chlamydia. In addition, it is helpful to know where the D&C was performed and what type of anesthesia was used. If the patient had not given the gestational age at which she had the procedure performed or the procedure type, that information should also be collected.

CLINICAL PEARL	STEPS 2/3

The risk for postabortal endometritis, which is one of the inflammatory conditions encompassed by the term pelvic inflammatory disease (PID), is increased several-fold when cervical chlamydia or gonococcal infections are present. It is unknown whether infection with bacterial vaginosis (BV)—a condition characterized by high numbers of pathogenic anaerobic bacteria in the vagina—at the time of surgical abortion increases the risk for infection. While BV is associated with PID, studies that have treated women for BV preoperatively have not found a reduction in postabortal infection. A diagnosis of candidiasis or trichomoniasis does not increase the risk for infection and should not prohibit the patient from receiving her abortion.

What are the next steps in the patient's evaluation?

Obtaining cervical cultures for gonorrhea and chlamydia may help identify the pathogen responsible for the infection, although negative cultures do not guarantee that an infection is not present. Potassium hydroxide (KOH) and normal saline preparations of the vaginal discharge can help identify yeast, trichomonas, or BV. Transvaginal ultrasound (TVUS) with color Doppler would be the best choice for evaluation of this patient. TVUS assesses for the presence of endometritis, abscess, and RPOC, so it is the first-line imaging modality in this case. Findings characteristic of RPOC include a thickened, heterogeneous endometrial echo complex (EEC) and/or an endometrial or intrauterine mass on grayscale ultrasound. If a pelvic abscess is suspected and TVUS findings are unclear, computed tomography (CT) can be obtained. Blood and uterine cultures are of low yield in the evaluation of this patient.

BASIC SCIENCE PEARL	STEP 1

RPOC are comprised of intrauterine tissue that develops following conception and persists following abortion. This tissue is derived from placental trophoblastic cells which invade and attach to the endometrium. These trophoblastic cells form chorionic villi, which are projections comprised of mesenchymal cores that invade the decidua basalis of the endometrium (Fig. 37.1). If a repeat D&C is performed, the pathologic diagnosis of RPOC is made if chorionic villi are found in the surgical specimen.

CLINICAL PEARL	STEPS 2/3

The addition of color Doppler flow to grayscale TVUS increases the accurate detection of RPOC by a factor of two (Fig. 37.2). This is because the detection of vascularity (active color flow in the tissue) within a thickened EEC or intrauterine mass is suggestive of RPOC. In contrast, avascularity within an ECC is suggestive of blood clots without RPOC.

Clinical, laboratory, and ultrasound findings are all used when making the diagnosis of RPOC.

The patient undergoes TVUS and a thickened, hypoechoic endometrium is seen. The surrounding myometrium is homogeneous, and a small, physiologic amount of free fluid is seen in the pelvis. When color Doppler flow is applied, increased vascularity within the endometrium is noted.

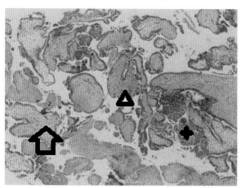

Fig. 37.1 Microscopy of a curettage specimen from a surgical termination of pregnancy. The photo shows finger-like chorionic villi mixed with maternal decidual tissue (purple staining tissue) and maternal red blood cells. *(From Fuchs N, et al. Clinical, surgical, and histopathologic outcomes following failed medical abortion. Int J Gynecol Obstet. 2012;117(3):234–238.)*

What is the most likely cause of this patient's symptoms?
All of the infectious causes previously discussed (endometritis, abscess, or RPOC) are in the differential diagnosis. The lack of a thickened, heterogeneous endometrium or intrauterine mass on TVUS makes RPOC lower on the differential. When pelvic abscess is present, clinical findings include higher fevers, abdominal rebound tenderness, severe abdominal or pelvic pain, and leukocytosis from 17,500 to 30,000/uL. TVUS findings characteristic of pelvic abscess include a complex adnexal cystic structure that often contains debris, fluid–fluid levels, and hyperechoic, thick walls, which this patient does not exhibit. In this patient, the findings are most consistent with a diagnosis of postabortal endometritis.

What factors lead to increased risk for postabortal endometritis?
Factors that are known to increase the risk for postabortal endometritis include an age younger than 20 years, a history of PID, and infection with gonorrhea and/or chlamydia at the time of surgery. This patient's age puts her at risk for postabortal endometritis, and her gynecologic history will have revealed whether she has any of the other listed risk factors. Most postabortal endometritis occurs in women who have no risk factors.

BASIC SCIENCE PEARL   **STEP 1**

Recent studies have demonstrated that fewer than 50% of cases of PID are attributable to *Neisseria gonorrhoeae* and *Chlamydia trachomatis*. Most ascending genital tract infections are polymicrobial and contain microorganisms found in the vagina, such as anaerobes *Gardnerella vaginalis, Haemophilus influenzae,* enteric gram-negative rods, and *Streptococcus agalactiae.* Cytomegalovirus (CMV), *Mycoplasma genitalium, Ureaplasma urealyticum,* and *Mycoplasma hominis* may also be associated with some cases of PID. Thus, antibiotic treatment should be broad spectrum.

Could this postabortal endometritis have been prevented?
Prophylactic antibiotics reduce the risk of postabortal endometritis by 40%. Currently, there are no published studies comparing different regimens of antibiotics, so the optimal regimen is unknown. Nitroimidazoles, such as metronidazole, and tetracyclines, such as doxycycline, have both been found to be effective. Doxycycline is inexpensive and can be given orally or parenterally. Nausea and emesis are the most common side effects of doxycycline ingestion, and these can be mitigated if doxycycline is taken with food. In current practice, preoperative administration of doxycycline appears to be most beneficial and is most commonly used.

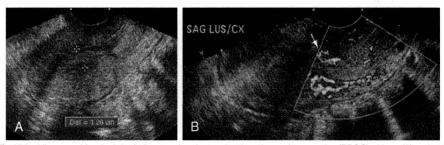

Fig. 37.2 Ultrasound *(sagittal view)* of uterus showing retained products of conception (RPOC) without (A) and with Doppler imaging (B) depicting thickened endometrial stripe and increased blood flow over the thickened portion of the endometrium, which together are suspicious for RPOC. *(From Durfee S. Retained products of conception. In: Gynecologic Imaging. Expert Radiology Series. Philadelphia: WB Saunders; 2011: 356–366.)*

How is postabortal endometritis treated?

Postabortal endometritis is treated in the same way that PID is treated, with broad-spectrum coverage that takes into account the pathogens most likely responsible. If the patient is stable and can be managed in the outpatient setting, a combination of ceftriaxone, doxycycline, and metronidazole can be used. If the patient meets any criteria for admission (i.e., tubo-ovarian abscess, sepsis, pregnancy, or fails outpatient management), parenteral regimens that include a third-generation cephalosporin such as cefotetan and doxycycline can be used. Treatment with gentamicin and clindamycin would also be acceptable. As this patient has a low-grade fever and no apparent signs of sepsis, she is a candidate for outpatient treatment with ceftriaxone, doxycycline, and metronidazole. If RPOC are seen on ultrasound, the patient should receive a dose of antibiotics and undergo repeat uterine aspiration. When the patient is unstable, unreliable, or unsuitable for follow-up, or a pelvic abscess is noted, the patient should be admitted to the hospital for parental antibiotics for at least 24 hours, and failure to improve in 48–72 hours would mandate surgical drainage. Surgical interventions can include radiologic-guided drainage of the abscess, laparoscopic surgery, or laparotomy.

> The patient received one dose of intramuscular ceftriaxone and a 2-week course of both doxycycline and metronidazole.

When should she follow up with her provider?

The patient should return to the clinic for evaluation in 3 days to ensure that the oral antibiotic regimen is working. If her fevers have not subsided or her pain is not significantly improved, consideration should be given to hospitalization where parenteral antibiotics can be administered and additional imaging or diagnostic laparoscopy can be performed.

> The patient misses her appointment 3 days later, but follows up a week later and reports that she has been taking the antibiotics as instructed and her pain is gone. You instruct her to finish the course of antibiotics, not resume sexual activity until she has reliable contraception, and to follow up in 1 month.

Why is it important to treat postabortal endometritis?

When postabortal endometritis is not treated, the patient is at increased risk for developing chronic pelvic pain, dyspareunia, secondary infertility, and sepsis, and is at increased risk for having future spontaneous abortions. The ascending genital tract infection leads to inflammation within the upper reproductive tract, resulting in damage to pelvic structures. As the morbidity associated with postabortal endometritis is high, it is extremely important to treat patients quickly once the diagnosis has been made.

Could this patient have had postabortal placement of an intrauterine device (IUD)?

Multiple studies have demonstrated that placement of an IUD immediately postabortion does not increase risk for infection even among high-risk patients, such as nulliparous adolescents who are at higher risk for postabortal infection.

> The patient returns to your office 1 month later and is counseled on postabortion contraception options. She opts to have an levonorgestrel IUD placed. Three months later, she has resumed sexual activity with her one male partner, is happy with this contraception, and is relieved that her risk of further unwanted pregnancy is now minimal.

BEYOND THE PEARLS

- Modern studies with adequate antibiotic prophylaxis show that less than 1% of women experience upper genital tract infection following medical or surgical induced abortion.
- Studies examining different vaginal preparations prior to induced abortion have demonstrated no difference between no vaginal preparation or using chlorhexidine digluconate in relation to occurrence of postabortal endometritis. This may be due to inability of the vaginal preparation to reduce numbers of bacteria in the endocervix.
- The effectiveness of preabortion antibiotics (such as doxycycline) in preventing postabortal endometritis is likely due to systemic administration, which may be more effective at eliminating bacteria from the endocervix than local vaginal preparation. Studies estimate that treating all patients with a perioperative dose of antibiotics would result in a 50% decrease in postabortal infections in the United States.

Case Summary

- A 19-year-old woman presents to the emergency room following induced abortion at 11 weeks' gestation with fevers, cramping, and an elevated white blood cell count. She was found to have postabortal endometritis based on her clinical presentation and findings on color Doppler ultrasound.
- The patient was sent home with antibiotics and had clinical improvement with resolution of pain. One month later, she is offered contraception options and receives a levonorgestrel IUD.

References

Achilles, S. L., & Reeves, M. F. (2011). Prevention of infection after induced abortion. *Contraception, 83*(4), 295–309.

Centers for Disease Control and Prevention (2015). Sexually transmitted diseases treatment guidelines, 2015. *MMWR, 64*(RR-03), 1–137.

Paul, M., Lichtenberg, S., Borgatta, L., Grimes, D. A., Stubblefield, P. G., & Creinin, M. D. (Eds.), (2011). *Management of unintended and abnormal pregnancy: comprehensive abortion care.* New York: John Wiley & Sons.

Sellmyer, M. A., Desser, T. S., Maturen, K. E., Jeffrey, R. B., Jr., & Kamaya, A. (2013). Physiologic, histologic, and imaging features of retained products of conception. *Radiographics, 33*(3), 781–796.

Shah C. (n.d.). *Endometritis.* Retrieved August 12, 2016, from https://sonoworld.com/CaseDetails/Endome tritis.aspx?ModuleCategoryId=572

Laura Anne Mihalko, MD ■ Frances Alba, MD

A 34-Year-Old Woman With Postoperative Flank Pain

A 34-year-old woman undergoes elective laparoscopic total abdominal hysterectomy for uterine leiomyomas. The next day on the gynecology floor, she develops right flank pain, nausea, and vomiting. She is afebrile, with a blood pressure of 140/86 mm Hg, a heart rate of 94/min, a respiration rate of 16/min, and oxygen saturation of 97% on room air. The patient's abdomen is soft, nondistended, and appropriately tender to palpation. Her incision sites are well approximated. She has mild right costovertebral angle tenderness. Her creatinine is 0.8 mg/dL; her white blood cell count is 12,000/µL. Her nausea improves slightly with ondansetron.

What is your differential diagnosis for this patient?

These symptoms can be due to side effects of the medications (such as anesthesia or opioids) or postoperative ileus. Her unilateral flank pain broadens the differential diagnosis to include musculoskeletal pain, pyelonephritis, nephrolithiasis, or acute urinary obstruction. Other less likely diagnoses include appendicitis, cholecystitis, renal infarction, or pleuritic chest pain due to pulmonary embolism. An infectious process is less likely because she is afebrile and has leukocytosis as expected for a postoperative state. In the setting of recent pelvic surgery, unilateral flank pain with nausea and vomiting is concerning for an iatrogenic ureteral injury with associated ipsilateral acute urinary obstruction. Unrecognized ureteral injury or obstruction can result in urinoma, abscess, ureteral stricture, urinary fistula, and, ultimately, loss of the kidney, so the index of suspicion should be kept high.

> This patient's symptoms are attributed to postsurgical pain and nausea secondary to opiate medications, and further investigation is not pursued. The flank pain, nausea, and vomiting improve somewhat, and she is discharged home on postoperative day 3.

BASIC SCIENCE PEARL   **STEP 1**

Flank or groin pain associated with urinary obstruction is proposed to be secondary to increased proximal intraluminal pressure within the ureter and renal pelvis. Stretching of the ureter wall and renal capsule occurs secondary to accumulation of urine and results in the sensation of pain through mechanoreceptors and the excitation of spinothalamic C fibers.

What diagnostic imaging techniques might have evaluated the patient's initial symptoms of flank pain, nausea, and vomiting?

A postoperative plain X-ray film of the abdomen and pelvis (kidney-ureters-bladder or KUB) is an appropriate initial choice to evaluate the gaseous bowel distention seen in postoperative ileus or to reveal radiopaque urolithiasis. A renal ultrasound would evaluate for the presence of hydronephrosis in the setting of acute ureteral obstruction and avoids ionizing radiation and the risks of intravenous (IV) contrast, so it is safe for pregnant patients or patients with renal failure or contrast allergy. If the level of clinical suspicion is high for ureteral obstruction or injury, the gold standard imaging technique is multiphasic computed tomography (CT) of the abdomen and pelvis with contrast. A triple-phase CT to evaluate the kidneys, ureters, and bladder is also known as a CT urogram (phase 1 without contrast, phase 2 with IV contrast, and phase 3 delayed by approximately 10 minutes to allow the kidneys to begin excreting the contrast dye into the collecting system). The third phase should display contrast within the renal pelvis, ureters, and bladder. If a patient is unable to receive IV contrast due to allergic reaction or renal insufficiency, a retrograde pyelogram in the operating room may be performed by fluoroscopy with cystoscopic retrograde injection of contrast through the distal ureteral orifices.

CLINICAL PEARL	STEPS 2/3

A CT urogram is a useful imaging modality in multiple clinical settings. Urolithiasis, renal masses, and renal cysts are seen on the initial noncontrast phase, and the contrast phase can identify benign and malignant renal masses. The third excretion phase can reveal hydronephrosis, ureteral obstruction, filling defects secondary to malignancies, or extravasation of urine due to injury at any level.

BASIC SCIENCE PEARL	STEP 1

An objective indicator of acute urinary obstruction is the presence of acute worsening of renal function. Obstruction of urine outflow causes increased pressure within the ureteral lumen. This increases pressure in the renal system and diminishes the pressure gradient across the glomerular basement membrane, interfering with renal filtration at the level of the glomerulus.

The patient returns to your clinic 1 month after surgery. She reports that she had persistent flank pain and nausea, but was otherwise doing well. Then, about 2 weeks ago, she developed constant urinary incontinence requiring many pads per day. She noted marked improvement in the nausea and right flank pain around the time that the incontinence began. She denies abdominal pain, dysuria, fevers, or chills. There are otherwise no new symptoms or changes reported, and her vital signs are within normal on exam today.

How do you classify the different types of urinary incontinence?
Urinary incontinence is defined as the involuntary loss of urine and is classified based on symptoms: stress incontinence, urge incontinence, mixed incontinence, and continuous incontinence. Stress urinary incontinence is leakage of urine during physical exertion or activities that increase abdominal pressure, such as coughing, sneezing, or exercise, whereas urge incontinence is associated with a sudden desire to urinate and inability to postpone voiding. Mixed incontinence is a combination of both stress and urge incontinence. Continuous incontinence is a constant leakage of urine that occurs without the sensation to void. It can occur when a nonfunctional bladder is filled to capacity and "overflows" or in the setting of a urinary fistula. A more complete history and physical will help to elicit the type of incontinence.

The patient describes continuous leakage of urine, even throughout the night. However, she does still have sensation to void and urinates normal volumes intermittently during the day. She reports that she will soak through a large pad within 2 hours. She is not sure if leakage is from the urethra because she "can't feel it coming out." Leakage is not associated with coughing, laughing, or sense of urgency. On speculum exam, her vaginal mucosa is moist, with rugae, and without abnormalities of the urethral meatus. The vaginal apex incision is intact, without evidence of granulation tissue at the incision or elsewhere in the vagina. After a few minutes of inspection, pooling of urine is noted in the dependent portion of the vagina, but no defects in the vaginal wall are seen. Her postvoid residual with ultrasound is 0 mL after a 150-mL void.

What is the most likely cause of the patient's urinary incontinence?
Stress incontinence is not consistent with this patient's presentation since the leakage of urine is unrelated to coughing, sneezing, laughing, or physical activity. The incontinence does not correlate with a sense of urgency to void, and overflow incontinence is unlikely in the setting of normal bladder emptying. It would be appropriate to check a urinalysis and possible urine culture, but a urinary tract infection is more likely to present with suprapubic pain, increased urinary frequency, and dysuria. This patient has the unique clinical feature of continuous urinary leakage that appears to be coming directly from the vagina. In the postsurgical setting, we keep suspicion high for a fistula, an abnormal connection between the urinary system and the vagina which bypasses the normal micturition pathway. A uretero-vaginal or vesico-vaginal fistula is high on the list for this patient's differential diagnosis.

What test can you do in the office to specifically evaluate this patient for a fistula?
The best in-office test for a urinary fistula is the "double-dye tampon test." This involves giving the patient 100 mg of phenazopyridine, a urinary analgesic agent that turns the urine bright orange. After 15–20 minutes, the bladder is catheterized and backfilled with 300 mL of methylene or indigo blue-dyed sterile saline. The catheter is removed, leaving the bladder full of blue fluid. A dry, white tampon is placed in the vagina, a pad is placed in the patient's underwear, and she is asked to walk vigorously for 10–15 minutes. The tampon and pad are then inspected to evaluate the presence and color of dye. If the top or sides of the tampon are dyed, there may be a fistula somewhere within the vagina: orange color alone indicates a uretero-vaginal fistula, whereas blue color indicates a bladder (vesico-vaginal) fistula. Blue dye on the string of the tampon (outside) or the pad but not on the upper tampon indicates that the patient may have leakage from her urethra.

> The patient undergoes the double-dye tampon test and returns with a dry pad. However, when the tampon is removed, the top of the tampon is bright orange and there is no blue dye.

What was the sequence of events that led to the formation of this patient's fistula?
The most likely sequence of events in this patient began with an unrecognized iatrogenic distal ureteral injury or bladder injury during her hysterectomy. The location of the distal ureter within the pelvis places it at risk for laceration, transection, avulsion, crush injury, and devitalization during pelvic surgery. The patient's initial flank pain and nausea were likely secondary to acute right ureteral obstruction. Relief of the flank pain that coincided with the onset of constant urinary leakage per vagina suggests the ultimate relief of obstruction via fistula formation. Given the results of her tampon test, we have more suspicion that she has a uretero-vaginal fistula.

CLINICAL PEARL   **STEPS 2/3**

The most common urinary tract fistula is a vesico-vaginal fistula occurring as a result of a bladder injury during pelvic surgery. Similarly, iatrogenic injury to the ureter is the most common cause of uretero-vaginal fistulae. Fistula formation from hysterectomy is fortunately rare (0.2%). Iatrogenic ureteral injury during major gynecologic surgery has an incidence of approximately 0.2%–0.4%, with a higher incidence seen with laparoscopic approach. During hysterectomy, the ureter can be injured at the pelvic brim during ligation of the infundibulo-pelvic ligament, at the level of the cervix during dissection or ligation of uterine vessels, or more distally during closure of the vaginal cuff.

What patient and surgical factors lead to an increased risk of fistula formation?

In the industrialized world, most urinary fistulae are iatrogenic and can occur from any part of the urinary tract. There are several patient-specific and surgical factors that can lead to fistulae formation: inadequate nutrition, a history of obstetrical trauma, pelvic malignancy or pelvic radiation, any prior abdominal or pelvic surgery, and other factors that distort anatomy such as obesity, pelvic inflammatory disease, and endometriosis. Intraoperative bleeding within the pelvis may require use of large clips or suture ligation, leading to inadvertent damage to the distal ureter or bladder. Retained foreign bodies, ischemic injury and tissue necrosis from cautery, disruption of blood supply, and infection can also lead to impaired healing and breakdown at the surgical site. Please note that the majority of fistulae form in patients who have none of these risk factors, so one must keep the index of suspicion high.

BASIC SCIENCE PEARL   **STEP 1**

It is vital to know the anatomy of the ureter while performing pelvic surgery. The distal ureter begins as it traverses anterior to the common iliac artery. Upon entering the true pelvis, the ureters travel posterior to the ovaries along the pelvic side wall. The ureters then course anteromedially in the medial leaf of the broad ligament, are crossed anteriorly by the uterine artery, and pass in front of the vagina just lateral to the cervix to enter the bladder posteriorly at the trigone.

What other imaging would be merited on suspicion of a vesico-vaginal or uretero-vaginal fistula?

All patients suspected of having a bladder fistula should undergo cystoscopy to attempt direct visualization. The appearance of a fistula can vary from bullous edema to a mature, well-demarcated opening in the bladder wall. Consider biopsy of the fistula tract if there is any concern or potential for malignancy. During cystoscopy, the bilateral ureteral orifices should be observed for efflux of urine. The previously discussed CT urogram is an appropriate imaging technique to evaluate a uretero-vesical fistula. A cystogram evaluates the bladder by retrograde instillation of contrast dye through a catheter with multiple X-ray images of the bladder (anterior/posterior and lateral views). The bladder must be completely distended for an accurate test, and a postvoid film should always be included. Another option is to obtain a voiding cystourethrogram (VCUG), a cystogram that includes more images obtained as the bladder fills and during the voiding phase. Contrast within the vagina can be seen during cystogram or VCUG in the presence of a fistulous tract. Finally, retrograde pyelography in the operating room is an excellent test to diagnose ureteral injury.

> The patient undergoes cystoscopy in the office, and the bladder appears normal. The bilateral ureteral orifices are in the normal anatomic position; efflux of clear urine is seen from the left ureter, but there is no efflux from the right side ureter. A CT urogram demonstrates mild right-sided hydroureteronephrosis (dilation of the urinary collecting system) from the kidney down to the uretero-vesical junction (UVJ). At the UVJ, there is a small amount of contrast extravasation. There is clear contrast spill to the vagina, and you explain to the patient that these findings strongly suggest a uretero-vaginal fistula.

How do you approach treatment of uretero-vaginal fistula?

Upon diagnosis of a urinary fistula, immediate intervention to control the fistula is essential because patients with fistulae are burdened with constant wetness, odor, skin irritation, urinary infections, and the expense of pads or diapers. Specifically for uretero-vaginal fistulae, goals

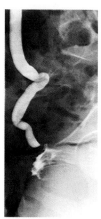

Fig. 38.1 Intravenous urography (IVU) showing pelvis with ureteral dilation proximal to an obstruction distally. This obstruction resulted in an uretero-vaginal fistula, and here you can see contrast spilling into the vagina. *(From Ginsberg D. Ureterovaginal fistula. In: Raz S, Rodríguez LV, eds.* Female urology. *Philadelphia: Saunders; 2008:821–4, fig. 84.1.)*

of care should include preservation of renal function and prevention of sepsis. If immediate surgical repair is not undertaken, urinary drainage and diversion is established with a ureteral stent or percutaneous nephrostomy tube placement. If a partial ureteral disruption is suspected, ureteral stenting in a retrograde fashion with cystoscopy may be attempted, but complete ureteral occlusion mandates percutaneous nephrostomy tube placement. Repair of the ureter depends on the location of the injury, although the distal ureter is most often injured during pelvic surgery. Associated inflammation and scarring of the distal ureter precludes primary reanastomosis of the ureteral ends, so surgical correction should reimplant the healthy proximal ureteral end into the bladder. The timing of this operative repair depends on many factors, but, in general, if the injury is not repaired intraoperatively or within 1 week of surgery, it is best to provide drainage as just discussed and repair the ureter in a delayed fashion after 2–3 months. Robotic, laparoscopic, and open abdominal approaches have all been shown to have efficacious outcomes. Overall success of surgical repair of uretero-vesical fistulae is greater than 90%.

> The patient undergoes placement of a right percutaneous nephrostomy tube, resolving her urinary incontinence. Two months later, she undergoes open right ureteral reimplantation with a urologic specialist. The ureter is traced as far distally as possible, and the healthy proximal end is implanted into the dome of the bladder. The percutaneous nephrostomy tube is removed at the time of surgery, and a ureteral stent and percutaneous drain are left in place. During her postoperative hospitalization, the percutaneous drain output is scant and serosanguineous, and the drain is removed prior to discharge on the second postoperative day.

How do you follow this patient after discharge?
The patient still has an indwelling ureteral stent that should be removed in the clinic after 3–4 weeks with outpatient cystoscopy. There is a small risk for development of a stricture at the site of the uretero-vesical anastomosis or vesico-ureteral reflux. Therefore, an outpatient follow-up visit should monitor for signs and symptoms of ureteral obstruction or reflux, and kidney function

should be checked with a basic metabolic panel. A few months after surgery, it is reasonable to perform a renal ultrasound to ensure resolution of the hydronephrosis.

> The patient returns for uncomplicated office stent removal 3 weeks later, and her creatinine is normal at that time. She has a renal ultrasound 3 months after surgery that is normal, indicating no ureteral strictures. She denies any leakage or pain and is happy to be feeling better and without symptoms.

BEYOND THE PEARLS

- The ureter can be easily visualized during surgery by searching for its characteristic vermiculation ("worm-like" motion) as it crosses the bifurcation of the common iliac vessels at the level of the pelvic brim.
- In the setting of acute unilateral ureteral obstruction, urine output and, for a time, markers of renal function like creatinine, may remain normal due to contralateral renal compensation.
- Factors to consider before the surgical repair of a fistula are nutritional status, the presence of infection or malignancy, urinary obstruction, or a foreign body. These factors should be modified prior to operation if possible, balancing this against the burden on the patient.
- Key principles for surgical repair of the ureter include spatulation of the ureter, a tension-free anastomosis, repair over an indwelling ureteral stent, maintenance of blood supply, and placement of a closed suction drain in the area of, but not directly overlying, the repair.

Case Summary

- A 34-year-old woman presents 3 days after laparoscopic hysterectomy with right flank pain, nausea, and vomiting resulting from an iatrogenic ureteral injury that goes undiagnosed.
- One month later, the patient has developed constant, severe urinary incontinence. History and physical reveal urine pooling in the vagina, and a double-dye tampon test and CT urogram are consistent with a right uretero-vaginal fistula located at the distal right ureter.
- The patient has temporary drainage of her kidney with a percutaneous nephrostomy tube, and she proceeds with ureteral reimplantation with retention of a stent.
- Three weeks after the surgery, her ureteral stent is removed in the clinic. Her renal ultrasound is normal 3 months later, and she has no complaints.

References

Adelman, M. R., Bardsley, T. R., & Sharp, H. T. (2014). Urinary tract injuries in laparoscopic hysterectomy: a systematic review. *Journal of Minimally Invasive Gynecology, 21*(4), 558–566.

Burks, F. N., & Santucci, R. A. (2014). Management of iatrogenic ureteral injury. *Therapy Advancement Urology, 6*(3), 115–124.

Gohanay, M., Yildiz, Y., & Tonguc, E. (2011). Abdominal, vaginal and total laparoscopic hysterectomy: perioperative morbidity. *Archives of Gynecology and Obstetrics, 284*, 385–389.

Hall, M. J., DeFrances, C. J., Williams, S. N., Golosinskiy, A., & Schwartzman, A. (2010). National hospital discharge survey: 2007 summary. *National Health Statistics Reports, 26*(29), 1–20.

Hwang, J. H., Lim, M. C., & Joung, J. Y. (2012). Urologic complications of laparoscopic radical hysterectomy and lymphadenectomy. *International Urogynecology Journal, 23*(11), 1605–1611.

Teeluckdharry, B., Gilmour, D., & Flowerdew, G. (2015). Urinary tract injury at benign gynecologic surgery and the role of cystoscopy: a systematic review and meta-analysis. *Obstetrics and Gynecology, 126*, 1161–1169.

Wein, A. J., Kavoussi, L. R., Novick, A. C., Partin, A. W., & Peters, C. A. (2012). *Campell-Walsh urology* (10th ed. rev.). Philadelphia: Elsevier/Saunders.

Sara Petruska, MD

A 35-Year-Old Woman With an Abnormal Pap Smear

A 35-year-old G2P2 female presents regarding her recent abnormal Pap smear. Two weeks ago, she was seen for her annual examination and was without complaints; her last Pap was normal 3 years ago. She has no abnormal bleeding, discharge, or pelvic pain, and her menstrual cycles are regular on oral contraceptives. She is considering another pregnancy in 1–2 years. You tell her that her Pap demonstrates low-grade squamous intraepithelial lesion (LSIL).

TABLE 39.1 ■ Who Needs Papanicolaou (Pap) Smear Screening?

Under age 21	No Pap screening, regardless of age at coitarche (first sexual intercourse)
Age 21–29	Screening with Pap every 3 years
	Human papilloma virus (HPV) testing should not be used for screening but may be used as a reflex test for ASCUS Pap
Age 30–64	Pap with HPV (co-testing) every 5 years is preferred
	Pap alone every 3 years is acceptable
65 and over	Stop if no history of cervical intraepithelial neoplasia (CIN) 2/3 in the past 20 years *and* 3 consecutive negative Paps or 2 consecutive negative HPV tests in the past 10 years (most recent within 5 years)
After hysterectomy	If the cervix has been removed and the patient has no history of CIN 2 or worse in the past 20 years, Pap screening is not indicated
Prior history of CIN 2/3, adenocarcinoma in situ or cervical cancer	Screening should continue for 20 years after last positive test for these conditions, even if this extends screening past age 65

What are the risk factors for an abnormal Pap smear?

Patients at increased risks for abnormal Pap smears and cervical dysplasia are those with tobacco use, early coitarche (age at first sexual intercourse), prior abnormal Pap smears, multiple partners or sexual partners who have had multiple past partners, immunosuppression, lower socioeconomic status, oral contraceptive use, poor nutrition, history of human papilloma virus (HPV) or other sexually transmitted infections, and lack of regular access to screening.

She reports a remote history of an abnormal Pap smear "many years ago," with normal Pap smears since. She denies new sexual partners and is monogamous with her husband. She is a heavy smoker.

CLINICAL PEARL	**STEPS 2/3**

HPV is a sexually transmitted infection that a majority of sexually active women will contract at some point, most in the first few years after coitarche. Most commonly, the immune system successfully clears the virus, but patients may continue to carry the virus at undetectably low levels. Patients can also reactivate HPV viral infection after several normal Pap smears or develop cervical dysplasia without new infection, so an abnormal Pap is not an indication of a new exposure. High-risk types are 16, 18, 31, 35, and 45. Oncogenes E6 and E7 allow high-risk types of HPV to transform host cells and can be tested for in certain clinical situations. Low-risk HPV types can cause genital condyloma (warts) but cannot transform cells and lead to cervical cancer.

TABLE 39.2 ■ How Papanicolaou (Pap) Smears Are Interpreted

Pap Smear Result	What Does the Cytologist See?	What Does this Mean?	What Are Options for the Next Step?
Normal cytology, HPV negative	Normal cells, negative test for HPV	There is no evidence of dysplasia or of HPV infection	Repeat Pap at the next recommended interval
Normal cytology, HPV positive	Normal cells, positive test for HPV	The HPV virus is present, but there is no evidence that it changed the host's cells (no dysplasia)	Repeat Pap with HPV test in 1 year
Atypical squamous cells of uncertain significance (ASCUS)	Some changes suggestive of atypia (larger and darker nuclei, higher nuclear to cytoplasmic ratio) without definitive evidence of dysplasia	The cells look slightly abnormal, but the cytopathologist is unable to say why. Possible causes could be dysplasia, cervicitis, vaginitis, or atrophy	For women over 25, test for HPV (if negative, dysplasia is not present, and, if positive, colposcopy is indicated). For patients under age 25, repeat the Pap in 1 year.
ASC-H (atypical squamous cells, high grade)	Equivocal features suggestive of but not sufficient to diagnose HSIL	Markedly abnormal cells are present, with outcomes for these patients closer to those of patients with HSIL than those with LSIL	Colposcopy is indicated (even if HPV test is negative)
Low-grade squamous intraepithelial neoplasia (LSIL)	Mild atypia is definitively seen	The patient is at risk for dysplasia, but the severity of the dysplasia is still uncertain	Colposcopy is indicated (even if HPV test is negative)
High-grade squamous intraepithelial neoplasia (HSIL)	Marked atypical features are definitively seen	The patient has a higher chance of severe dysplasia than if her Pap was LSIL, but her diagnosis is still uncertain	Colposcopy is indicated (even if HPV test was negative)

HPV, Human papilloma virus.

How do providers manage abnormal Pap smears?

Guidelines for management are released by the American Society for Cytopathologists and Colposcopists (ASCCP). Cervical cancer screening guidelines evolve rapidly, so physicians should refer to the most current set of guidelines. The last set of guidelines was released in 2013 and are available at www.asccp.org in the clinical practice section or via the ASCCP phone application. In guidelines, management strategies are designated as "preferred," "acceptable," or "unacceptable." Another guideline revision is anticipated in 2017.

You review with the patient that colposcopy is indicated for further evaluation of her Pap smear. The patient wonders what she will feel during the colposcopy.

How would you describe a colposcopy experience to a patient?

For colposcopy, a speculum is placed in the vagina and the cervix is inspected by a colposcope, a microscope with 10–40× magnification to view the cervix. The colposcope itself does not touch the patient. Application of solutions to the cervix, like acetic acid (vinegar), may burn or tingle. If a biopsy is needed, most patients feel a poorly localized, menstrual-like cramp or no discomfort during the biopsy. This is because the cervix has visceral innervation, unlike the somatic innervation of the distal vagina and vulva.

How would you prepare yourself, the examiner, to perform a colposcopy?

Prior to the patient being in the room, sit in the examiner's stool with good posture and position the binoculars for ease of viewing. Once the patient is in the room and positioned with her buttocks just past the edge of the table in lithotomy, the table height should be adjusted, a speculum placed, and the cervix brought into view. The colposcope is moved to within 15 cm of the cervix to bring the cervical epithelium into focus and allow sufficient space for instruments. Some colposcopes focus by adjustment knobs; others by moving the scope itself.

What is the transformation zone (TZ), and what is its role in colposcopy?

The TZ is that portion of the cervix where stratified squamous epithelium on the external rounded portion of the cervix (the "portio"), which appears shiny and smooth, transitions to the redder and "rough-looking" columnar epithelium of the internal cervix. The TZ must be fully visualized all the way around and any lesions fully seen in order to have an "adequate" colposcopy, which may require movement of the cervix with cotton swabs. Dysplastic lesions begin within the TZ, so if part of the TZ or a lesion is not seen, unseen lesions or a higher grade within a seen lesion cannot be excluded.

How do solutions applied to the cervix highlight lesions or dysplasia on colposcopy?

After observing the cervix for leukoplakia, raised masses, or abnormal vasculature, you may apply a solution to highlight the TZ and patches of dysplasia or carcinoma. Acetic acid (3%) reacts with the higher protein and nuclear concentration of metaplastic cells (creating a thin white line at the TZ) and will turn dysplastic areas bright white. Alternatively, 5% Lugol's iodine solution, which stains glycogen in healthy tissues brown, will cause areas of carcinoma or dysplasia to appear pale because these areas contain less glycogen than healthy tissues. Note, however, that ectropion, endometrium, and columnar epithelium also appear pale with application of Lugol's solution.

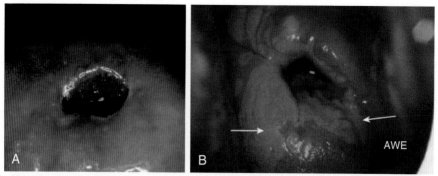

Fig. 39.1 Normal colposcopic view of adult cervix with typical squamocolumnar junction visible (A) and a cervix with dysplasia showing an acetowhite lesion when stained with acetic acid (B). *(From (A) Spitzer M. Colposcopy: pitfalls and tricks of the trade. In: Apgar B, Brotzman G, Spitzer M, eds. Colposcopy. 2nd ed. Philadelphia: Saunders; 2008:521–30, fig. 27-10; (B) Newkirk GR. In: Pfenninger and Fowler's procedures for primary care. Philadelphia: Saunders; 2011:919–35, fig. 137-4.)*

You explain the colposcopy procedure, and the patient agrees to proceed. After acetic acid is applied, colposcopic exam demonstrates two separate areas of acetowhite change at 12 o'clock and 6 o'clock on the portio of the cervix. No abnormal vascularity is noted.

What if no lesions are seen on the colposcopic view of the cervix?

In this situation, a discrepancy exists between the level of changes seen on Pap smear (LSIL) and the colposcopic examination, so one must suspect that more dysplastic lesions may exist in unseen regions of the cervix. In such situations, an endocervical curettage (ECC) should be obtained. A small curette is placed within the cervical canal and rotated while applying pressure to the canal walls to remove small strips of tissue. An endocervical brush is then used to collect the specimen.

What descriptors are used to describe colposcopic lesions, and what is most concerning?

Low-grade lesions (cervical intraepithelial neoplasia [CIN] 1) typically have acetowhite change with a translucent appearance and have feathery borders that resemble a coastline. Higher-grade lesions (CIN 2–3) are more opaque white with straighter borders. Vascular punctation, or a dotted pattern, represents capillary loops within subepithelial papillae. Vascular mosaicism, or a tiling pattern, is created by networks of capillaries running parallel to the epithelial surface. Both punctation and mosaicism may appear fine and regular, associated with low-grade changes, or may be coarse and irregular, suggesting high-grade disease. Extremely irregular vessels, such as comma-shaped segments and corkscrews, are seen with microinvasive or invasive carcinoma and so are most concerning. A green filter on the light can highlight vascular changes. A biopsy should be obtained from any areas that appear abnormal. Visualizing the lesion does not give the diagnosis, but it allows you to target biopsy sites.

How is a cervical biopsy performed?

The biopsy forceps is a long, slender instrument with two small blades forming jaws at the tip. They have a straight, or inactive, blade that is inserted into the external os and held parallel with the axis of the cervix, while the articulating, or active, blade is pressed against the portio of the cervix over the target lesion. After the handle is squeezed, the forceps are removed and the biopsy specimen (usually 2–3 mm in size) is retrieved. The wooden handle of a cotton-tip swab can be used to move the biopsy specimen from the jaws of the forceps to a formalin-filled cup. It is best to retrieve the specimen without contacting the formalin.

You perform biopsies of both lesions and obtain an ECC, and she tolerates these procedures well. She asks you to reach her by cell phone when you receive her results.

BASIC SCIENCE PEARL	**STEP 1**

CIN 3 and squamous carcinoma in situ are functionally the same, both indicating a full thickness dysplasia without evidence of invasion.

What different results might be seen on cervical biopsy?

A biopsy might show no evidence of malignancy or dysplasia but could show cervical inflammation, cervicitis, or metaplasia. A biopsy may also show HPV effect, such the presence of koilocytes,

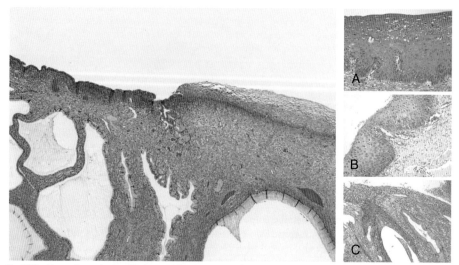

Fig. 39.2 Normal cervical pathology at the squamocolumnar junction on histology (*left panel*) with the right panel showing CIN 1 (A), CIN 2 (B), and CIN 3 (C) and increasing abnormality of the nucleus and structure in the epithelial layers. *(From (A) Michael H, Kerr SE.* Comprehensive cytopathology, *4th ed. Philadelphia: Saunders; 2015:119–65, fig. 8-1; (B) Litjens RJNTM.* Hum Pathol. *2014;45(2):221–6, figs. A, B, C.)*

without dysplastic changes. If dysplasia is seen, it may be described as CIN 1, CIN 2–3, CIN 3, squamous carcinoma in situ (CIS), invasive squamous cell carcinoma, adenocarcinoma in situ, or invasive adenocarcinoma. Extension into endocervical glands is not invasion, because it represents lateral spread of dysplasia on the epithelium as it invaginates into gland spaces. However, this finding is associated with recurrence after excision.

What types of treatment are available?
The cervix can be ablated with cryotherapy or laser, or the dysplasia can be excised using a loop excisional electrosurgical procedure (LEEP) or cold knife cone (CKC). Ablation or a LEEP can be performed in the office or in the operating room based on available equipment. Because of the increased sidewall retraction needed and risk of bleeding with CKC, this procedure is performed in the operating room.

Which types of dysplasia should be treated?
CIN 1 is likely to resolve on its own in an average of 18 months, but persistence for 24 months should be treated by either excision or ablation. For ablation to be acceptable, as it does not provide a pathological specimen, the colposcopy must have been adequate, the ECC negative or CIN 1, and the patient must have no history of past dysplasia treatment. If the colposcopy was inadequate, the ECC shows CIN 2–3 or ungraded dysplasia, or if the patient had prior treatment, the patient requires an excisional procedure. While CIN 2 may resolve spontaneously in younger women, CIN 2 should be treated in women over 25. CIN 3 should be treated by ablation or excision for women of any age, with ablation again reserved for patients with adequate colposcopies and with normal cells or CIN 1 on ECC. Adenocarcinoma in situ should also be treated with excision. If an invasive cervical cancer is noted on colposcopic biopsy, excision with CKC, cystoscopy, and proctoscopy should be performed in the operating room to allow for staging and treatment planning.

Your patient's results return showing CIN 3 with a negative ECC. After reviewing the options, she requests an office LEEP. You perform the LEEP, and the pathology demonstrates CIN 3 with negative endocervical and ectocervical margins. At her 2-week follow-up visit, she is healing well. She understands that, per current guidelines, she should have Pap and HPV co-testing in 12 and 24 months.

BEYOND THE PEARLS

- For patients with ASCUS/HPV+ Pap and LSIL Pap, colposcopy detects high-grade dysplasia 15% of the time, whereas 50% have no visible lesion. Therefore, you can advise an LSIL patient that there is a 50% chance that she will have a biopsy at the time of colposcopy and an 85% chance that her follow-up will be a repeat Pap in 1 year.
- Failure to ensure adequate follow-up for abnormal Pap smears and biopsy specimens opens patients to unnecessary risk and gynecologic practices to medicolegal pitfalls. Make sure that you counsel each patient on how her next step will be communicated to her, when she should expect to hear about her results, and what she should do if she is not contacted. Clearly document this counseling in your notes.
- The ability of colposcopy to detect dysplasia depends more on the number of biopsies taken than on the experience of the colposcopist, so multiple biopsies increase sensitivity if multiple areas are affected.
- Document thoroughly how well a patient tolerates the colposcopy procedure in your notes, because this will help you to plan how she may tolerate an office procedure for treatment of dysplasia, such as an ablation or a LEEP.

Case Summary

- A 35-year-old woman with a Pap smear showing an LSIL comes for follow-up.
- She undergoes colposcopy, and the findings are consistent with an adequate colposcopy and acetowhite changes on acetic acid staining, so a biopsy is taken.
- The biopsy is consistent with cervical intraepithelial neoplasia (CIN) 3, and she undergoes a LEEP. You recommend that she have a repeat Pap and HPV testing 12 and 24 months from now.

References

ASCUS-LSIL Triage Study (ALTS) Group (2003). Results of a randomized trial on the management of cytology interpretations of atypical squamous cells of undetermined significance. *American Journal of Obstetrics and Gynecology*, *188*(6), 1383–1392.

Massad, L. S., et al. (2013). 2012 updated consensus guidelines for the management of abnormal cervical cancer screening tests and cancer precursors. *Journal of Lower Genital Tract Disease*, *17*, S1–27.

Pretorius, R. G., Belinson, J. L., Peterson, P., et al. (2015). Which colposcopies should include endocervical curettage? *Journal of Lower Genital Tract Disease*, *19*, 278–281.

Saslow, D., Solomon, D., Lawson, H. W., et al. (2012). American Cancer Society, American Society for Colposcopy and Cervical Pathology, and American Society for Clinical Pathology screening guidelines for the prevention and early detection of cervical cancer. *Journal of Lower Genital Tract Disease*, *16*, 1–29.

Tanya E. Franklin, MD, MSPH

A 28-Year-Old Woman With a History of Pulmonary Embolism Who Desires Contraception

A 28-year-old G0 female presents as a new patient for her annual examination, Pap smear, and contraception counseling. She denies any complaints, and her menstrual cycles are regular with a normal flow. She is engaged to be married next year to her male partner, is currently sexually active, and hopes to start a family in 3–5 years. She has no past surgical history and no known drug allergies. The patient is obese, with a body mass index (BMI) of 35 kg/m², and she has a pertinent past medical history of a pulmonary embolus (PE).

What are the risk factors for venous thromboembolism (VTE)?
Risk factors for VTE are obesity, pregnancy, increasing age, immobility, trauma, surgery, combined hormonal contraception (CHC) or hormone therapy, malignancy, acute medical illness, nephrotic syndrome, inflammatory bowel disease, selective estrogen receptor modulators, heart or respiratory failure, varicose veins, central venous catheterization, and inherited or acquired thrombophilia.

Three years ago, the patient reported an episode of shortness of breath and chest pain that resulted in her evaluation and the diagnosis of a PE. At the time, she was on combined oral contraception (COC). She wants to prevent pregnancy now and therefore is eager to begin contraception as soon as possible.

What medical and social history questions should be asked to determine the best contraceptive method for this patient?
Prior history of thrombosis in the patient and her family raises suspicion for a familial thrombophilic syndrome, which could increase her risk of a repeat VTE if she uses certain types of hormonal contraception. The patient's weight, physical activity, and tobacco use can also increase her risk of recurrent PE. Close attention to any medications or medical conditions that could reduce the efficacy of a contraceptive method is also important in this patient.

What tests should be ordered to evaluate for familial thrombophilic syndrome?
To evaluate for familial thrombophilic syndrome, one should test for factor V Leiden mutation, prothrombin G2010 A mutation, protein C, protein S, and antithrombin deficiency. Antiphospholipid antibodies (APAb) should also be evaluated to test for systemic lupus erythematosus and antiphospholipid antibody syndrome (APAS). Most common thrombophilias can be tested for by a thrombophilia panel, which evaluates factor V Leiden mutations, prothrombin gene mutation, protein C and S, antithrombin activity, and, in some cases, will test for APAb levels.

BASIC SCIENCE PEARL	STEP 1

Estrogen increases hepatic production of the coagulation factors, including factor VII, factor X, and fibrinogen. This is the mechanism by which exogenous estrogen use increases VTE risk.

CLINICAL PEARL	STEPS 2/3

Among women with thrombophilic mutations, CHC users have a 2–20 times higher risk for VTE than do nonusers. Therefore, CHCs are contraindicated in this population.

The patient reports that she was evaluated by a hematologist following her PE. She had testing with a thrombophilia panel and was found to be heterozygous for factor V Leiden but had no other coagulation abnormalities or known thrombophilias.

CLINICAL PEARL	STEPS 2/3

Factor V Leiden is the most common cause of activated protein C resistance. It is the most common thrombophilic condition, with a prevalence in Caucasians of 5%. Women may be heterogenous (one normal gene copy and one mutated copy) for factor V Leiden mutations or homogenous, with two mutated gene copies. As one would guess, the homogenous state is more severe and has a higher risk of VTE.

How should this patient be counseled regarding contraception recommendations?

The US Medical Eligibility Criteria (US MEC) provides guidance on contraception use in the setting of certain medical conditions and patient characteristics. The medical conditions are classified as category 1, 2, 3, or 4 to categorize the safety of each contraceptive method. Category 1 means the medical condition has no contraindications for use of that contraceptive method, while category 2 indicates that the advantages of the contraceptive method generally outweigh the theoretical or proven risks and can be used. Category 3 denotes that the theoretical or proven risk usually outweighs the advantages of the contraceptive method, so the method is not recommended in the medical condition unless other more appropriate methods are not available or unacceptable for use. Category 4 means the medical condition represents an unacceptable health risk for that contraceptive method and should never be used in that population. The risk of a recurrent VTE in this patient with a given contraceptive method is based on the presence of one or more risk factors for recurrent VTE. The patient's VTE should also be categorized based on the presence of an acute or recent VTE with anticoagulation therapy in the past 3 months.

What are the recommendations for a family history of VTE?

If the patient does not have a personal history of VTE, it is reasonable to assess family history. However, even with a family history of VTE in a first-degree relative, CHCs are a category 2 and not contraindicated.

What should you tell the patient about hormone-containing methods?

The patient should be counseled about all contraceptive methods and advised to avoid all CHC methods. CHC options include the pill, the transdermal patch, and the vaginal ring. COCs include a pill that includes both estrogen and a progestin. The transdermal patch is a thin plastic patch that is placed on the skin for contraception and is changed weekly; it contains both estrogen and progestin. The vaginal ring, which also contains both estrogen and progestin, is a small plastic ring that is inserted once a month for contraception. The progestin-only pill (POP) is a

TABLE 40.1 ■ The US Medical Eligibility Criteria (US MEC) for the Use of Common Contraceptive Methods in Patients With a Personal or Family History of Venous Thromboembolism (VTE)

	Cu-IUD	LNG-IUD	Implant	DMPA	POP	CHC
History of DVT/PE, not receiving anticoagulation therapy						
i. Higher risk for recurrent DVT/PE	1	2	2	2	2	4
ii. Lower risk for recurrent DVT/PE	1	2	2	2	2	3
Acute DVT/PE	2	2	2	2	2	4
DVT/PE and established anticoagulant therapy for at least 3 months						
i. Higher risk for recurrent DVT/PE	2	2	2	2	2	4a
ii. Lower risk for recurrent DVT/PE	2	2	2	2	2	3a
Family history (no personal history)	1	1	1	1	1	2

Methods of contraception are denoted as intrauterine devices (IUDs) such as the copper-(Cu) or levonorgestrel-containing (LNG) IUD, depot medroxyprogesterone acetate (DMPA), implantable contraception (Implant), progestin-only pills (POP), and combined hormonal contraceptives (CHC). *DVT*, Deep venous thrombosis; *PE*, pulmonary embolism.

aCHC may be considered in the case where it is being used to prevent blood loss from menses or risk of bleeding ovarian cysts.

birth control pill that doses only 35 µg of norethindrone daily. Strict compliance is necessary for efficacy, and patients should be advised that optimal use is taking it at a similar time every day.

BASIC SCIENCE PEARL   **STEP 1**

CHCs contain both ethinyl estradiol plus some formulation of progestin such as desogestrel, drospirenone, levonorgestrel, norethindrone, norgestimate, or norgestrel. CHC contraception works by preventing follicle maturation, thinning the endometrial lining, thickening the cervical mucus, and suppressing luteinizing hormone (LH) to prevent ovulation.

The patient was advised to use a progestin-only contraceptive method or a nonhormonal method of contraception. The patient has a very irregular schedule and does not think she can be compliant.

What other reliable, progestin-only options are available for this patient?
The patient was counseled on long-acting reversible contraceptives (LARC). LARC are long-term methods of birth control and include injections, subdermal implants, and intrauterine devices (IUDs). Depot medroxyprogesterone acetate (DMPA) is a progestin-only injection given every 3 months. The IUD is a contraceptive device inserted into the uterus by a health care provider. The hormonal IUD is a levonorgestrel-containing (LNG) IUD that is effective for 3–5 years, and the copper-containing nonhormonal IUD (Cu-IUD) is effective for 10 years. The subdermal implant, a progestin-only method effective for 3 years, is a contraceptive device inserted under the skin of the upper arm by a health care provider.

Since the patient desires pregnancy prevention for 3–5 years, she decides to have the 5-year LNG-IUD. You counsel her that because the LNG-IUD is a category 2 method for her, and she is scheduled for quick follow-up, she can have the IUD placed. The patient takes a nonsteroidal antiinflammatory drug (NSAID) 1 hour prior to placement, and the IUD is inserted without complication. She returns in 6 weeks for a string check, and she denies any issues surrounding sexual intercourse, pelvic pain, or severe bleeding. She is planning a knee arthroscopy in 1 month, and she is worried about VTE risks around this surgery.

TABLE 40.2 ■ US Medical Eligibility Criteria (US MEC) Categories for Common Contraceptive Methods

	Cu-IUD	LNG-IUD	Implant	DMPA	POP	CHC
Major surgery						
i. With prolonged immobilization	1	2	2	2	2	4
ii. Without prolonged immobilization	1	1	1	1	1	2
Minor surgery without immobilization	1	1	1	1	1	1

Methods are shown regarding surgery being planned in light of woman's current contraception method, with numbers designating the US MEC categories.

Methods of contraception are denoted as intrauterine devices (IUDs) such as the copper-(Cu) or levonorgestrel-containing (LNG) IUD, depot medroxyprogesterone acetate (DMPA), implantable contraception (Implant), progestin-only pills (POP), and combined hormonal contraceptives (CHC).

CLINICAL PEARL   **STEPS 2/3**

There is no contraindication to IUD placement in adolescents and nulliparous women, and actually very little evidence suggests that it is technically more difficult in these populations. In fact, LARC methods, including IUDs, should be encouraged in all appropriate candidates, including nulliparous women and adolescents, due to the reliability, safety, and ease of use of these methods.

What recommendations should be given to patients with thrombophilias and contraceptive management in the perioperative period?

PE is a major cause for surgery-related deaths. The risk of unintended pregnancy as well as the risk of VTE should be discussed with the patient. If the patient is considered to be at high risk for VTE, stopping CHC 1 month or more before major surgery should be considered. A progestin-only method such as a POP, DMPA, subdermal etonogestrel implant, or IUD can be used until the risk of thromboembolic disease has returned to baseline. If a brief surgical procedure is planned and the assessed perioperative risk of VTE is low, then CHC discontinuation is not necessary. This patient is having a minor orthopedic surgery but may have prolonged immobilization; if she were using CHC, she would have to consider an alternative contraceptive around the surgery, but her LNG-IUD can be continued safely.

BEYOND THE PEARLS

- Although COC users experience a fourfold increased risk of thromboembolism, this risk remains lower than the increased risk of VTE during pregnancy.
- In addition to exogenous estrogens, age, history of VTE, pregnancy, obesity, surgery, air travel, and familial thrombophilic syndromes can increase risk of VTE.
- Women currently on anticoagulation therapy are at risk of severe bleeding or anemia from ruptured ovarian cysts or menses, so these women should consider CHC methods to control ovarian cyst formation and menstrual blood loss. In well-anticoagulated women, CHC does not increase recurrent thrombosis, and a different risk–benefit ratio is considered on a case-by-case basis. Therefore, COC use can be considered to prevent ovarian cysts or excess menstrual blood loss in well-anticoagulated women.
- Other contraindications to estrogen-based contraception are impaired liver function, estrogen-dependent cancers such as endometrial and breast malignancy, undiagnosed vaginal bleeding, and known or suspected pregnancy.

Case Summary

- A 28-year-old woman presents as a new patient for her annual gynecologic examination and contraception counseling. She has a history of PE.
- The patient has had testing for thrombophilias and is heterozygous for factor V Leiden. She is counseled that she is at risk for recurrent thromboembolism and that a progestin-only method or a nonhormonal method of contraception is recommended.
- The patient opts to have an LNG-IUD placed and has it inserted without incident; she is happy with its use 6 weeks later.
- She is planning an upcoming arthroscopy surgery, and is counseled that, although she is at high risk of a recurrent thrombotic event in the postoperative period, she can continue her LNG-IUD safely around the surgery to prevent pregnancy.

References

American College of Obstetricians and Gynecologists (ACOG) (2006). ACOG practice bulletin number 73: use of hormonal contraception in women with coexisting medical conditions. *Obstetrics and Gynecology, 107*(6), 1453–1472. Reaffirmed 2011.

American College of Obstetricians and Gynecologists (ACOG) (2007). ACOG practice bulletin number 84: prevention of deep vein thrombosis and pulmonary embolism. *Obstetrics and Gynecology, 110*(2 Pt 1), 429–440. Reaffirmed 2016.

Curtis, K. M., Jatlaoui, T. C., Tepper, N. K., et al. (2016). U.S. selected practice recommendations for contraceptive use, 2016. *Morbidity and Mortality Weekly Report (MMWR) Recommendations and Reports, 65*(4), 1–66.

Hatcher, R. A., Trussell, J., Nelson, A. L., et al. (2011). *Contraceptive technology* (20th revised ed.). New York: Ardent Media.

Ambareen Jan, MD

A 56-Year-Old Woman With Menopausal Symptoms

A 56-year-old woman presents to your office for her annual gynecologic visit. Her last menstrual cycle was 14 months ago. She expresses that she has hot flushes at least three times a day, and these are regularly waking her from sleep,. For the past 2 months she has been experiencing painful intercourse, decreased libido, and vaginal dryness.

What history is necessary in a patient with these symptoms?
When taking a history and physical on a postmenopausal patient, it is essential to obtain a thorough gynecologic history. This includes questions about the last menstrual cycle, menstrual pattern, any postmenopausal bleeding, sexual activity, painful intercourse, and gynecologic surgeries and infections. It is also necessary to obtain the patient's medical and surgical history along with current medications.

The patient has a history of well-controlled diabetes treated with metformin. She had a normal mammogram and Pap smear 12 months ago. She has a monogamous male sexual partner and no former history of sexual dysfunction. She has no personal or family history of breast or ovarian cancer. She is a current smoker (10 cigarettes a day) but denies illicit drug or alcohol use. Her blood pressure is 119/80 mm Hg, heart rate is 89/min, and temperature is 37°C (98.6°F). Her vaginal exam is remarkable for decreased rugae and excoriations. A vaginal culture is sent for analysis.

How is menopause defined, and what are the associated symptoms?
Menopause is defined as amenorrhea (lack of menses) for more than 1 year. Symptoms include hot flushes, night sweats, atrophy of the vagina, decreased libido, mood swings, and sleep disturbances. These symptoms are in correlation with a decrease in circulating estrogen after the number of ovarian follicles decrease secondary to age. Up to 80% of women may experience hot flushes during menopause, but far fewer seek treatment for these symptoms. This patient reports hot flushes and sexual symptoms, with no medical history that clearly explains these. Therefore, she is highly likely to be suffering from postmenopausal symptoms.

CLINICAL PEARL   **STEPS 2/3**

Vasomotor symptoms can sometimes be attributed to certain medications. Hot flushes are the most common side effect of the medications tamoxifen and raloxifene (selective estrogen receptor modulators), which are used in the treatment of breast cancer. Vaginal dryness and decreased libido can be caused by β-blockers or certain antidepressants. There can also be a psychological component such as depression, previous sexual trauma, or stress.

What are the physical exam findings in a postmenopausal patient?

A comprehensive physical exam should be performed on all patients. Decreasing estrogen levels can cause hair loss, brittle nails, and thinning of the skin. On the pelvic exam, lack of estrogen in vaginal tissues manifests as decreased rugae, pallor and thinning of vaginal epithelium, attenuations of the labia minora, and possible excoriations, consistent with this patient's exam.

What laboratory evaluation is indicated in a patient with menopausal symptoms?

The patient should have an evaluation of follicle stimulating hormone (FSH) and luteinizing hormone (LH) levels, which measure the hypothalamic hormones that stimulates follicle development, ova release, and menstruation in premenopausal women. FSH will be greater than 30 IU/L in menopausal women, and LH will be greater than 40 IU/L. The patient should also be tested for thyroid disease or hypoglycemia as these may cause sweating and vasomotor symptoms that can be mistaken for vasomotor symptoms of menopause; this patient is at risk for both disorders based on her age and medical history.

BASIC SCIENCE PEARL   **STEPS 1/2/3**

The pituitary gland exhibits a negative feedback mechanism in response to a decrease in circulating estrogen levels and releases FSH and LH. Therefore, in postmenopausal women, the FSH and LH levels are elevated. FSH is the preferred test in diagnosing menopause when clinical or menstrual history are not useful or inadequate.

The patient's vaginitis profile is negative for bacterial vaginosis, yeast, and trichomoniasis. FSH and LH levels are 60 IU/L and 50 IU/L, respectively, and her glucose and thyroid-stimulating hormone (TSH) are normal. With no evidence of infection, and lab results consistent with ovarian failure, a diagnosis of menopause is given.

What is the treatment of menopause, and when should it initiated?

Hormone replacement therapy (HRT) should be offered to patients with menopausal symptoms in which HRT is not contraindicated. HRT should also be offered to patients who undergo bilateral oophorectomy before menopause or premature ovarian failure. Vasomotor symptoms, commonly known as "hot flashes," (or "flushes") are the primary reason patients are started on HRT. Typically, severe vasomotor symptoms are treated with systemic (oral or transdermal) estrogen therapy with or without progestins. In women experiencing only vulvar or vaginal symptoms, local or vaginal estrogen therapy is the preferred method of treatment because oral therapy does not address vulvar or vaginal symptoms as effectively. Side effects of oral or systemic HRT include elevated blood pressure, irregular uterine bleeding, breast tenderness and/or swelling, bloating, nausea, headaches, and mood swings. HRT slightly increases cardiovascular events (CVEs) and thrombotic events (TEs). There is significant controversy about this risk, but past studies have also reported an increased risk of breast or endometrial hyperplasia or cancer with certain types of HRT, so women need to be adequately counseled about these risks.

CLINICAL PEARL   **STEPS 2/3**

In patients who still have a uterus, oral estrogen along with progesterone can be given for vasomotor symptom treatment. Progesterone is given to prevent effects of unopposed estrogen, including endometrial hyperplasia or cancer. In patients without a uterus (posthysterectomy), one should consider estrogen alone as the combination of progesterone and estrogen was found to be associated with breast cancer, whereas estrogen therapy alone was not associated with an increased risk of breast cancer in past trials.

TABLE 41.1 ■ Systemic Hormone Replacement Therapy (HRT) Regimens Commonly Used in Clinical Practice

Manner of Administration	Medications Contained	Advantages for Patients
Oral estrogen therapy	Conjugated estrogen 0.3–0.635 mg/day or Estradiol 0.45–2 mg/day	• Easy to take; inexpensive • No increased breast cancer risk • Possible to take if no uterus
Oral estrogen with progestin therapy (progestin oral or injected)	One of above estrogens with Medroxyprogesterone acetate (MPA) 5–10 mg/day for 12–14 consecutive days per month or Depot MPA (injected) every 3 months	• Easy to take if oral only • Lowered breast cancer risk • Protects uterus
Transdermal estrogen therapy	One spray 0.06% estradiol gel daily or One sachet 0.1% estradiol gel daily or Transdermal film 0.025–0.1 mg released per day, one application/week	• No oral use • First-pass effect
Transdermal combined therapy (estrogen and progestin)	Estradiol 0.045 mg/levonorgestrel 0.015 mg released per day, one application/week or Estradiol 0.05 mg/norethindrone 0.14–0.25 mg released per day, one application/week	• No oral therapy • Apply once weekly • Protects uterus

When is hormone replacement therapy contraindicated?

Contraindications include breast and endometrial cancer, a genetic mutation predisposing the patient to breast cancer (such as BRCA), a history of CVEs or TEs such as myocardial infarction or stroke, chronic liver disease, hypertriglyceridemia, and age over 60. Smoking alone is not an absolute contraindication, but smokers with additional comorbidities that that increase their risk of CVEs or TEs should avoid HRT.

Given the patient's relative contraindication of smoking and diabetes, both of which are risk factors for CVEs, she is counseled on lifestyle changes and smoking cessation. She is prescribed vaginal estrogen, which has less systemic risks, for her vaginal and sexual symptoms.

What are alternatives to HRT for postmenopausal symptoms?

Lifestyle modifications may be helpful for vasomotor symptoms; these include smoking cessation, weight loss, avoiding synthetic fabrics, layering clothing, cooling drinks or fans, decreasing room temperature, and dietary changes such as avoiding aggravating foods (e.g., spicy foods and caffeine). For patients in whom systemic HRT is contraindicated, the serotonin-norepinephrine reuptake inhibitor (SNRI) venlafaxine and some selective serotonin reuptake inhibitors (SSRIs) can be given as alternatives to treat vasomotor symptoms.

CLINICAL PEARL	STEPS 2/3

Other alternatives to HRT that are acceptable but have limited data include clonidine, gabapentin, and herbal remedies such as black cohosh, ginseng, St. John's wort, and ginkgo biloba.

The patient returns to the clinic after 4 weeks. She has made lifestyle changes and decreased smoking to two cigarettes per day. Her hot flushes are now once a day, and her vaginal dryness has decreased with improved sexual function, but she still is very bothered by hot flashes. Because the patient has systemic effects that have not resolved with lifestyle changes, oral estrogen is now discussed. Oral estradiol and medroxyprogesterone is initiated after counseling, and she plans to return in 1 month.

Are there advantages to HRT other than symptom control?

Past studies indicate that oral HRT also significantly decreases the risk of colon cancer and negative outcomes of osteoporosis, such as hip or vertebral fracture. Patients who become menopausal at younger ages may also have lowered mortality from HRT. Stroke, coronary artery disease, and peripheral vascular disease increase after menopause, and changes in the vaginal epithelium increase susceptibility to urinary tract infections (UTIs). Adequate and appropriate treatment of estrogen deficiency can prevent these negative effects.

BASIC SCIENCE PEARL	STEP 1

Estrogen plays a large role in regulating bone health by inhibiting the RANK ligand. The RANK ligand is responsible for activating osteoclasts, which break down bone. Therefore, when estrogen decreases in postmenopausal women, these patients are more prone to osteopenia and osteoporosis.

CLINICAL SCIENCE PEARL	STEPS 2/3

Screening for osteoporosis with DEXA scan begins at age 65. The FRAX risk assessment tool helps to identify patients who may be at an increased risk for bone disease and require early screening. It includes age, sex, BMI, previous fragility fracture, parental hip fracture, alcohol intake, smoking status, corticosteroid use, rheumatoid arthritis, and other secondary causes of osteoporosis.

The patient returns in 1 month and reports she had only one hot flush this month and has returned to comfortable sexual intercourse. Her blood pressure is 120/75 mm Hg, her vaginal exam shows healthy, rugated tissue, and she reports no negative side effects from her vaginal or oral estrogen. She plans to follow-up for her next gynecologic exam.

When should the patient consider stopping her estrogen?

There are no specific recommendations for how long patients can be on HRT, but it should be continued as long as benefits outweigh risks for the individual, and plans to continue or discontinue should be addressed at each gynecologic visit. In general, HRT should be administered at the lowest dose possible for the shortest duration as treatment is most beneficial for younger patients at the early onset of symptoms.

BEYOND THE PEARLS

- A well-known study called the Women's Health initiative is the primary study quoted in discussions of the risks and benefits of HRT. There were two arms of the study: an estrogen plus progestin (E+P) arm for women with a uterus and an estrogen-only (EO) arm in women without a uterus. In each arm women were randomized to either receive hormone or placebo. The results demonstrated that in the E+P arm, there was an increased risk of breast cancer, an increase in stroke, TEs, and CVEs, and a decreased risk of colon cancer and hip fractures. In the EO arm, there was also an increase in TEs, but there was no increased risk of CVEs or breast cancer.
- Patients should be adequately warned that "bioidentical hormones" or herbal remedies, both of which are highly marketed to women for menopausal symptoms, are not regulated

BEYOND THE PEARLS—cont'd

for purity or rigorously tested for effectiveness. Just because these products are labeled "natural" does not mean they are without dangers or side effects. For example, there is no consistent evidence that soy products increase estrogen levels significantly, and herbal medications such as black cohosh can cause significant liver toxicity.

- Women who are considering ovarian removal at the time of a hysterectomy for benign disease should be counseled that removal of ovaries before age 65 is associated with earlier mortality and morbidity, so women without increased risk of ovarian or breast cancer should have preservation of the ovaries considered before age 65.

Case Summary

- 56-year-old woman presents to the office with amenorrhea for 1 year and symptoms of hot flushes, dyspareunia, decreased libido, and vaginal dryness. Her follicle stimulating hormone (FSH) and luteinizing hormone (LH) levels are elevated, and physical exam shows vaginal thinning and excoriations.
- Due to current smoking, she is started on lifestyle changes and provided with advice for smoking cessation along with vaginal estrogen. She returns in 4 weeks with improved vaginal symptoms but continued bothersome vasomotor symptoms. She has decreased her smoking.
- After counseling on risks and benefits, she is started on systemic hormone replacement therapy (HRT) with an appropriate response to therapy and resolution of her symptoms.

References

American College of Obstetricians and Gynecologists (2014). ACOG Practice Bulletin No. 141: management of menopausal symptoms. *Obstet Gynecol, 123*(1), 202–216.

Katz, V., Lobo, R., Lentz, G. M., & Gershenson, D. M. (2007). *Comprehensive gynecology* (5th ed.). Philadelphia, PA: Elsevier, 1039–1065.

Parker, W. H., Broder, M. S., Chang, E., Feskanich, D., Farquhar, C., Liu, Z., et al. (2009). Ovarian conservation at the time of hysterectomy and long-term health outcomes in the nurses' health study. *Obstet Gynecol, 113*, 1027–1037.

Shifren, L. J., & Gass, M. L. S. (2014). North American Menopause Society (NAMS) Recommendations for Clinic Care of Midlife Women Working Group. *Menopause, 21*(10), 1038–1062.

The Women's Health Initiative Study Group. (1998). Design of the Women's Health Initiative clinical trial and observational study. *Control Clin Trials, 19*, 61–109.

Nita Desai, MD, MBA

A 22-Year-Old Woman With Painful Menses

A 22-year-old woman presents to your office with painful menses. She experienced menarche at age 12, and her menses became painful by age 15. Menses occur at 28- to 30-day intervals, and bleeding lasts for 4–6 days with moderate flow. Her pain begins 2–3 days before the onset of bleeding and tapers in intensity once she starts bleeding. Her pain is located in the central aspect of the lower abdomen, radiates to her low back, is described as "crazy-intense cramping" by the patient, and is associated with bloating and loose bowel movements. The pain is minimally improved with nonsteroidal antiinflammatories and a heating pad and is aggravated by wearing tight clothing. In the past, her pain has caused her to miss her college classes, and she is concerned how this may affect her new job, or worse, her ability to have children in the future. She has been sexually active for the past 2 years and notes occasional painful intercourse.

What is your differential diagnosis for this patient?

Although there are a plethora of causes of painful menses, when evaluating a patient with chronic, cyclic pain (chronic pain is defined as lasting 6 months or greater), the most likely culprits are adenomyosis (endometrial tissue that grows into the uterine wall), dysmenorrhea, endometriosis (endometrial tissue that grows anywhere outside the confines of the uterus), and chronic pelvic inflammatory disease (PID). When chronic pelvic pain consistently peaks prior to the onset of menstrual bleeding, such as in this patient, endometriosis should be high on the differential. Endometriosis, chronic PID, adenomyosis, and dysmenorrhea can all include intense cramping, usually beginning 2–3 days before the onset of bleeding; generalized abdominal pain and bloating; and associated fatigue, nausea, vomiting, and bowel movement or urinary changes.

CLINICAL PEARL   **STEPS 2/3**

Most patients with endometriosis have pain that peaks prior to the onset of menstrual bleeding and lessens as the bleeding begins. Dysuria and/or dyschezia are also more typically associated with endometriosis than with dysmenorrhea or chronic pelvic infection. A thorough history regarding the exact time of onset of pain and associated factors can help to narrow the diagnosis. A pain and menstrual diary may be helpful in illuminating this history.

What factors of the history can differentiate these three diagnoses on the differential?

Typically, adenomyosis will present as intense cramping associated with the onset of menstrual bleeding in conjunction with a heavy bleeding pattern. Physical examination can include an enlarged, tender, boggy uterus. Dysmenorrhea presents as recurrent, crampy, suprapubic pain at the onset or just prior to menstrual bleeding; other symptoms, such as radiating pain or nausea and fatigue, can be present, but the physical examination findings will typically be normal.

Endometriosis patients have cyclic, although sometimes noncyclic, pelvic pain with menstrual bleeding. These patients may also have associated dyspareunia, dyschezia (pain with bowel movements), and infertility. Physical exam can range from normal to findings of minimal mobility of uterus, adnexal masses, and uterosacral nodularity. Chronic PID typically presents as lower abdominal pain in a sexually active patient, and pelvic exam findings of cervical motion tenderness or pelvic organ tenderness would increase your suspicion for chronic PID.

CLINICAL PEARL   **STEPS 2/3**

Acute PID includes an oral temperature greater than 38.3°C (101°F) and abnormal cervical or vaginal mucopurulent discharge. Chronic PID is less consistent because it may present without vital sign changes, and cervical cultures may be negative.

On physical exam, the patient has normal vital signs and a soft, nontender abdomen. On speculum exam, there is no discharge or vaginal lesions. On bimanual exam, while her uterus and ovaries are freely mobile, they are also moderately tender to palpation. Additionally, there is fullness noted in the left adnexa.

What types of laboratory testing or imaging studies would be useful for this patient?
As with most patients, the clinical picture must guide subsequent testing. Adenomyosis can often be confirmed on ultrasound imaging, but endometriosis is less consistently seen. While magnetic resonance imaging (MRI) could further delineate a globular uterine wall or adnexal masses, it is expensive and is not confirmatory for endometriosis. Patients with dysmenorrhea, endometriosis, and chronic PID can all have normal ultrasound and laboratory results, so imaging should only be ordered to clarify the clinical picture and confirm adnexal masses and/or delineate their characteristics. For patients in whom chronic PID is suspected, vaginal or cervical cultures should be performed to confirm bacterial origin and to direct antibiotic therapy.

CLINICAL PEARL   **STEPS 2/3**

CA 125, a laboratory marker that is elevated in epithelial ovarian cancer and used to monitor therapy in these cancers, is also elevated in a plethora of benign conditions including endometriosis, liver cirrhosis, acute peritonitis, acute pancreatitis, acute PID, first trimester of pregnancy, and in healthy individuals without cause.

Transvaginal ultrasound (TVUS) imaging reveals a 6 cm smooth, anteverted uterus. The right ovary is 3 cm and appears normal, but the left ovary, also 6 cm in size, contains a 4 cm cyst. The cyst is described as a hypoechoic mass containing diffuse, homogenous, low-level internal echoes.

How do you next counsel your patient?
The description of this cyst is characteristic of an endometrioma. The fluid inside the cyst on TVUS is consistent with what is described as "chocolate fluid," which results from the degradation of the internal blood products within the cyst wall over time. Given the patient's clinical picture and the appearance of this adnexal mass, this patient likely has endometriosis. However, definitive diagnosis of endometriosis is only confirmed by histopathology, so surgical exploration is considered diagnostic as well as therapeutic (Fig. 42.1).

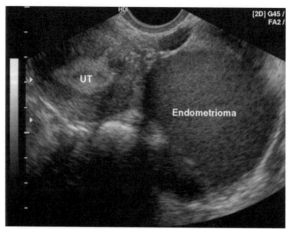

Fig. 42.1 Ultrasound appearance of an endometrioma, with excellent display of the homogenous, low-level echoes within the smooth, curving cyst wall. The endometrioma is adnexal in location, as it can be seen adjacent to the uterus (UT).

BASIC SCIENCE PEARL	STEP 1

Microscopically, endometriotic implants consist of endometrial glands and stoma with or without hemosiderin-laden macrophages.

CLINICAL PEARL	STEPS 2/3

Many other imaging appearances of endometriomas have been described, including anechoic cysts, solid-appearing masses, solid elements in a cyst with low-level internal echoes, and punctate echogenic foci in the wall of the cyst. The most common misdiagnoses of endometriomas by sonography are hemorrhagic and dermoid cysts.

What is the next step in management?

At this point in time, the patient should be counseled regarding treatment options, which include both medical and surgical choices. Conservative therapies for endometriosis include suppression of menstrual cycle, specifically ovulation, through use of oral contraceptive pills (OCPs), depot-medroxyprogesterone acetate (DMPA) or depot-leuprolide, and intrauterine devices (IUDs). All of these medications can improve symptoms and prevent future disease by interrupting the menstrual cycles but will not cure or reverse current lesions, such as large endometriomas. In patients in whom conservative therapies have failed or who desire pregnancy, surgery should be offered.

The patient decides that she would like to try DMPA at this time, because she is desperate for her pain and menses to stop. She has one injection of DMPA and repeats it 3 months later. Six months after starting this therapy, she comes to your office discouraged. She still has intermittent, crampy pelvic pain that occurs 3 days per month, and she is very bothered by the irregular spotting caused by her DMPA. She is now engaged to be married and wants to think about starting a family in the future. She asks if she can explore surgical therapy. A repeat TVUS shows her former ovarian cyst is unchanged in appearance.

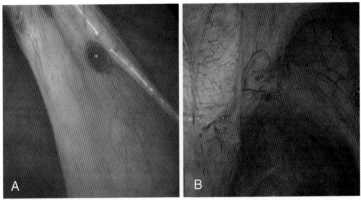

Fig. 42.2 Laparoscopic views of endometriosis lesions in the pelvic peritoneum. The left panel (A) shows a round, red, vascular lesions of the "vesicular" type, and the right panel (B) shows a "powder-burn" lesion type.

What surgical options should you discuss with her?

Surgery for endometriosis can be divided into two broad categories: "clean up" or "take out." Most patients will see improvement of pain with fulguration or excision of endometriosis lesions, including endometriomas. In those patients who have completed childbearing, definitive treatment in the form of hysterectomy, with or without bilateral salpingo-oophorectomy, can be considered. Surgery can be performed via minimally invasive techniques such as laparoscopic or robotic-assisted laparoscopy or through laparotomy, although minimally invasive techniques are preferred due to faster recovery and less pain. The patient should also be counseled about the risks of surgery, particularly as patients with endometriosis may have intraabdominal adhesions that can increase the risk of bleeding, organ injury, or a longer or more complicated surgery. She should also be counseled about the fact that endometriosis can recur after surgical treatment and offered options to prevent endometriosis after any planned surgery (Fig. 42.2).

> The patient elects to proceed with surgical treatment. She undergoes a laparoscopic lysis of adhesions and left ovarian cystectomy. Pathology of peritoneal biopsies in the pouch of Douglas is consistent with endometriosis, and the pathology of the ovarian cyst is benign and consistent with an endometrioma. Postoperatively, the patient was started on to prevent endometriosis recurrence. Four months postoperatively, the patient's pain and dyspareunia have completely resolved.

What is long-term follow-up for this patient?

In general, provided there are no contraindications, the patient can use OCPs until she is ready to conceive. Ideally, all medical options should be exhausted prior to considering primary or repeat surgery unless there is a clinical indication to do so. Endometriosis is primarily a disease of reproductive-aged women, so as the patient ages, pain is less likely to be due to endometriosis.

BEYOND THE PEARLS

- Epidemiologic reports estimate 176 million women are affected with endometriosis worldwide, and 1 in 10 women in the United States.
- Early diagnosis and intervention are key factors in the prevention of severe disease in endometriosis, which can lead to severe pain and infertility.

- While imaging can be helpful endometriosis, it is not required for diagnosis and therefore should be ordered sparingly.
- Most patients have improvement of pain with fulguration of endometriosis lesions, but excision should be considered in patients in whom fulguration was not previously successful or in patients with deep infiltrating endometriosis (DIE). The delimitation of DIE is made in the operating room by the surgeon.
- Exhaustion of medical options is preferable prior to surgical intervention; however, evidence demonstrates that patients see the most long-term relief when both modalities are used in conjunction with one another.

Case Summary

- A 22-year-old woman presents to your office with chronic, cyclic pelvic pain since 3 years after menarche (age 15). She is suspected of having endometriosis based on clinical history, physical exam with tender pelvic organs, and ultrasound findings showing a 4 cm ovarian cyst with low-level, homogenous internal echoes.
- The patient attempts DMPA therapy for 6 months but is not pleased with the outcome and wants to explore surgical therapy for definitive diagnosis and management. She undergoes a laparoscopic left ovarian cystectomy. Her pathology is consistent with endometriosis.
- Postoperatively, she uses oral contraceptive pills (OCPs) for suppression, and her symptoms improve dramatically.

For Further Reading

American College of Obstetricians and Gynecologists (2010). ACOG Practice bulletin number 114: Management of endometriosis. *Obstetrics & Gynecology, 116*(1), 223–226.

Asch, A. B., & Levine, M. D. (2007). Variations in appearance of endometriomas. *Journal of Ultrasound in Medicine, 26*, 993–1002.

European Society of Human Reproduction and Embryology (ESHRE) (2007). *Guideline for the diagnosis and treatment of endometriosis.* www.eshre/eu.

Fleisher, M., Dnistrian, A., Sturgeon, C., Lamerz, R., & Witliff, J. (2002). *Practice guidelines and recommendations for use of tumor markers in the clinic. Tumor markers. Physiology, pathobiology, technology and clinical applications.* Washington: AACC Press, 33–63.

Muyldermans, M., Cornillie, F. J., & Kininckx, P. R. (1995). CA 125 and endometriosis. *Human Reproduction Update, 1*(2), 173–187.

Osayande, A. S., & Mehulic, S. (2014). Diagnosis and initial management of dysmenorrhea. *American Family Physician 89*(5), 341–346.

CASE 43

Kara A. Ehlers, MD ▪ Kelly Pagidas, MD

A 26-Year-Old Woman With Irregular Menses

A 26-year-old woman presents with irregular menstrual cycles since she started menses at age 11, and the length of time between periods has lengthened over the past 3 years.

What additional information would you want to know from the patient?

It is important to obtain more detailed information about her menstrual cycles. You will ask her the first day of her last menstrual period (LMP), how frequently her cycles occur, the number of days she bleeds and how many pads or tampons she uses per day when her cycles occur, whether she is soaking pads or clothes, and if she experiences pain with her menses. It is vital to know if the patient is sexually active, as irregular bleeding can be secondary to a pregnancy, which must be ruled out. Inquire about previous surgeries, particularly pelvic surgeries, and if her menstrual pattern changed around the time of these procedures. Review her medical conditions and medications; thyroid disease, coagulation problems, weight changes, and medications such as antidepressants, corticosteroids, hormonal therapies, and herbal supplements can all change menstrual patterns. Last, ask about relevant symptoms such as coarse, dark, terminal hairs distributed in a male pattern (hirsutism), acne, and milky breast discharge (galactorrhea) that may indicate certain endocrine disorders.

What is the differential diagnosis for irregular menstrual bleeding?

In 2011, the International Federation of Gynecology and Obstetrics (FIGO) presented a new classification system for uterine bleeding abnormalities, and the American College of Obstetricians and Gynecologists (ACOG) supports this classification system for the differential diagnosis of abnormal uterine bleeding (AUB). The new system is known as the PALM-COEIN system (*P*olyp, *A*denomyosis, *L*eiomyoma, *M*alignancy and hyperplasia, *C*oagulopathy, *O*vulatory dysfunction, *E*ndometrial, *I*atrogenic, and *N*ot yet classified respectively). The most common cause of irregular menses is ovulatory in origin (AUB-O in the PALM-COEIN), and the most common cause of AUB-O is an endocrine imbalance such as polycystic ovarian syndrome (PCOS), where the mechanism of the AUB is primarily unopposed estrogen.

The patient has been having bleeding episodes every 3–4 months, which last up to 2 weeks, and she uses 5–10 pads per day. She denies breast discharge, but does report problems with acne, coarse facial hair, and a 50-pound weight gain over 3 years.

What should you look for in the physical exam?

In your thorough physical and pelvic exam, signs to look for include hirsutism and acne, thyroid enlargement or masses, visual deficits (which can indicate a pituitary mass), galactorrhea, acanthosis nigricans (a sign of insulin resistance), increased body mass index (BMI) or truncal obesity,

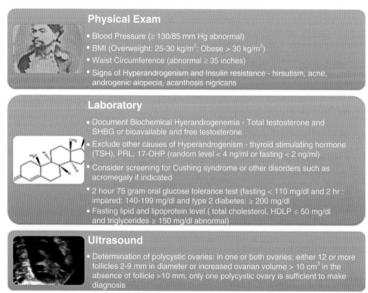

Physical Exam

- Blood Pressure (≥ 130/85 mm Hg abnormal)
- BMI (Overweight: 25-30 kg/m²; Obese > 30 kg/m²)
- Waist Circumference (abnormal ≥ 35 inches)
- Signs of Hyperandrogenism and Insulin resistance - hirsutism, acne, androgenic alopecia, acanthosis nigricans

Laboratory

- Document Biochemical Hyerandrogenemia - Total testosterone and SHBG or bioavailable and free testosterone
- Exclude other causes of Hyperandrogenism - thyroid stimulating hormone (TSH), PRL, 17-OHP (random level < 4 ng/ml or fasting < 2 ng/ml)
- Consider screening for Cushing syndrome or other disorders such as acromegaly if indicated
- 2 hour 75 gram oral glucose tolerance test (fasting < 110 mg/dl and 2 hr : impared: 140-199 mg/dl and type 2 diabetes: ≥ 200 mg/dl
- Fasting lipid and lipoprotein level (total cholesterol, HDLP ≤ 50 mg/dl and triglycerides ≥ 150 mg/dl abnormal)

Ultrasound

- Determination of polycystic ovaries: in one or both ovaries; either 12 or more follicles 2-9 mm in diameter or increased ovarian volume > 10 cm³ in the absence of follicle >10 mm; only one polycystic ovary is sufficient to make diagnosis

Fig. 43.1   Recommended evaluation for polycystic ovarian syndrome.

and signs of Cushing syndrome such as moon facies, buffalo hump, bruising, or purple abdominal striae. A pelvic exam would rule out clitoral enlargement or structural lesions of the cervix, vagina, and uterus. Laboratory evaluation and imaging should be guided on findings and suspicion of comorbidities (Fig. 43.1).

CLINICAL PEARL   **STEPS 2/3**

A finding of an enlarged clitoris (clitoromegaly) is rare in PCOS, and its presence necessitates a workup for an androgen-producing tumor (adrenal or ovarian) or congenital adrenal hyperplasia. There is no androgen level that is pathognomonic for an androgen-secreting tumor, but total testosterone of 200 ng/dL or greater or dehydroepiandrosterone (DHEAS) levels of 700 µg/dL or greater are suspicious.

What is the pathophysiology of hirsutism, and what are some common causes?

Hirsutism results from conversion of villus hairs to dark, coarse terminal hairs from excess androgens (hyperandrogenism). The most common cause in women is PCOS, with idiopathic hirsutism being second. Other causes include late-onset congenital adrenal hyperplasia, an androgen-producing ovarian tumor, exogenous steroid use, and Cushing syndrome.

BASIC SCIENCE PEARL   **STEP 1**

Both the adrenals and ovaries contribute to the circulating level of androgens in women. The adrenals primarily secrete DHEA or dehydroepiandrosterone sulfate (DHEAS), both of which are 90% of adrenal origin. These weak androgens serve as prohormones for more potent androgens such as testosterone and dihydrotestosterone (DHT), with DHT being most potent. The ovary is the primary source (makes 75%) of testosterone.

TABLE 43.1 ■ Diagnostic Criteria that Must Be Met for the Diagnosis of Polycystic Ovary Syndrome (PCOS) as per Various Expert Guidelines

Signs and Symptoms	National Institutes of Health Criteria 1990[a]	Rotterdam Consensus Criteria 2003[b]	Androgen Excess Society 2006[c]
Hyperandrogenism[d]	Required	Possible criteria	Required
Oligo- or amenorrhea[e]	Required	Possible criteria	Possible criteria
Polycystic ovaries on ultrasound		Possible criteria	Possible criteria

[a]Both required.
[b]Two of the three required.
[c]Hyperandrogenism required plus one of the two other criteria.
[d]Hyperandrogenism can be by biochemical (elevated androgens on laboratory testing) or clinical (signs on physical exam) criteria.
[e]Menses less often than every 40 days (oligomenorrhea) or no menses for ≥3 months (amenorrhea).

The patient weighs 93 kg (205 lbs) and is 1.63 M (5′4″) tall (BMI 35.2 kg/m²). Her blood pressure is 130/85 mm Hg. Physical exam is significant for coarse hair on her upper lip and chin as well as her upper chest and abdomen. She is also noted to have a darkening of the skin behind her neck. Her pelvic exam reveals normal external genitalia, cervix, and uterus.

How would you make a diagnosis of PCOS?
Women with PCOS commonly present with menstrual irregularities and infertility, but may also present with comorbidities such as diabetes, weight problems, or hirsutism, which is present in 70% of women with PCOS. PCOS is the most common endocrine disorder in women, with at least 6%–10% prevalence by the National Institute of Health (NIH) diagnostic criteria and up to 15% by Rotterdam criteria (Table 43.1). The essential diagnostic criteria include hyperandrogenism, oligo- or amenorrhea, and polycystic ovaries by ultrasound. All diagnostic schemes require more than one sign or symptom and clarify that PCOS is a diagnosis of exclusion.

The patient's laboratory work shows a free testosterone (fT) of 7.0 pg/mL, DHEAS of 450 μg/dL, thyroid stimulating hormone (TSH) of 2.3 mIU/L, prolactin level of 10 ng/mL, 17-OHP of 1.5 ng/mL, and a fasting glucose of 90 mg/dL and 2 hour glucose of 130 ng/mL. A transvaginal ultrasound (TVUS) reports ovarian volume of 15 cm³ per ovary. She is given the diagnosis of PCOS.

What comorbidities are associated with PCOS, and how can you screen for them?
Comorbidities such as obesity, metabolic syndrome, and endometrial malignancy should be screened for routinely in women with PCOS, starting from the initial presentation. Women with PCOS have long periods of unopposed estrogen, which thickens the lining of the uterus, contributing to AUB and placing them at risk for precancerous changes in the endometrium. The endocrine imbalances and prevalence of an elevated BMI in women with PCOS also puts them at increased risk of metabolic syndrome, nonalcoholic fatty liver disease, and mood disturbances such as depression. Hypertension screening is easily done by office blood pressure assessment, diabetes or insulin resistance is screened for with the 2 hour glucose tolerance test (glucose levels alone are not adequate in patients with PCOS), and fasting lipid panels are performed to screen for hyperlipidemia.

CLINICAL PEARL   **STEPS 2/3**

The diagnosis of metabolic syndrome requires 3 out of 5 different physical and laboratory findings: a waist circumference of 35 inches or more (for women), elevated fasting blood sugar of 100 mmol/dL or more, elevated blood pressure of 135/85 mm Hg or higher, reduced high-density lipoprotein (HDL) to less than 50 mg/dL, or a high triglyceride level of 150 mg/dL or more. Metabolic syndrome is associated with cardiovascular and cerebrovascular accidents, peripheral vascular disease, and early death.

You counsel the patient that she has a normal lipid profile and glucose screening, although she has prehypertension. Our patient would like to have more regular and predictable menses. She is currently single and does not "want to be pregnant now."

What PCOS therapies are available to patients who do not currently desire pregnancy?
The most important factor, regardless if the patient is seeking pregnancy now or in the future, is lifestyle modification with a focus on optimizing weight through a healthy diet and exercise. For patients with PCOS, weight reduction as low as 5% can lead to a decrease in serum testosterone and spontaneous resumption of menses and ovulation. Other treatment goals for PCOS women include avoidance of irregular or heavy bleeding, decrease in acne and hirsutism, and prevention and early treatment of comorbid diseases. Combination low-dose oral contraceptive pills (OCPs) are an excellent option for women with PCOS who do not desire pregnancy. First, OCPs regulate the menstrual cycle and protect the endometrium from long periods of unopposed estrogen. Also, OCPs increase sex hormone binding globulin, which decreases unbound androgens and improves hirsutism and acne. As OCPs should not be used in smokers over age 35 or patients with uncontrolled hypertension, this patient with prehypertension will be carefully monitored if she opts to start on OCPs. Other hormonal treatments such as progesterone-only contraceptives (POPs), a levonorgestrel intrauterine device (IUD), or injectable long-acting medroxyprogesterone (Depo-Provera) have the benefit of improving bleeding and protecting the endometrium from unopposed estrogen. However, these progesterone-only alternatives do not decrease androgens in the manner of combined OCPs.

How would you manage hirsutism in a woman with PCOS?
Antiandrogen medications for hirsutism include spironolactone, flutamide, and finasteride, all of which appear to have similar efficacy, but none of which is approved by the U.S. Food and Drug Administration (FDA) for hirsutism. Antiandrogens are teratogenic, so the patient must be counseled on the importance of contraception if using these medications. Topical eflornithine, an inhibitor of ornithine decarboxylase, is FDA approved for hirsutism treatment in women, with approximately 60% reporting improvement after 6 months. Medical therapy for hirsutism is often underwhelming and takes more than 6 months, so patients should be aware that both medical therapy and mechanical removal of hair (shaving, plucking, waxing, depilatory creams, etc.) may be necessary.

BASIC SCIENCE/CLINICAL PEARL   **STEPS 1/2/3**

Spironolactone is an aldosterone antagonist that also antagonizes the androgen receptor in hair follicles, inhibits ovarian and adrenal steroidogenesis, and directly inhibits 5-α-reductase activity. These mechanisms make it an excellent choice for hirsutism treatment in PCOS. However, spironolactone does not decrease current hair growth and, as a diuretic, has the potential side effects of orthostatic hypotension and hyperkalemia.

The patient elects for levonorgestrel IUD placement at this time, as her acne and abnormal hair growth are not that bothersome to her at this time. Two years later, she returns to your office stating that she removed her levonorgestrel IUD 6 months ago as she is recently married and would like to start a family. Her menstrual cycles remain infrequent (every 40–45 days). She has continued a diet and exercise regimen and has remained stable at a weight of 72.5 kg (160 lbs) (BMI 27.5 kg/m²).

What therapies are available for PCOS patients who currently desire pregnancy?

As infertility in PCOS is caused by lack of consistent ovulation, the two therapies most commonly used for PCOS infertility are induction agents: clomiphene citrate and letrozole. Clomiphene citrate, a selective estrogen receptor agonist (SERM), works by binding to estrogen receptors in the pituitary and preventing the normal negative feedback loop, leading to the pituitary releasing more gonadotropins. Although clomiphene is typically first-line, recent randomized controlled trials have reported that the use of letrozole is associated with a higher cumulative live birth rate and ovulation rate in infertile women with PCOS. Injectable gonadotropins can also be used to stimulate follicular development in PCOS women, but daily injections are a barrier for some patients, and gonadotropins carry a higher risk of multiple gestation and ovarian hyperstimulation syndrome (OHSS) than oral induction agents.

The patient is started on clomiphene citrate and notes a positive ovulation predictor kit with subsequent positive home pregnancy test on her third cycle. An ultrasound reports a single live intrauterine gestation at 8 weeks. Her current weight is 81.6 kg (180 lbs) (BMI 30.9 kg/m²), as she gained weight during her treatment cycles.

What are some important recommendations that you want to review with her?

The importance of weight control during pregnancy must be emphasized, as obese women are at increased risk of gestational diabetes, preeclampsia, cardiac dysfunction, Caesarean section, and birth defects. Her recommended weight gain during pregnancy should be only 5-10 kg (11–20 lbs). Excessive weight during pregnancy is associated with higher risk of retaining the excess weight postpartum, which would worsen her PCOS.

BEYOND THE PEARLS

- Women with PCOS have an increased risk of obstructive sleep apnea (OSA) independent of BMI, so are 9–30 times more likely to have OSA than BMI-matched controls. Clinicians can use a validated screening tool for OSA (such as the Epworth Sleepiness Scale) and refer those who screen positive for formal sleep studies.
- In women with PCOS, the drug metformin is used primarily as an adjunct with ovulation induction agents to treat insulin resistance. However, there is no evidence for improved live birth rates or decreased pregnancy complications with metformin use in PCOS.
- OHSS is a life-threatening complication of infertility treatments that results from the development of a large number of ovarian follicles. These follicles produce excess vascular endothelial growth factor (VEGF), which increases vascular permeability with massive fluid shifts to the extravascular space and a hypercoagulable state resulting from hemoconcentration, hypovolemia, and elevated estrogen levels. OHSS can lead to hypovolemic shock, respiratory failure from pulmonary edema, pulmonary emboli, or renal failure from microthrombi in renal tubules. Treatment is supportive and involves restoring fluid balance and preventing thrombotic events.

Case Summary

- A 26-year-old woman presents with irregular menses since menarche with an increase in the interval between menses in the past few years. Her physical exam is remarkable for the presence of hirsutism, acanthosis nigricans, elevated blood pressure, and elevated body mass index (BMI). Her laboratory profile is only notable for an elevated testosterone and dihydroepiandrosterone (DHEAS), and an ultrasound demonstrates polycystic ovaries. She is given the diagnosis of polycystic ovarian syndrome (PCOS).
- She does not desire pregnancy presently, and her hirsutism is not problematic for her. She opts to use a progesterone-containing intrauterine device (IUD) and initiates a diet and exercise regimen.
- She returns in 2 years and desires to become pregnant. She has lost weight and has been able to maintain it. She pursues oral ovulation induction agents and conceives after her third cycle; you review with her the importance of avoiding excess weight gain during the pregnancy.

References

American College of Obstetricians and Gynecologists (ACOG) (2009). Practice bulletin 108: polycystic ovary syndrome. *Obstetrics and gynecology*, *114*(4), 936–949 Reaffirmed 2015.

American College of Obstetricians and Gynecologists (ACOG) (2013). Practice bulletin 136: management of abnormal uterine bleeding associated with ovulatory dysfunction. *Obstetrics and gynecology*, *122*(1), 176–185 Reaffirmed 2015.

American College of Obstetricians and Gynecologists (ACOG) (2015). Practice bulletin 156: obesity in pregnancy. *Obstetrics and gynecology*, *126*(6), e112–e126.

American Society of Reproductive Medicine (ASRM) (2015). Practice committee document obesity and reproduction: a committee opinion. *Fertility and Sterility*, *104*(5), 1116–1126.

Fauser, B. C. J. M., Tarlatzis, B. C., Rebar, R. W., et al. (2012). Consensus on women's health aspects of polycystic ovary syndrome (PCOS): the Amsterdam ESHRE/ASRM-Sponsored 3rd PCOS Consensus workshop group. *Fertility and Sterility*, *97*, 28–38.

Hoffman, B. L., Schorge, J. O., Schaffer, J. I., et al. (2012). Polycystic ovarian syndrome and hyperandrogenism. In B. L. Hoffman, J. O. Schorge, & J. I. Schaffer (Eds.), *Williams gynecology* (2nd ed.). New York: McGraw-Hill.

Legro, R. S., Brzyski, R. G., Diamond, M., et al. (2014). Letrozole versus clomiphene for infertility in the polycystic ovary syndrome. *The New England Journal of Medicine*, *371*(2), 119–129 2014.

Adrienne Gentry, MD ▪ Kelly Pagidas, MD

A 25-Year-Old With Recurrent Pregnancy Loss

A 25-year-old woman who had a positive pregnancy test in her doctor's office earlier today is admitted overnight secondary to vaginal bleeding and menstrual cramps. In the office, she was told that she is "having a miscarriage". She is scheduled today for a suction dilation and curettage (D&C). The patient is very tearful and distraught because this her third pregnancy loss.

What additional information do you want from this patient?

It is important to obtain more detailed information about her current pregnancy. You would want to know the date of her last menstrual period (LMP) and if her menses are regular in order to calculate an estimated gestational age. You also want to know how her doctor came to the diagnosis of a "miscarriage": particularly, if an ultrasound was done, was the pregnancy in the uterus, and was a gestational sac, a fetus, or both visualized? All of this information will help you to formulate and categorize the type of loss and rule out ectopic pregnancy. You also want to expand on her pregnancy history and know the number of her miscarriages or if she had other pregnancies ending in birth, elective termination, or intrauterine demise. If former pregnancies ended in spontaneous abortion (miscarriage), you want to know the gestation age when they occurred, how they were diagnosed, and whether or not she passed the pregnancy spontaneously or required medical or surgical intervention. This will help identify if the patient meets criteria for the definition of recurrent pregnancy loss (RPL) and narrow down the possible cause. You want to find out whether or not the patient has any medical conditions, is a smoker, abuses alcohol, uses illicit drugs, or if she takes any medication that could be contraindicated in pregnancy. Let us go back to our patient.

CLINICAL PEARL   **STEPS 2/3**

RPL is a disease that is quite distinct from sporadic pregnancy loss and infertility. The American Society of Reproductive Medicine (ASRM) defines RPL by the presence of two or more failed pregnancies before the 20th week of gestation, and the pregnancies must be documented by ultrasonography or histopathological examination. This definition excludes ectopic, molar, or preclinical (biochemical) pregnancy.

BASIC SCIENCE/CLINICAL PEARL   **STEPS 1/2/3**

Of clinically recognized pregnancies, 10% end in spontaneous miscarriage. However, fewer than 5% of women will experience two consecutive losses, and only 1% will experience three or more losses. Pregnancy loss can be further subcategorized into *embryonic loss*, defined as a loss at less than 7 weeks of gestation, with or without the presence of fetal cardiac activity on ultrasound, or *fetal loss*, defined as loss at more than 7 weeks of gestation and the presence of fetal cardiac activity prior to the loss. Embryonic loss is far more common than fetal loss (6:1).

The patient's LMP was 8 weeks ago and she has regular cycles. Yesterday, her doctor performed an ultrasound and noted a gestational sac, a yolk sac, and a fetal pole in the uterus measuring 6 weeks without fetal cardiac activity. This is her third spontaneous pregnancy loss; her two previous losses were documented by ultrasound at 7 weeks and 9 weeks, respectively, and were passed with the assistance of misoprostol use. She asks you if it would be worthwhile to send the tissue from the suction D&C for testing.

What would be your working diagnosis based on the information that you have on hand?
Because all her losses appear to have occurred prior to 10 weeks of gestation, and all were documented by ultrasound, she meets the criteria for RPL and warrants an evaluation. Evaluation of the products of conception (POC) for cytogenetic analysis is controversial. There is a clear psychological benefit to the patient or couple in analyzing the POC because knowledge of a genetically abnormal pregnancy that could not have been viable may be a relief. However, there are limitations with regard to cytogenetic analysis of POCs, including the possibility of maternal tissue contaminating the specimen.

What are common causes of RPL?
The gestational age at pregnancy loss may guide us toward a cause, although there is a great degree of overlap. Embryonic losses (<7 weeks gestation) are most commonly associated with chromosome anomalies (primarily trisomies), which increase in prevalence with increasing maternal age. Fetal losses (>7 weeks), on the other hand, are more often genetically normal. The etiology of RPL is multifactorial, with the exception of clear genetic abnormalities. The major categories of possible etiologies for RPL (Fig. 44.1) are grouped under parental causes, fetal causes, and unexplained. It is also important to note that each loss is an independent event, attributed to possibly different factors. Only 50% of women who undergo an evaluation for RPL get a definite diagnosis.

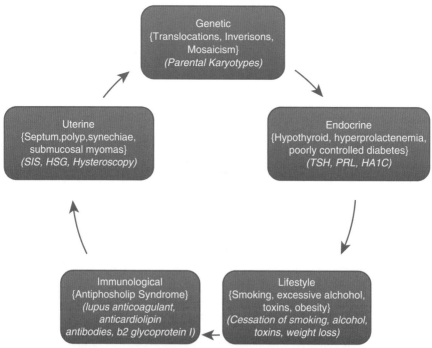

Fig. 44.1 Etiology and evaluation of recurrent pregnancy loss.

CLINICAL PEARL	STEPS 2/3

The risk of sporadic miscarriage in women younger than 35 years of age is estimated to be 9%–12% (50% in women over age 40). If POCs are sent for cytogenetic analysis and the karyotype reveals a 46, XX (a normal female karyotype), testing should be done to differentiate between fetal chromosomes versus maternal contamination. Chromosomal abnormalities are seen in approximately 50% of clinical losses and 70% of preclinical losses. The most common cause of chromosomal abnormalities in embryos is parental translocations.

The patient undergoes an uncomplicated suction D&C and elects to have the tissue sent for cytogenetic analysis. She sees you in the office 3 weeks postprocedure and wants to know her results and recommended next step. The tissue cytogenetics show trisomy 14.

What testing would you recommend for this patient for her RPL?
The workup should first include peripheral karyotypes of both parents. You also want to rule out maternal factors such as possible uterine causes and endocrine causes. Uterine imaging, such as saline infusion sonogram (SIS), a hysterosalpingogram (HSG), or hysteroscopy, evaluates for inherited and acquired uterine abnormalities (uterine septum, submucosal polyps or myomas, and intrauterine synechiae). Thyroid-stimulating hormone (TSH) and prolactin (PRL) testing is recommended. If this testing is normal, a workup for antiphospholipid syndrome (APS, Fig. 44.2) is merited. Let us review our patient's workup.

BASIC SCIENCE PEARL	STEP 1

The negative effects of antiphospholipid antibodies on pregnancy appears to be directed at the trophoblast. It acts as an inhibitor of cytotrophoblast differentiation and invasion, induces apoptosis of the syncytiotrophoblast, and initiates maternal inflammatory pathways on the syncytiotrophoblast.

The patient completes the workup that you recommended. Both the patient and her partner have normal parental karyotypes; SIS imaging and her TSH and PRL are normal. However, her anticardiolipin antibodies (ACA) and her β2 glycoprotein levels are greater than the 99th percentile.

What do you recommend next?
We can be reassured that we have not identified a genetic, uterine, or endocrine cause, but we are concerned that the patient may have APS. However, to make the confirmatory diagnosis of APS, we need to repeat her laboratory work 10–12 weeks later to ensure that the results were not transient as pregnancy itself can cause elevated antiphospholipid antibodies.

You repeat her levels in 12 weeks and the titers are again greater than the 99th percentile for ACA and β2 glycoprotein. She asks you how long she needs to wait before she starts trying to get pregnant again and what she can do to lower her risk of another miscarriage.

How would you advise her on trying to get pregnant again?
Historically, patients who had a miscarriage were told that they needed to wait a minimum of 3 months before they started trying to get pregnant again. However, recent data demonstrate that there is no difference in the risk of another loss if women conceive within 3 months of a recent loss. You would advise her that, based on her history and laboratory test results, she has a diagnosis of APS. You would also recommend that she starts on low-dose aspirin prior to conception. Once a viable pregnancy is confirmed, she should start anticoagulation with the use of twice-daily unfractionated heparin.

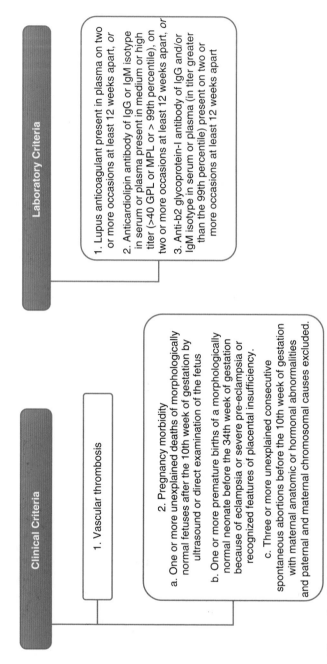

Fig. 44.2 Diagnostic criteria for antiphospholipid antibody syndrome (APS). For APS to be diagnosed, one of the clinical criteria and one of the laboratory criteria must be met.

CLINICAL PEARL STEPS 2/3

The use of twice-daily unfractionated heparin and low-dose aspirin is superior to aspirin alone in minimizing the risk of another pregnancy loss in the background of APS. The live birth rate is 74% compared to 43%, respectively. There is no indication to screen for inherited thrombophilias in women with RPL in the absence of a personal history of a vascular thrombosis as anticoagulation in pregnancy is not associated with an improvement in the live birth rate.

She is started on low-dose aspirin, and she conceives 2 months after her suction D&C. She is started on twice-daily unfractionated heparin once ultrasounds performed at 7 weeks and 10 weeks of gestation report a live intrauterine gestation with appropriate interval fetal growth and consistent with her gestational age by her LMP.

BEYOND THE PEARLS

- Women with recurrent pregnancy loss have a good prognosis for a live birth; greater than 70% of women will have a successful pregnancy outcome even if no workup or treatment is initiated, so reassurance is important from the outset.
- RPL carries with it an enormous psychological burden on women/couples, including depression, anxiety, and feelings of anger, grief, and guilt. Providing both psychological support and counseling has been associated with a positive outcome.
- Peripheral parental karyotypes are warranted in the evaluation of RPL to detect balanced structural chromosomal abnormalities (balanced reciprocal and Robertsonian translocations). These are seen in about 2%–5% of couples with RPL.
- Recurrent false-positive serologic tests (VRDL) for syphilis are seen in women with positive ACA.
- If a parental structural chromosomal translocation is identified, the use of in vitro fertilization (IVF) and preimplantation genetic diagnosis (PGD) has not been associated with an improvement in the live birth rate.
- Data are lacking for the routine screening for infections such as *Ureaplasma urealyticum, Mycoplasma hominus, Listeria monocytogenes, Chlamydia trachomatis, Toxoplasma gondii*, rubella, cytomegalovirus, and herpes virus in women with RPL. Some of this testing was formerly designated by the ToRCH acronym (Toxoplasma, rubella, cytomegalovirus, herpes simplex), and some women with RPL still receive a ToRCH workup.

Case Summary
- A 25-year-old woman is admitted for a suction dilation and curettage (D&C) for a spontaneous pregnancy loss at 8 weeks of gestation diagnosed by ultrasound.
- She has had two other prior pregnancy losses that occurred at less than 10 weeks of gestation and meets the criteria for recurrent pregnancy loss (RPL).
- She undergoes a suction D&C, and cytogenetic analysis of the products of conception (POCs) reveals trisomy 14.
- Her clinical history and laboratory work for RPL are consistent with antiphospholipid syndrome (APS).
- She desires to reinitiate attempts at pregnancy as soon as possible. She is started on low-dose aspirin prepregnancy. She conceives 2 months after her suction D&C, and she is started on twice-daily unfractionated heparin once a viable, intrauterine gestation is confirmed.

References

American College of Obstetricians and Gynecologists (ACOG) Practice Bulletin (No. 132). (2012). Antiphospholipid syndrome. *Obstet Gynecol*, *120*, 1514–1521.

Practice Committee of the American Society of Reproductive Medicine (2013). Definitions of infertility and recurrent pregnancy loss: a committee opinion. *Fertil Steril*, *99*, 63.

Practice Committee of the American Society of Reproductive Medicine (2012). Evaluation and treatment of recurrent pregnancy loss: a committee opinion. *Fertil Steril*, *98*, 1103–1111.

Yen & Jaffe's (2014). Reproductive endocrinology: physiology, pathophysiology and clinical management. In Strauss, J. F., & Barbieri, R. L., (Eds.), *Female infertility and male infertility* (7th ed.). Philadelphia: Elsevier Saunders.

Yelena Dondik, MD ■ Kelly Pagidas, MD

A 17-Year-Old Girl With Absent Menses

A 17-year-old girl presents to the office because she is concerned that she has not had her menstrual period yet. She is starting college in the fall and is concerned that she still looks "like a child."

What other questions do you want to ask this patient?

First, you want to clarify if she has never had any menstrual bleeding (primary amenorrhea) or if she had menses previously and they have since stopped (secondary amenorrhea). Primary amenorrhea merits workup by age 15 if there are secondary sexual characteristics (SSC), no menses by age 13 if SSC are absent (no breast development), or if no menses has occurred by 3 years after breast development. Regarding her complaints about her appearance, you want to get a description of her breast development and pubic and axillary hair growth. You want to document how tall she is compared to her peers and family members, her neonatal and childhood development, any medications she is taking, any recent stress, change in her weight, diet and exercise habits, breast symptoms such as discharge or pain, and any neurological symptoms such as headaches or visual changes or breast discharge.

CLINICAL PEARL   **STEPS 2/3**

The median age of onset of puberty in females is currently reported at 9.5–9.7 years, with the median age of menarche at 12.4 years. The sequence of pubertal maturation is typically (1) growth acceleration, (2) breast development (thelarche), (3) pubic hair development (pubarche), (4) growth spurt, and (5) onset of menses (menarche).

How should one approach the diagnosis in primary amenorrhea?

In the absence of pregnancy, primary amenorrhea is due to either a genetic condition causing gonadal dysfunction or an anatomic abnormality of the outflow tract. One simple way to think about primary amenorrhea is to break it into three basic considerations. The first is evidence of estrogen production by the ovaries, displayed by the presence or absence of breast development. Second, we consider the presence of a uterus, which is evident on pelvic exam and/or ultrasound. For example, Müllerian agenesis would be suspected in the presence of normal SCC with the absence of the uterus. Third, we look for evidence of gonadal function using a follicle stimulating hormone (FSH) level.

CLINICAL PEARL   **STEPS 2/3**

The most common cause of primary amenorrhea is gonadal dysgenesis secondary to Turner syndrome or Swyer's syndrome (43% of primary amenorrhea), followed by Müllerian agenesis (15%), and physiologic delay of puberty (14%).

She states that she never has seen any menstrual bleeding at all, not even "spotting." The patient buys bras "in the kid's section of the store," she is shorter than all the girls in her class, and she does not shave. She denies headaches, vision changes, galactorrhea, past medical or surgical problems, or a family history of delayed puberty.

What would be the most likely cause of amenorrhea in our patient?

Our working diagnosis is primary amenorrhea without estrogen production because her lack of SCC is highly suggestive of gonadal dysfunction or failure. Her other diagnosis could be physiological delay of puberty (also known as constitutional delay), but this is usually associated with a family history of delayed puberty.

What are the physical exam findings to look for when evaluating primary amenorrhea?

A physical exam, focusing on breast and pubic hair development assessed by Turner staging, guides our differential. As noted earlier, breast development is a sign of functioning gonads, and a pelvic exam assesses for presence of a uterus or vagina. Assessment of any skin changes, such as presence or excess of hair, acanthosis nigricans, and acne, can aid in the diagnosis (Fig. 45.1).

CLINICAL PEARL   **STEPS 2/3**

Androgen insensitivity is a rare disorder with karyotype 46 XY, which represents approximately 5% of primary amenorrhea. Serum testosterone in these patients will be in the normal male range or slightly elevated, and the patients will have no pubic hair.

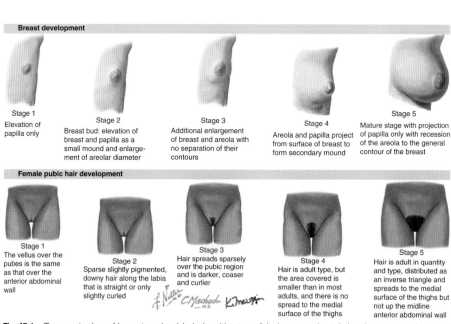

Breast development

Stage 1
Elevation of
papilla only

Stage 2
Breast bud: elevation of
breast and papilla as a
small mound and enlarge-
ment of areolar diameter

Stage 3
Additional enlargement
of breast and areola with
no separation of their
contours

Stage 4
Areola and papilla project
from surface of breast to
form secondary mound

Stage 5
Mature stage with projection
of papilla only with recession
of the areola to the general
contour of the breast

Female pubic hair development

Stage 1
The vellus over the
pubes is the same
as that over the
anterior abdominal
wall

Stage 2
Sparse slightly pigmented,
downy hair along the labia
that is straight or only
slightly curled

Stage 3
Hair spreads sparsely
over the pubic region
and is darker, coaser
and curlier

Stage 4
Hair is adult type, but
the area covered is
smaller than in most
adults, and there is no
spread to the medial
surface of the thighs

Stage 5
Hair is adult in quantity
and type, distributed as
an inverse triangle and
spreads to the medial
surface of the thighs but
not up the midline
anterior abdominal wall

Fig. 45.1 Tanner staging of breast and pubic hair, with stage 0 being no pubertal development and stage 5 being adult development. *(From Calabria AC, Langdon DR. Netter's pediatrics. Philadelphia: Elsevier; 2011: 416–21, fig. 67-3.)*

On physical exam, the patient is noted to be 4'11" and 125 lbs. She has Tanner Stage 1 breast and pubic hair development, and she has a broad chest with widely spaced nipples. On pelvic exam, a normal vagina and cervix are present, and a small uterus is palpable.

What labs should be part of her initial workup?

After exclusion of pregnancy, the next step is to measure the FSH, thyroid-stimulating hormone (TSH), and prolactin (PRL) levels. These three tests will identify most amenorrhea causes (Fig. 45.2).

The patient's FSH level is 68 mIU/mL, and her TSH and PRL are in the normal range.

What additional workup would you like to order for this patient?

A level of greater than 30 mIU/mL in the presence of persistent amenorrhea is considered indicative of gonadal failure. Gonadal failure (agenesis or dysgenesis) often has a genetic cause, and your next step with this patient would be a karyotype. Turner syndrome, which is monosomy X (45, X karyotype) or 45, X mosaicism associated with a milder clinical presentation such as secondary amenorrhea, can be clearly diagnosed with a karyotype.

Karyotype testing of our patient reveals 45 XO; she is diagnosed with Turner syndrome.

What physical exam findings are commonly seen in Turner syndrome?

Patients with Turner syndrome commonly have short stature and lack of breast development. Skin manifestations include extra folds of skin on the neck giving the appearance of a short "webbed" neck (seen in about 30% of females with Turner syndrome), a low hairline at the back of the neck, multiple pigmented nevi, and lymphedema (puffiness or swelling) of the hands and feet. Skeletal abnormalities such as a "shield" chest with widely spaced nipples, cubitus valgus (a forearm that angles farther away from the body when extended), shortened fourth metatarsals, and Madelung deformity of the forearm (congenital subluxation of the distal ulna) are also common features in Turner syndrome (Fig. 45.3).

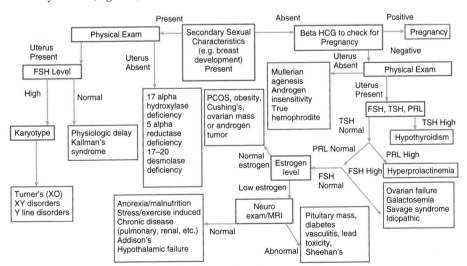

Fig. 45.2 Decision tree for primary amenorrhea.

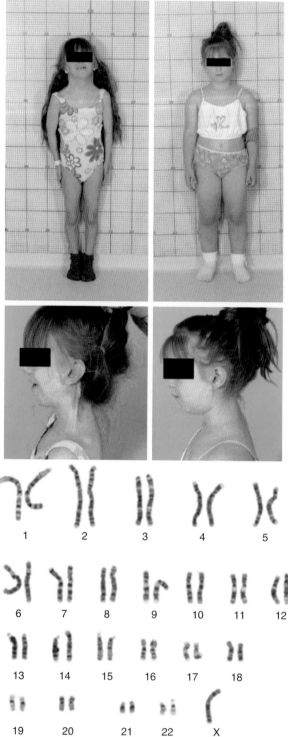

Fig. 45.3 Girls with Turner syndrome and the karyotype associated with this are shown. The girl on the left had an earlier diagnosis due to small jaw (micrognathia and webbed neck). The girl on the right panels had delayed diagnosis due to less stigmata, but had short stature that led to her chromosome investigation. The bottom panel shows the karyotype associated with Turner syndrome, with only one X chromosome visualized. *(From Saenger P, Bondy CA. Pediatric endocrinology. Philadelphia: Elsevier; 2013:664–96.e1. (A) fig. 16-6; (B) fig. 16-2.)*

What other medical conditions are associated with Turner syndrome in adults, and how should you screen for them?

One-third of patients with Turner syndrome are born with a heart defect, most commonly coarctation of the aorta or abnormalities of the aortic valve. Of Turner syndrome children, 5%–10% have aortic coarctation that needs immediate surgical correction, and 30% have a bicuspid aortic valve. These cardiac defects can be life-threatening, especially during pregnancy and even after surgical correction. Consultation with an experienced cardiologist is prudent, and evaluation typically will include echocardiography and an electrocardiogram (ECG). High blood pressure, kidney malformations, and skeletal malformations are also seen. A high incidence of osteoporosis plagues Turner patients, due to lack of estrogen from their nonfunctioning or "streak" ovaries, so bone mineral density screening is warranted. Turner syndrome women are also at twice the risk of developing type II diabetes, and hypothyroidism is seen in approximately 30% secondary to Hashimoto's thyroiditis. Screening with fasting glucose level and TSH (if not performed during the amenorrhea workup) is recommended.

> The patient has a cardiac evaluation and is noted to have a mild form of aortic coarctation that does not require surgical intervention. Her blood pressure is 116/63 mm Hg, and her fasting glucose is 67 mg/dL (normal). A skeletal survey and renal imaging are normal. While reassured by her normal findings, she is concerned about her sexual development given her Turner syndrome.

What treatment options are available for her?

Any form of premature ovarian insufficiency requires estrogen replacement therapy (ERT), both to prevent bone loss and premature coronary heart disease and also to establish menses and SSC. Progestins are used concurrently to prevent the risks of endometrial hyperplasia and cancer from unopposed estrogen exposure. When Turner syndrome is diagnosed in childhood, the use of low-dose anabolic steroid with growth hormone (GH) has been shown to increase final adult height compared to those who had a delay in the start of therapy. In our patient, it would be prudent to initiate ERT to induce breast development and consider the use of GH, as she is still short in stature and likely not at full height. Girls with Turner syndrome may start a low-dose of estrogen at age 11–12 to induce puberty, and patients older than 15 years may be started with adult doses to achieve a target estradiol concentration of 100 pg/mL. A simple way to administer hormones is through oral contraceptive pills (OCPs), or patients may use an estradiol patch or estradiol pills with monthly administration of medroxyprogesterone.

> The patient is started on hormone replacement and GH therapy. She continues combined OCPs for 3 years and has monthly menses, buys adult bras, and gains 1.5 inches in height. The patient is dating a young man she met in college, and they plan to become engaged their senior year. She is concerned about her future fertility potential.

How would you counsel this patient about attempting pregnancy in the future?

Because Turner syndrome is due to ovarian dysgenesis, only 2%–5% of women with Turner syndrome have the potential for spontaneous pregnancy, usually those with mosaicism. When pregnancies do occur in Turner syndrome patients, they are associated with high rates of spontaneous abortion and chromosomal abnormalities. In vitro fertilization (IVF) with donor oocytes is a treatment option for Turner patients, and pregnancy rates with IVF in these patients are equivalent to the general population. However, any Turner patients desiring pregnancy require a cardiovascular evaluation because the risk of death from aortic rupture or dissection during pregnancy or postpartum is as high as 2%. Due to this, pregnancy is absolutely contraindicated in Turner patients with a cardiac anomaly. The options of adoption and surrogacy should be discussed to build a family with a patient like this one.

BEYOND THE PEARLS

- Menopause occurring before the age of 40 is defined as primary ovarian insufficiency (POI), and occurs in 1% of women (0.1% younger than age 30). About 12% of women with POI have structural abnormalities of the X chromosome. A "premutation" in the fragile X gene (FMR1), defined as 55–200 CGC repeats, is associated with POI.
- Patients with XY karyotype cells (i.e., Turner mosaic with XY cells) are at some risk of gonadoblastoma and dysgerminoma, so surgical gonadectomy is offered to these women with consideration of their goals and desires integrated with their diagnosis and genotype.
- Classic Turner syndrome karyotype (45, X) is the most common human chromosomal abnormality occurring in zygotes (0.8%), but fewer than 3% of these fetuses survive to term.
- Some women with Turner syndrome have visual-spatial or mathematics learning issues, even though Turner patients have normal overall intelligence and language skills.
- Short stature is seen in all patients with Turner syndrome (45, X) and 80% of mosaic patients, with the average height being less than 58 inches. This is partially due to the loss of the SHOX gene on the X-chromosome, a gene important for long bone growth. Loss of the SHOX gene is also the reason for the Madelung deformation of the wrist and/or forearm.
- 46, XY gonadal dysgenesis (GD) is a result of abnormal testis development in utero. In pure-complete GD (previously called Swyer syndrome), there is only a fibrous streak which does not secrete androgens, so these individuals are phenotypically female.

Case Summary

- A 17-year-old girl presents with primary amenorrhea and no breast or pubic hair development. Her physical exam is remarkable for short stature, a broad chest, lack of secondary sexual characteristics, but a normal vagina and uterus. Her laboratory profile is notable for an elevated FSH.
- A karyotype is done and confirms the diagnosis of Turner syndrome (45, X0). You start her on estrogen and progestin therapy to induce puberty, as well as growth hormone treatment in an attempt to optimize her height potential.
- She returns in 3 years and wants to discuss fertility options, and you review with her the cardiac risks in pregnancy with Turner syndrome.

References

Practice Committee of the American Society of Reproductive Medicine. (2008). Current evaluation of amenorrhea. *Fertility and Sterility*, *90*(5), S219–S225.

Reindollar, R. H., Byrd, J. R., & McDonough, P. G. (1981). Delayed sexual development: a study of 252 patients. *American Journal of Obstetrics and Gynecology*, *140*(4), 371–380.

Reindollar, R. H., Novak, M., Tho, S. P., & McDonough, P. G. (1986). Adult-onset amenorrhea: a study of 262 patients. *American Journal of Obstetrics and Gynecology*, *155*(3), 531–543.

Strauss, J. F., & Barbieri, R. L. (Eds.). (2014). *Yen and Jaffe's reproductive endocrinology: physiology, pathophysiology, and clinical management* (3rd ed.). New York. Elsevier Saunders.

Virginia Mensah, MD ■ Kelly Pagidas, MD

A 33-Year-Old Woman With Infertility and Endometriosis

A 33-year-old woman is seen in your office for her annual gynecological exam. On her review of systems, she reports that she has been trying to get pregnant with her one male partner for the past 3 years without success. She is very tearful and is embarrassed to talk about it.

What additional questions would you want to ask this patient?

Before you ask further questions, it is important to acknowledge her sadness and the normalcy of such feelings and to assure her that she is not alone in experiencing difficulty in becoming pregnant. The inability to conceive (infertility) affects 10%–15% of couples in their reproductive years. A detailed history should be elicited from our patient, targeting questions that can lead to possible causes for her inability to conceive and plan future workup. You want to know the date of her last menstrual period, her menstrual regularity, if she experiences pain with menses, and if she has had prior pelvic surgery, pelvic infections, or exposure to or treatment for sexually transmitted infections (STIs). You should ask this patient what methods she is using for timing and frequency of coital activity. It is also important to get information on her partner, targeting his history of STIs, and genital surgeries or trauma. Most importantly, you also want to know if either of them have had a prior pregnancy or child together or with another partner. A detailed medical history is also warranted for the patient and partner because many medical conditions are associated with infertility. Inquire if she/he is a smoker, beyond a social drinker, uses illicit drugs, or if she/he is on any medication that is contraindicated in prepregnancy.

CLINICAL PEARL   **STEPS 2/3**

Although infertility is defined as failure to achieve a successful pregnancy after 12 months, earlier evaluation and treatment may be justified based on medical history and physical findings. Evaluation is warranted after 6 months for women older than 35 years. In women older than 40 years, based on expert opinion, immediate evaluation and treatment is warranted.

BASIC SCIENCE PEARL   **STEP 1**

Fecundability is the probability of achieving a pregnancy in one menstrual cycle. In healthy young couples, this is approximately 0.25. Fecundability is highest during the first 3 months of attempts, at 0.25 (25%), followed by 0.15 (15%) for the next 9 months. Approximately 80% of couples will conceive within the first 6 months. Because about 10% of all clinical pregnancies result in a spontaneous miscarriage, fecudability is distinct from *fecundity*, which is the probability of achieving a pregnancy that results in a live birth in one menstrual cycle.

CLINICAL PEARL   **STEPS 2/3**

The age decline in female fertility is secondary to a natural decrease in both oocyte number and quality. The decline is gradual after the age of 32 years but decreases at a more rapid pace after the age of 37 years. The age-related decline in female fertility is also associated with a significant increase in the rate of aneuploidy and spontaneous miscarriage.

The patient confirms that she has regular periods every 29 days. She experiences menstrual pain for the first 2 days, relieved with ibuprofen. She is using ovulation predictor kits and, when it turns positive, only has sexual intercourse that day and 2 days later. She has never had any surgeries or STIs. Her partner is healthy, and he reports no history of surgeries, genital trauma, or infection. Neither report any prior pregnancies or children. She asks you if it would be worthwhile for her and her partner to stop smoking.

What would be your working diagnosis based on this information?

By the history alone, there does not appear to be any obvious cause of infertility. She does have painful menses (dysmenorrhea), which may suggest pelvic disease or endometriosis. The American Society of Reproductive Medicine (ASRM) defines infertility as the inability to conceive after 12 months of regular, unprotected intercourse. Therefore, this couple's inability to get pregnant for 3 years and lack of any prior pregnancies meets the criteria for primary infertility. Therefore, an infertility workup is warranted. Regarding the patient's question about smoking cessation, we would strongly recommend that both partners stop smoking as smoking is associated with female and male infertility and poor pregnancy outcomes.

CLINICAL PEARL   **STEPS 2/3**

The *ovulatory* or *fertility window* is defined as the 6-day interval preceding and ending on the day of ovulation. A woman's peak fecundability is observed when coital activity occurs within 2 days prior to ovulation and greatest when it occurs the day prior to ovulation. The highest fecundity was associated with daily intercourse (37% per cycle) compared to 15% per cycle if intercourse occurs only once weekly.

CLINICAL PEARL   **STEP 2/3**

Common myths that need to be debunked are that frequent intercourse adversely affects sperm quantity. Data support that abstinence intervals as short as 2 days are associated with normal sperm counts, and intervals of greater than 5 days have a negative impact. In men with normal semen parameters, quality and quantity remain normal even with daily ejaculation. In men with oligospermia, sperm counts may even be higher with daily ejaculations. Sperm morphology is also not affected with frequent ejaculations, although after 10 days or more of abstinence some deterioration is noted.

What are common causes of infertility?

The etiology of infertility is either male-factor, female-factor, or a combination of both. Female factors include ovulatory dysfunction, tubal disease, pelvic disease/endometriosis, or unexplained (Fig. 46.1). Ovulatory dysfunction can be due to oligo- or anovulation, as in women with polycystic ovarian syndrome (PCOS), other endocrine diseases (e.g., thyroid dysfunction, hyperprolactinemia), or older maternal age. Male-factor infertility is primarily due to abnormal spermatogenesis secondary to genetic, structural, hormonal, or idiopathic causes.

Primary infertility diagnosis in couples

- Ovulatory Disorders
- Male Factor
- Tubal Disease
- Unexplained
- Endometriosis
- Other

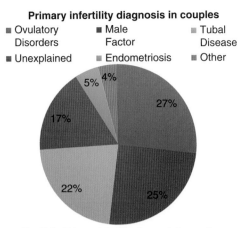

Fig. 46.1 Primary infertility diagnosis in couples.

What testing would you recommend to this patient?

The classic workup for female infertility consists of evaluation of ovarian function, tubo-uterine integrity, and evaluation of spermatogenesis in the male partner, if the women has a male partner involved (Fig. 46.2). In the presence of regular menstrual cycles, it is not necessary to confirm that ovulation is occurring monthly, and ovarian reserve screening is recommend only in women older than 35 years of age or to predict the success of certain gonadotropin treatments. The presence of tubal disease and uterine abnormalities is evaluated with imaging such as a hysterosalpingogram (HSG). Evaluation of the male consists of semen analysis to assess the quality and quantity of the sperm.

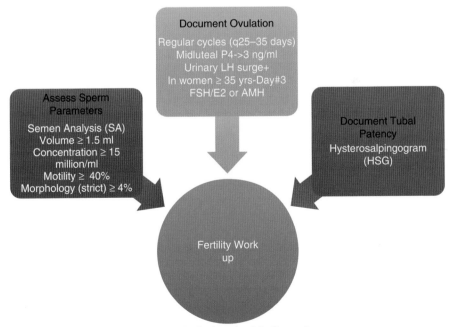

Fig. 46.2 Evaluation of an infertile couple.

Our patient undergoes a HSG that demonstrates a normal uterine cavity and bilateral fill and spill of both fallopian tubes. Her day 3 follicular stimulating hormone (FSH) and estradiol are 5.5 mIU/mL and 30 pg/mL, respectively. Her anti-Mullerian hormone (AMH) level is 3.0 ng/mL. Her partner has a semen analysis that demonstrates 50 million sperm/mL with a 30% motility and 6% normal morphology.

What would you recommend for this patient?

Given that her workup is normal, there is no evidence of tubal disease, and her ovarian screen parameters are appropriate for her age, our working diagnosis is unexplained infertility. Her partner has a normal sperm count, but the sperm motility is low, so there could be a mild male-factor component. It is recommended to repeat the semen analysis to ensure that this was not an isolated finding. She has dysmenorrhea, but the possibility of endometriosis can only be determined by diagnostic laparoscopy, which is reserved for use in selected cases where there might be benefit for concurrent surgical treatment of advanced endometriosis or adhesions, and hormonal treatment of endometriosis in patients trying to conceive is not indicated because it would further delay achieving a pregnancy.

You review the possibility of the presence of endometriosis, given her dysmenorrhea, but she wisely declines surgical intervention as her symptoms are mild and relieved with nonsteroidal antiinflammatory drugs (NSAIDs). The repeat semen analysis on her partner is normal with 70% motility.

What would you discuss next with this patient?

Even though the patient is young, the 3-year duration of infertility warrants discussion of the spectrum of infertility options in order to consider prompt initiation of treatment. In the presence of tubal patency and adequate sperm, superovulation and intrauterine insemination (IUI) would be appropriate first-line treatments. In vitro fertilization (IVF) is an option that would decrease her time to conception (Table 46.1), but she does not have to bypass less invasive treatments. You ask your patient what options she would like to pursue.

TABLE 46.1 ■ The 2013 Centers for Disease Control (CDC) Assisted Reproductive Data in Women Using Their Own Oocytes

<35 years	35–37 years	38–40 years	41–42 years	43–44 years	>44 years
39.9%	31.6%	21.1%	11.1%	5.2%	1.6%

Live birth rate per IVF cycle by maternal age.

The patient decides to undergo three treatment cycles of superovulation and IUI using clomiphene citrate, but following this treatment she still has not become pregnant.

What do you recommend next for this patient?

Because it is common for couples to require 3–4 infertility treatment cycles to achieve a pregnancy, you should encourage and reassure your patient and her partner. We can consider an additional three cycles of superovulation IUI with clomiphene citrate or consider use of gonadotropins with

IUI, but this has an elevated risk of higher order multiple gestation. We can re-explore the option of ruling out endometriosis with consideration of surgical treatment if advanced disease is noted, or consider moving to IVF. IVF is associated with the shortest time to conception compared to the other treatments, and the risk of multiple gestation can be minimized by following the recommendation of transferring only a single embryo.

> The patient completes her first IVF treatment cycle. Twenty oocytes are aspirated and result in eight embryos, one of which is transferred at the blastocyst stage and five of which are able to be cryopreserved for future use. A β-human chorionic gonadotropin (hCG) level drawn 15 days after the oocyte retrieval is positive, and an ultrasound performed at 8 weeks of gestation reports a live intrauterine gestation with a crown rump length consistent with her gestational age by her embryo transfer date.

BEYOND THE PEARLS

- Lifestyle changes that enhance a couple's fertility include smoking cessation, reduction of caffeine and alcohol, maintaining normal weight, stress reduction, avoidance of excessive exercise, and intercourse during the fertile window.
- Women attempting pregnancy need to be on at least 400 µg of folic acid daily.
- The diagnosis of infertility for a woman or couple is associated with depression, anxiety, and feelings of anger, grief, and shame. Because stress and infertility are associated, providing both psychological support and embarking on stress-reducing methods is associated with positive outcomes for fertility treatment compliance and success.
- Infertility tests that are not part of the routine workup include culture of mycoplasma, postcoital testing, endometrial biopsy, and antisperm antibody testing.

Case Summary

- A 33-year old woman presents for her annual exam and concurrently reports inability to conceive for the past 3 years. She and her partner meet the criteria for primary infertility.
- The couple's infertility workup is unremarkable except for a mild decrease in sperm motility, but subsequent semen analysis is normal. The patient reports a history of mild dysmenorrhea but declines laparoscopy, so her evaluation is consistent with unexplained infertility with the possibility of endometriosis.
- The couple initiates conservative infertility treatment cycles with superovulation using clomiphene citrate and IUI. After three failed treatments, the patient undergoes her first IVF treatment cycle. A single blastocyst embryo is transferred and 8 week ultrasound confirms a single, viable intrauterine gestation.

References

Practice Committee of the American Society for Reproductive Medicine. (2013). Definitions of infertility and recurrent pregnancy loss: a committee opinion. *Fertility and Sterility*, *99*(1), 63.

Practice Committee of the American Society for Reproductive Medicine. (2015). Diagnostic evaluation of the infertile female: a committee opinion. *Fertility and Sterility*, *103*(6), e44–e50.

Practice Committee of the American Society for Reproductive Medicine. (2015). Diagnostic evaluation of the infertile male: a committee opinion. *Fertility and Sterility*, *103*(3), e18–e25.

Practice Committee of the American Society for Reproductive Medicine. (2012). Endometriosis and infertility: a committee opinion. *Fertility and Sterility*, *98*(3), 591–598.

Practice Committee of the American Society for Reproductive Medicine. (2013). Optimizing natural fertility: a committee opinion. *Fertility and Sterility*, *100*(3), 631–637.

The American College of Obstetricians and Gynecologists Committee on Gynecological Practice and the Practice Committee of the American Society for Reproductive Medicine. (2014). Female age-related fertility decline. Committee Opinion No. 589. *Fertility and Sterility, 101*(3), 633–634.

Yen, Jaffe's. (2014). Reproductive endocrinology: physiology, pathophysiology and clinical management. In J. F. Strauss, & R. L. Barbieri (Eds.), *Female infertility and male infertility* (7th ed.). Philadelphia: Elsevier Saunders.

CASE 47

Braden Barnett ■ John D. Carmichael

A 22-Year-Old Woman With Amenorrhea

A 22-year-old woman presents for outpatient evaluation of 3 months with no menstrual periods. Menarche was at age 12 years. Menses were previously regular, occurring monthly and lasting for 4 days. She has completed several home pregnancy tests over the past 3 months that are consistently negative.

What is the difference between primary and secondary amenorrhea?

Amenorrhea, or lack of menstruation, is classified as primary or secondary. Primary amenorrhea, defined as no pubertal development by age 13 years or no menarche within 5 years of breast budding or by age 15, is usually related to chromosomal or anatomic abnormalities. Secondary amenorrhea, or lack of previously normal menses for 3 months or lack of previously irregular menses for 6 months, is almost always related to an acquired hormonal abnormality.

The patient denies any recent changes to her eating or exercise routine, weight, hair, or skin. She does note a few months of clear to milky discharge from her nipples that is described as "a few drops" each day, and her breasts are non-painful. She reports mildly decreased libido, but denies hot flashes, dyspareunia, headaches, vision changes, or galactorrhea. The remaining review of systems is negative.

CLINICAL PEARL   **STEP 2/3**

There are three types of nipple discharge: lactation, physiologic nipple discharge (galactorrhea), and pathologic nipple discharge. In the absence of breastfeeding, lactation would be expected to cease by 6 months postpartum. Pathologic nipple discharge is characterized by the presence of blood, so any nipple discharge that tests negative for blood and is not associated with lactation is defined as physiologic nipple discharge.

How is galactorrhea related to hyperprolactinemia?

Galactorrhea is frequently caused by hyperprolactinemia. While galactorrhea is a good predictor of elevated prolactin levels, the absence of galactorrhea does not predict normal prolactin levels.

Your patient has no previous past medical or surgical history and takes no medications. She is in graduate school and is sexually active in a monogamous relationship. She uses condoms for contraception and has never been pregnant.

What medications can cause amenorrhea?

Oral contraceptives can cause amenorrhea for up to several months, as can androgenic drugs such as danazol. Drugs that induce hyperprolactinemia (opioids and certain antipsychotics, antiemetics, antidepressants, and antihypertensives) are common causes of amenorrhea, so should be asked about in the history (Table 47.1).

> Physical examination reveals a healthy appearing woman without hirsutism or acne. Her body mass index is 23 kg/m². The thyroid, breast, and pelvic examinations are normal. Visual fields testing is normal.

What are the next steps in evaluation?

As with all patients presenting with amenorrhea, ruling out pregnancy the first step. After this, the workup for secondary amenorrhea focuses on acquired hormonal abnormalities (thyroid-stimulating hormone [TSH], prolactin, and follicle-stimulating hormone [FSH], and luteinizing hormone [LH]). Since the patient has no history of intrauterine surgery, acquired uterine outflow obstruction (Asherman syndrome) is unlikely.

CLINICAL PEARL   **STEPS 2/3**

Scar tissue within the uterine cavity, usually the result of intrauterine trauma associated with a surgical procedure (e.g., curettage for pregnancy complications), can lead to intrauterine adhesions (synechiae). Asherman syndrome is the presence of intrauterine adhesions with symptoms such as infertility or amenorrhea.

If the TSH level is abnormal, then thyroid disease must be evaluated and treated appropriately. If the TSH is normal and the prolactin is elevated, then an evaluation for hyperprolactinemia should commence. If the TSH and prolactin are normal, the gonadotropins (LH and FSH) are low or normal, and uterine outflow obstruction is not suspected, then hyperandrogenism should be considered. Hirsutism, acne, and male pattern baldness can all be seen in hyperandrogenic women. If any of these are present, the workup should include early morning serum levels of 17-hydroxyprogesterone (to screen for late-onset congenital adrenal hyperplasia due

---

TABLE 47.1 ■ **Drug Classes That Can Cause Hyperprolactinemia With Example Drugs That Have Moderate to High Frequency of Increasing Prolactin Levels**

Anesthetics
Anticonvulsants
Antidepressants (tricyclics [e.g., clomipramine] more than selective serotonin receptor inhibitors)
Antihistamines
Antihypertensives (methyldopa, verapamil)
Cholinergic agonists
Catecholamine depletors
Dopamine receptor blockers (e.g., metoclopramide)
Dopamine synthesis inhibitors
Estrogens
Neuroleptics/antipsychotics (cause hyperprolactinemia by dopamine [D_2] blockade)
First-generation antipsychotics: Haloperidol, fluphenazine, chlorpromazine, prochlorperazine
Second-generation antipsychotics: Risperidone, paliperidone, asenapine
Neuropeptides
Opiates and opiate antagonists

to 21-hydroxylase deficiency) and testosterone. Patients with hyperandrogenism should also be screened for features of Cushing syndrome (round facies, plethora, striae that are wide and violaceous, dorsocervical or supraclavicular fat deposition, central obesity).

The patient has normal laboratory work except an elevated prolactin level (Table 47.2).

TABLE 47.2 ■ Laboratory Tests in Our Presenting Patient

Laboratory Results	Reference Range
Prolactin = 523 ng/mL	<20 ng/mL
LH = 0.8 mU/mL	Follicular or luteal phase, 5–22 mU/mL; midcycle peak, 30–250 mU/mL
FSH = 1.3 mU/mL	Follicular or luteal phase, 5–20 mU/mL; midcycle peak, 30–50 mU/mL
TSH = 1.6 µU/mL	0.5–5.0 µU/mL

LH, Luteinizing hormone; *FSH,* follicle-stimulating hormone; *TSH,* thyroid-stimulating hormone.

What are causes of hyperprolactinemia?
Elevated prolactin can be caused by physiologic causes (nipple stimulation, intercourse, pregnancy/lactation, exercise, or stress), medication-related, hypothalamic-pituitary disease (prolactinomas, co-secretion from somatotroph adenoma, and disease of the pituitary stalk), and other causes (untreated/undertreated hypothyroidism, macroprolactinemia, chronic renal failure, chest wall injury, polycystic ovarian syndrome [PCOS], epileptic seizures).

What if the patient is taking a medication that may elevate her prolactin?
If the patient is not taking any drugs that could cause hyperprolactinemia, the next step is to obtain a magnetic resonance imaging (MRI) of the sella turcica of the cranium to evaluate for a pituitary mass or secretory mass. In a patient with suspected drug-induced hyperprolactinemia, it is recommended to discontinue the medication for 3 days and then remeasure the prolactin level, pursuing a sella MRI only if the hyperprolactinemia persists. If the medication cannot be discontinued and relation of the drug to prolactin is unclear, then a sella MRI is indicated.

CLINICAL PEARL	STEPS 2/3

With the exceptions of metoclopramide, risperidone, and phenothiazines (chlorpromazine, prochlorperazine), medication-induced hyperprolactinemia generally is less than 100 ng/mL.

What are secretory or pituitary tumor causes of hyperprolactinemia?
Lactotroph adenomas (prolactinomas) are the most common type of secretory pituitary tumor, but prolactin can also be co-secreted from somatotrophic (growth hormone [GH]) producing pituitary adenomas. Hyperprolactinemia is much more mild in conditions causing loss of dopamine inhibition via hypothalamic-pituitary stalk damage ("stalk effect") from granulomas, irradiation, Rathke's cleft cysts, trauma, craniopharyngiomas, germinomas, metastases, meningiomas, or suprasellar pituitary mass extension. There is a strong positive correlation between prolactinoma size and prolactin elevation. A prolactin level of higher than 500 ng/mL is usually only seen with macroprolactinomas, and a prolactin level of higher than 200 ng/mL in the absence of another secondary cause (pregnancy, medications, chronic renal failure) will virtually guarantee the presence of a prolactinoma on MRI. If a sellar mass of larger than 1 cm is present, but the prolactin is less than 100 ng/mL, stalk effect from a nonprolactinoma tumor is more likely.

An MRI with and without contrast demonstrates a 1.6-cm sellar mass consistent with a pituitary macroadenoma confined to the sella. It shows upward extension and convexity of the diaphragma sella, but no cavernous sinus invasion or optic chiasm contact. The diagnosis is a lactotroph macroadenoma (macroprolactinoma).

What is the next step in management?

Treating asymptomatic microprolactinomas with dopamine agonists is generally not recommended. However, dopamine agonists should be initiated in patients with macroprolactinomas (regardless of symptoms) or symptomatic microprolactinomas. This patient is symptomatic (amenorrhea) so warrants therapy. These drugs will lower prolactin levels, decrease tumor size, and restore gonadal function. Even in patients with neurologic sequelae such as visual field deficits, a dopamine agonist is the first step in treatment and may avoid surgery. The available dopamine agonists are cabergoline, which is dosed twice weekly, and bromocriptine, which is taken once or twice daily.

CLINICAL PEARL   **STEPS 2/3**

Despite very few head-to-head comparisons, cabergoline is favored over bromocriptine due to higher biochemical efficacy (lowering prolactin levels), better structural efficacy (tumor shrinkage), and lower incidence of unpleasant side effects (mainly headaches, dizziness, and nausea).

How long should the patient continue her dopamine agonist?

Patients should be treated with a dopamine agonist for at least 2 years, as long as therapy appears to be effective. After 2 years of therapy, the dosage of the dopamine agonist can be tapered and possibly discontinued in patients with normal prolactin levels and tumor shrinkage.

What are contraindications to dopamine agonist therapy?

Uncontrolled hypertension is a contraindication to dopamine agonist therapy, as is any known history of cardiac valvular disorders. Although 3 mg of cabergoline per day in Parkinson's patients has been associated with cardiac valve regurgitation, most prolactinoma patients develop no issues and standard doses of cabergoline do not require echocardiographic screening.

How should women be counseled about prepregnancy planning?

The risk for the mother with a prolactinoma is growth of the tumor during the pregnancy, and women who receive only medical management prior to conception have a 31% risk of symptomatic pituitary tumor enlargement in pregnancy. Bromocriptine crosses the placenta, but the incidences of congenital malformations, abortions, or long-term harmful effects are not increased in patients taking bromocriptine during pregnancy. Cabergoline has been studied much less. Women of childbearing age should be counseled about the risks and discontinue dopamine agonist therapy once they discover a pregnancy, but need not avoid desired pregnancy while taking a dopamine agonist.

The patient initiates cabergoline, and her prolactin normalizes, her tumor shrinks considerably, and her amenorrhea resolves. Two years later, she returns to clinic reporting a positive home pregnancy test, and she stopped her cabergoline after the test 1 week prior.

How are prolactinomas monitored during pregnancy?

Pregnant women with prolactinomas should undergo clinical examination each trimester, screening for symptoms of new or worsening headaches and changes in vision, which should trigger formal visual field testing and a pituitary MRI without gadolinium contrast. Measuring prolactin levels is not helpful during pregnancy, as they increase up to 10 times during pregnancy.

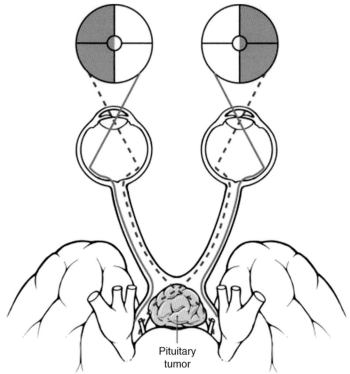

Fig. 47.1 Bitemporal hemianopia as caused by the effect of a sellar mass.

The patient does well during the first trimester, but in the second trimester reports new and severe headaches. Visual field testing shows a bitemporal hemianopia. Her MRI shows the prolactinoma has grown to 1.1 cm with mild optic chiasm compression (Fig. 47.1).

How are growing, symptomatic prolactinomas treated during pregnancy?
Dopamine agonist therapy is preferred to surgical management during pregnancy, and bromocriptine is preferred given the larger body of literature supporting its safe use. Surgical debulking, preferably in the second trimester, is reasonable if dopamine agonist therapy fails.

The patient is started on low-dose bromocriptine with excellent response in her symptoms and visual field test. She delivers a healthy baby, and, after breastfeeding, she restarts cabergoline with good response.

BEYOND THE PEARLS

- Once a patient is known to have a structural abnormality in the hypothalamic or pituitary region, pituitary hormones (adrenocorticotropic hormone [ACTH], TSH, LH/FSH, GH) are not useful to measure their hormonal axes. Target hormones (cortisol, free thyroxine [FT4], estradiol/testosterone, insulin-like growth factor [IGF-1]) should be ordered instead.
- Occasionally, a macroprolactinoma may initially demonstrate a normal or only mildly elevated prolactin level. This falsely low value is due to the "hook effect." In a two-site

Continued

BEYOND THE PEARLS–Cont'd

sandwich assay, an extremely high level of prolactin can bind both the capturing antibodies and the signaling antibodies. This effect can be overcome by repeating the assay after diluting the sample by 1:100. Many newer methods have compensated for the hook effect, so the laboratory should be consulted in this clinical situation.

- The pituitary gland may double in volume during a normal pregnancy and postpartum due to lactotroph hypertrophy. This must be considered when interpreting MRI results during pregnancy, and one should restrict treatment to patients with visual compromise or symptoms.
- Prolactinomas larger than 4 cm, or "giant prolactinomas," can be particularly aggressive. They may grow large enough to cause hydrocephalus or even a spontaneous cerebrospinal fluid (CSF) leak from the nose. While an external drain may be necessary as a temporizing measure, the initial management remains dopamine agonist therapy.
- Very rarely, pituitary carcinomas, which are defined by the presence of metastasis, may develop. Most such malignancies arise from corticotroph (ACTH-producing) tumors or prolactinomas. Surgery and dopamine agonist therapy are the treatment for lactotroph carcinomas, and radiation and chemotherapy may also be required.

Case Summary

- A 22-year-old woman with no medical history presents with 3 months of amenorrhea. She has a normal physical exam, and lab testing shows elevated prolactin.
- An MRI reveals a 1.6 cm sellar mass, and she is diagnosed with a lactotroph macroadenoma (macroprolactinoma).
- The patient is placed on a standard dose of cabergoline with biochemical and structural resolution. She becomes pregnant and suffers recurrence of her macroprolactinoma but responds well to bromocriptine therapy.

References

Dekkers, O. M., Lagro, J., Burman, P., et al. (2010). Recurrence of hyperprolactinemia after withdrawal of dopamine agonists: systematic review and meta-analysis. *The Journal of Clinical Endocrinology and Metabolism, 95*(1), 43–51.

Dinç, H., Esen, F., Demirci, A., et al. (1998). Pituitary dimensions and volume measurements in pregnancy and postpartum. MR assessment. *Acta Radiologica, 39*(1), 64–69.

Klein, D. A., & Poth, M. A. (2013). Amenorrhea: an approach to diagnosis and management. *American Family Physician, 87*(11), 781–788.

Melmed, S., Casaneuva, F. F., Hoffman, A. R., et al. (2011). Diagnosis and treatment of hyperprolactinemia: an Endocrine Society clinical practice guideline. *The Journal of Clinical Endocrinology and Metabolism, 96*(2), 273–288.

Schade, R., Andersohn, F., Suissa, S., et al. (2007). Dopamine agonists and the risk of cardiac-valve regurgitation. *The New England Journal of Medicine, 356*(1), 29–38.

Valassi, E., Klibanski, A., & Biller, B. M. (2010). Potential cardiac valve effects of dopamine agonists in hyperprolactinemia. *The Journal of Clinical Endocrinology and Metabolism, 95*(3), 1025–1033.

Kylie G. Fowler, MD ■ Lauren Damle, MD

A 3-Year-Old Girl With Vaginal Discharge

A 3-year-old girl is brought to your clinic by her mother for evaluation of foul-smelling vaginal discharge. Her mother reports the discharge has been present for the past 2 weeks, and recently she had two episodes of light pink spotting on her underwear. She reports her daughter is also experiencing "itching down there."

How is the prepubertal genital tract different from older pubertal females?

Due to the lack of estrogen, the prepubertal vagina is atrophic and has a higher pH than the post-pubertal vagina, and it is more susceptible to irritation and inflammation. The prepubertal vulva also lacks labial fat pads and protective hair. Poor hygiene can become a problem as young girls become independent with toilet training, especially because of the close proximity of the vagina to the anus.

BASIC SCIENCE PEARL	STEP 1

Between approximately 6 weeks after birth and the onset of puberty, estrogen levels are low in the female child, resulting in atrophic vaginal tissue and a vaginal pH of 6.5–7.5 (normal vaginal pH following puberty is 3.8–4.5).

When a prepubertal child presents with vaginal discharge, what do you need to know about her history?

In addition to onset and duration of symptoms, the clinician should inquire about associated pain, itching, and physical signs that the parents may have noticed such as erythema or rash. The quantity, color, and consistency of discharge should be obtained. The clinician should also review where the girl is in the process of toilet training and who is helping maintain hygiene. The patient can be asked to demonstrate how she wipes in the clinic. Additional history should review bathing habits, soaps and detergents, what kind of underwear the patient wears, and if there are other types of clothing worn that could lead to vulvovaginal irritation such as swim suits, leotards, or leggings. A complete developmental, medical, and surgical history should be obtained, as well as a history of any recent illness in the patient or family. Specific history of atopic dermatitis or allergies should be obtained and medications reviewed. It is important to ask who cares for the child, including adults at home, day care providers, or baby sitters. The clinician should ask the child's parents about enuresis, behavioral changes, nightmares, headaches, or nonspecific abdominal pain, which may suggest abuse or other social stressors. The parents should be asked directly if there is any suspicion of abuse. While vulvovaginal symptoms are common in this population, it is important to screen for child abuse.

CLINICAL PEARL   **STEPS 2/3**

Physicians are mandated reporters of child abuse. If physical or sexual abuse is suspected, then it is legally mandatory to report the concerns to local child welfare authorities. If the parent or guardian with the child is not the suspected abuser, that person should be informed that there is a concern for possible abuse and that the issue will be investigated by trained authorities. Information on mandated reporting, reporting guidelines, and state-by-state reporting phone numbers and resources can be found at www.childwelfare.gov.

The patient's mother gives some additional details about the vaginal discharge: she reports it is yellow and green with a foul odor and has been present every day for the past 2 weeks. The mother has also noticed redness of the labia. The patient has been scratching her vulva occasionally, but she does not complain of pain. She been toilet trained for the past 6 months, and her parents or daycare workers assist with hygiene. She wipes from front to back and needs full assistance with wiping after bowel movements. She takes daily baths and enjoys "bath bombs" that fizz and turn the water different colors; otherwise, Dove gentle soap is used and scent-free laundry detergent. She participates in dance class and wears tights and leotards once a week for 1 hour; otherwise, she wears cotton underwear. The patient has met all developmental milestones, has no past medical or surgical history, and does not take any medications. She has no known allergies and has had no recent illness. The patient is cared for at home by her mother and father and lives with one younger brother who is 12 months old and healthy. Her parents work out of the home; during this time, she is in daycare. Her mother has no concerns about abuse at the daycare and feels her daughter enjoys being there.

What is the differential diagnosis of vulvovaginal symptoms in a prepubertal child?

The differential for vulvovaginal symptoms in a prepubertal child is broad. It includes "nonspecific" vulvovaginitis, which often results from poor hygiene or vulvovaginal irritants and is the most common cause of vulvovaginal symptoms in this age group. Specific infections are sometimes found, often resulting from respiratory pathogens, hence the importance of asking about recent illness in the family. In cases of recurrent vulvovaginitis, an occult infection with pinworms should be considered as a contributor to the symptoms. Additional causes may include foreign bodies in the vagina such as toilet paper, beads, hair pins, crayons, or even batteries. Vulvar dermatoses can also cause symptoms of vulvovaginitis in this age group.

BASIC SCIENCE PEARL   **STEP 1**

Specific vulvovaginitis results from a known pathogen, such as Group A β-hemolytic streptococcus. Infections with Group A β-hemolytic streptococcus may be accompanied by pharyngeal or skin infections and can result in scarlet fever. Other specific pathogens include *Haemophilus influenza*, *Staphylococcus aureus*, *Neisseria meningitidis*, and *Streptococcus pneumoniae*. Occasionally, enteric organisms such as *Shigella* and *Yersinia* can result in a bloody, mucopurulent vaginal discharge. *Candida* species rarely cause infection in prepubertal girls secondary to the higher vaginal pH.

Following a thorough history, how will you perform a physical exam?

Vital signs, height, weight, and body mass index (BMI) should be obtained when the child presents to clinic. A basic physical exam including skin, head and neck, chest wall, lungs, heart, and abdomen may be obtained with the patient sitting on the lap of a parent or sitting on the examination table with the parent nearby. Talk to the child and involve her in the basic exam to comfort and reassure her. Prior to the gynecologic exam, it is important to explain the exam to both the child and her parents, emphasizing that no instrumentation will be used as this is an exam of the external genitalia only. Reassure the patient and parents that the exam will not hurt. Ask for permission from the child and parent before proceeding with the exam. Once permission has been obtained, the patient can be placed supine on the examination table and asked to make her legs "like a frog" or "like a butterfly" (Fig. 48.1). If the child is especially nervous, this position can be obtained while lying on a parent.

CLINICAL PEARL   **STEPS 2/3**

Before doing a gynecologic exam on a very young patient, the differences between "good and bad touch" should be reviewed with the patient. Remind the child that the genital area is private and no one should see or touch it without her permission. Discuss your role in her health care and that sometimes doctors need to examine the genital region in order to make her feel better (Fig. 48.1).

Once positioned, gentle downward and outward pressure may be placed on the buttocks in order to visualize the labia majora, labia minora, clitoris, urethra, hymen, and lower vagina. Alternatively, the anatomy can be examined by gently gripping the labia majora and providing outward traction. If more complete visualization of the vagina and cervix is required, this can be achieved with the knee-chest position. The patient is positioned prone with her head resting to one side, knees bent to support her weight, and her buttocks in the air. A sheet can provide additional coverage and comfort.

What tests should you obtain?

In patients with the initial presentation of nonspecific vulvovaginitis without any vaginal bleeding, no testing is necessary. If there is discharge, bleeding, or symptoms on examination that suggest a specific vulvovaginitis, vaginal cultures should be obtained. A small swab can be inserted into the vagina for sampling, with care to avoid the hymen, and the swab can be premoistened with sterile saline to improve comfort. Be sure to explain the swab to the child and let her feel a sample swab demonstrating the softness of the material. The sample will then be placed in a specified specimen tube for laboratory culture. If sexual abuse is suspected, testing for *Neisseria gonorrhea* and *Chlamydia trachomatis* should be performed. Whenever possible, an expert in child abuse should evaluate a patient who discloses a history of abuse or for whom there is strong suspicion of abuse.

> The patient has a normal general physical exam with the following genitourinary findings: normal female external genitalia without lesions or rashes, Tanner stage I, intact patent hymen, and minimal amount of gray-green, malodorous discharge seen at vaginal introitus. There is a small amount of toilet paper visualized in the lower vagina.

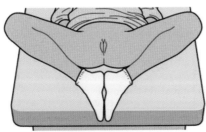

Fig. 48.1 The "frog leg" position for gynecologic examination of a young, prepubertal girl. *(From Sach CJ, Wheeler M. Roberts and Hedges' clinical procedures in emergency medicine. Philadelphia: Elsevier; 2014: 1188–1203.e1, fig. 58–12.)*

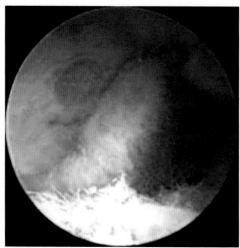

Fig. 48.2 Vaginoscopy showing a foreign body in a prepubertal young girl. *(From Merritt DF. Genital trauma in the pediatric and adolescent female. Obstet Gynecol Clin. 2009 Mar 1;36(1):85–98, fig. 1.)*

How should the foreign body found on physical exam be removed?

Often small amounts of toilet paper or other small foreign bodies can be flushed from the vagina while the patient is in clinic. Saline can be flushed into the vagina using a small catheter (a pediatric, 12-French Foley catheter works well). The saline should be slightly warmed, and all steps of the procedure should be explained in detail to the patient and her parents. The child should be allowed to feel and see the catheters. If the toilet paper can be easily seen, a small moistened cotton swab may be gently inserted into the vagina and twirled to grasp and remove it. If the foreign body is unable to be removed in the office setting, the child may require an examination under anesthesia and vaginoscopy. A rigid or flexible cystoscope is placed into the vagina with care to avoid damaging the hymen. While pinching the labia closed the vagina is distended with sterile water or saline to allow for visualization of the vagina and cervix. Once the foreign body is identified, it can be removed with a narrow forceps or flushed out with the distention media. Confirmation of complete removal can be made afterward with vaginoscopy. Vaginoscopy is also a useful diagnostic step in the evaluation of diagnosis recurrent or refractory vulvovaginitis, vaginal bleeding, or persistent discharge (Fig. 48.2).

How would the evaluation change if the parents reported continued vaginal bleeding and no foreign object was found in the vagina?

The differential diagnosis of prepubertal vaginal bleeding includes trauma, foreign object in the vagina, infection, urethral prolapse, vulvar dermatoses, precocious puberty, hormone-secreting tumors, and genitourinary tract malignancies. If the external genital exam is normal without signs of trauma or dermatologic pathology and a foreign object is not clearly seen, further investigation must be performed. Vaginoscopy as previously described is useful for excluding a foreign object and assessing for genital tract malignancies (sarcoma botryoides is the most common in this age group). A pelvic ultrasound can also be performed to assess for size of uterus and any ovarian pathology. Labs should also be sent for assessment of precocious puberty, which include luteinizing hormone (LH), follicle-stimulating hormone (FSH), estradiol, and thyroid panel.

> The decision is made to use a small pediatric Foley catheter and warm saline to flush the toilet paper from the patient's vagina. The procedure was successful, and yields a large amount of wadded, pink-stained toilet paper, and the patient does well with the procedure.

What after-care information should be provided to the patient's parents?

The patient's parents should be advised on basic vulvovaginal hygiene care for their daughter as she continues to grow and gain more independence. Because of the hypoestrogenic state of the genitalia of prepubertal girls, this area is especially susceptible to irritants. Young girls should sit in warm water at night and allow gentle motion of the water to naturally cleanse the vulva and vagina. No soap is necessary in this area. Bubble baths, "bath bombs," and heavily scented products should be avoided. To avoid vaginal voiding (urine refluxing into the vagina and causing irritation), patients should be taught to void with their knees wide open or even to sit backward on the toilet. Wiping should be taught in a front-to-back manner. Underwear should be made of breathable cotton, and extended periods of tight and/or moist clothing (like leotards or wet swimsuits for several hours) should be avoided.

BEYOND THE PEARLS

- Urethral prolapse, or prolapse of the urethra mucosa through the external meatus, is a common cause of prepubertal vaginal bleeding. It has the appearance of a ring of dark red beefy tissue and can be easily confused with trauma to the inexperienced gynecologist. It is aggravated by chronic constipation. It is treated by frequent sitz baths and sometimes with a short course of topical estrogen. Refractory cases should be referred to a urologist.
- Lichen sclerosus is a vulvar dermatosis that can masquerade as vulvar trauma or even sexual abuse and can occasionally be seen in prepubertal girls. The classic figure-of-eight pattern of hypopigmentation of the skin is noted on exam, and girls may display ecchymosis, petechia, or small lacerations that result in bleeding. Treatment is topical clobetasol or an other high-potency steroid ointment. Biopsies are not generally recommended in prepubertal girls as malignancy risk is low.
- Testing for sexually transmitted infections in children requires special considerations. A urine sample for a nucleic acid amplification test (NAAT) can be used as a screening tool. However, if positive, a confirmatory culture from the vagina must be obtained. For chlamydia trachomatis, a second NAAT that targets a different gene sequence can be used as a confirmatory test. In cases of *Neisseria gonorrhoeae*, isolates of bacteria must be cultured to confirm *N. gonorrhoeae* as other *Neisseria* species may be present in children, such as *N. meningitidis*.

Case Summary

- A 3-year-old girl presents with 2 weeks of foul-smelling discharge and two episodes of vaginal spotting. She is otherwise healthy and has no "red flags" for infection or abuse.
- A careful history is obtained and an age-appropriate physical exam reveals a foreign body in the vagina, which is removed with a gentle flush of warm saline through a pediatric catheter placed in the vagina.
- Following resolution of the foreign body, education and guidance is provided regarding vulvovaginal hygiene and care for prepubertal girls.

References

Cemek, F., Odabas, D., Senel, U., & Kocaman, A. T. (2016). Personal hygiene and vulvovaginitis in prepubertal children. *Journal of Pediatric and Adolescent Gynecology, 29*(3), 223–227.

Emans, J. S. (2012). Office evaluation of the child and adolescent. In J. S. Emans, & M. R. Laufer (Eds.), *Pediatric and adolescent gynecology* (6th ed) (pp. 1–20). Philadelphia: Lippincott Williams & Wilkins.

Emans, J. S. (2012). Vulvovaginal problems in the prepubertal child. In J. S. Emans, & M. R. Laufer (Eds.), *Pediatric and adolescent gynecology* (6th ed) (pp. 42–60). Philadelphia: Lippincott Williams & Wilkins.

McGreal, S., & Wood, P. (2013). Recurrent vaginal discharge in children. *Journal of Pediatric and Adolescent Gynecology, 26*(4), 205–208.

Stricker, T., Navratil, F., & Sennhauser, F. H. (2003). Vulvovaginitis in prepubertal girls. *Archives of Disease in Childhood, 88*(4), 324–326.

Lauren Damle, MD

A 15-Year-Old Concerned About Not Having Her Period

A 15-year-old girl presents to the office with concerns that her menstrual period has not started yet. She recalls that her breast development started at age 11 and pubic hair growth started at age 12. Her older sister experienced menarche at age 13 and her mother around age 12. She denies any significant medical or surgical history. She is an active athlete who is on the cross country and volleyball teams, but she denies restricting calories or negative feelings about her body image. During a confidential interview, she denies sexual activity.

When should delayed menarche be evaluated?
Absence of menstrual periods at age 15 should be evaluated, and primary amenorrhea (absence of menses by age 13 without sexual characteristics and age 15 with sexual characteristics) can be evaluated at an earlier age if there are concerns about other pathology such as signs of androgenization or evidence of an eating disorder. If more than 3 years have passed since onset of thelarche (breast budding) without onset of menarche, an evaluation is warranted.

What is the most common cause of primary amenorrhea?
The most common cause of primary amenorrhea, or delayed menarche, is constitutional delay. However, this is a diagnosis of exclusion. Other etiologies for delayed menarche must be evaluated and excluded before making a diagnosis of constitutional delay (Table 49.1). Asking about the patient's mother's and sisters' age of menarche is an important aspect of the family history.

CLINICAL PEARL	**STEPS 2/3**
The median age of menarche is 12.4 years; menarche prior to age 10 is considered premature.	

You perform a physical exam. Her vital signs show a temperature of 37°C (98.7°F), a heart rate of 61/min, blood pressure of 104/62, respiration rate of 14/min, height 1.6 m (5'5"), and a weight of 53 kg (117 lbs) (BMI of 19.5 kg/m², the 39th percentile for her age). She is a well-appearing female in no apparent distress. Her cardiovascular and pulmonary exams are unremarkable. Her abdomen is soft, nontender, and there are no palpable masses or hernias. Her breast exam reveals Tanner 4 development. Her genitourinary exam shows normal external genitalia without clitoromegaly, a normal urethral meatus and anus, but an absent vaginal opening.

What is the differential diagnosis in this case?
A patient with normal female secondary sexual characteristics and primary amenorrhea may have constitutional delay, hypothalamic amenorrhea due to excessive exercise or disordered eating, other endocrine dysfunction such as thyroid disease, or primary ovarian insufficiency. In this case, the finding of an absent vaginal opening narrows the differential diagnosis considerably. The

TABLE 49.1 ■ Disorders Associated With Primary Amenorrhea

Diagnosis	Secondary Sexual Characteristics	Internal Reproductive Structures	Labs	Karyotype
Mullerian agenesis/Mayer-Rokitansky-Kuster-Hauser (MRKH) syndrome	Female genitalia, normal breast development, normal pubic and axillary hair	Absent upper vagina, cervix, uterus, fallopian tubes (possible rudimentary uterine horn); ovaries present	Normal female estradiol and testosterone, pubertal FSH and LH	46, XX
Complete androgen insensitivity (CAIS)	Female genitalia, normal breast development, absent or sparse pubic and axillary hair	No Mullerian structures, intra-abdominal gonads, possibility of inguinal gonads	Elevated total serum testosterone and androgens	46, XY
Turner syndrome (TS)	Female genitalia, usually absent breast and pubic hair development but can be variable (usually mosaic TS)	Normal Mullerian structures; streak gonads	Elevated gonadotropins (FSH, LH), prepubertal estradiol levels	45, X (mosaic variations possible: 45, X/46, XX or 45, X/46, XY)
Swyer syndrome	Female genitalia, no breast development or pubic/axillary hair	Normal Mullerian structures; streak gonads	Elevated gonadotropins (FSH, LH), prepubertal estradiol levels	46, XY
Aromatase deficiency	Varying degrees of virilization of external genitalia	Normal Mullerian structures	Elevated androgens	46, XX (can present in normal 46, XY males as well)
Kallman syndrome	Female genitalia, absent pubertal development; characterized by anosmia (lack of sense of smell)	Normal Mullerian structures	Undetectable FSH, LH due to failure of hypothalamus to produce gonadotropins; prepubertal estradiol	46, XX (can present in 46, XY as well)
Obstructive anomalies (vaginal septum, imperforate hymen)	Female genitalia, normal breast development and pubic/axillary hair	Normal Mullerian structures; hematocolpos or hematometrocolpos	Normal pubertal FSH and LH, female estradiol levels	46, XX

FSH, Follicular stimulating hormone; *LH,* luteinizing hormone.

differential diagnosis includes Mullerian agenesis (lack of development of internal female reproductive structures), partial androgen insensitivity syndrome, or a structural anomaly of the vagina such as a low transverse vaginal septum, partial vaginal agenesis, or an imperforate hymen. Generally, a structural anomaly that causes obstruction of menstrual flow presents as cyclic abdominal pain due to the back up of menses into the upper vagina and uterus and a pelvic mass on exam or imaging. However, such anomalies can present prior to menarche and therefore be painless.

What is the next step in evaluation?
The suggested laboratory evaluation in this case would be follicle-stimulating hormone (FSH), luteinizing hormone (LH), estradiol, testosterone levels, and a karyotype. Imaging should also be performed. A pelvic ultrasound should be done to assess for internal Mullerian structures, and a renal ultrasound should be performed to confirm normal bilateral kidneys. Magnetic resonance imaging (MRI) may be indicated if small, rudimentary Mullerian structures cannot be visualized by transabdominal ultrasound. Laparoscopy is rarely indicated for diagnostic purposes.

> In our patient, results of the laboratory evaluation reveal pubertal levels of FSH (6.0 mIU/mL) and LH (7.1 mIU/mL), an estradiol level of 86 pg/mL, and total testosterone of 16 ng/dL. Her karyotype is 46, XX. A transabdominal pelvic ultrasound reveals normal bilateral ovaries with follicles but no identifiable uterus or cervix.

What is this patient's diagnosis, and what is the etiology?
The diagnosis is Mullerian agenesis, also known as Mayer-Rokitansky-Kuster-Hauser Syndrome (MRKH). Normal female levels of testosterone and 46, XX karyotype eliminate congenital androgen insensitivity syndrome (CAIS) from the differential. The ultrasound findings in MRKH confirm the absence or partial absence of Mullerian structures. The fallopian tubes, uterus, cervix, and upper vagina are all derived from the Mullerian ducts, so any of these structures may be undeveloped or absent in MRKH.

CLINICAL PEARL   **STEPS 2/3**

Prevalence of Mullerian agenesis is quoted as 1 in 4,000–10,000 females. CAIS is less common, with a prevalence of 1 in 13,000–40,000 live births.

What is the recommended treatment for this patient?
The primary goal for many women with MRKH is to create a functional vagina for the purpose of sexual intercourse. However, not all patients will have this goal, and patients must be emotionally ready and mature enough to participate in the process and maintain the neovagina prior to embarking on neovagina creation. Younger patients, like ours, may not yet be ready to create a vagina or have desire for sexual activity, and some patients may choose to never create a vagina. It is important to evaluate the patient's personal desires and expectations for treatment. First-line recommendation for the creation of a neovagina is the use of graduated-size dilators to open the potential vaginal space. This can be accomplished quickly or gradually over years, according to the patient's comfort level. The patient starts with short dilators, applies pressure to the space between the urethra and perineum for 20–30 minutes 2–3 times daily, and gradually works up to longer or wider dilators. The assistance of a trained pelvic floor physical therapist can be very helpful. Success of dilation to create a functional vagina varies from 75% to 95%. Surgical creation of a neovagina is offered if vaginal dilation is not successful. There are a variety of surgical techniques including split skin grafts from the leg (Abbe-McIndoe procedure), pelvic peritoneum (Davydov procedure), or bowel vaginoplasty. A procedure called the Vecchietti procedure uses an

olive-shaped dilator attached to tension sutures placed laparoscopically and tractioned through abdomen to create a vagina within a few days. Even after surgical creation of a neovagina procedure, regular vaginal dilation is still necessary to maintain patency.

CLINICAL PEARL	STEPS 2/3

Mullerian agenesis may be associated with urinary system anomalies, particularly congenital absence of one kidney. Any patient diagnosed with Mullerian agenesis should also have a renal ultrasound to assess for congenital renal anomalies. Renal anomalies are present in 30% of women with MRKH.

What are this patient's fertility options?

Adoption and gestational carrier are options for this patient in the future. Women with MRKH have functional gonads and the ability to have genetic children using a gestational carrier. In the future, uterine transplantation may be a reality for some women with Mullerian agenesis, but currently this is considered experimental.

BASIC SCIENCE PEARL	STEP 1

The internal female reproductive system is embryologically derived from the paired Mullerian (paramesonephric) ducts. The ducts arise on the lateral aspect of the Wolffian (mesonephric) ducts, which in males give rise to the epididymis, ductus deferens, and seminal vesicles when Mullerian-inhibiting substance (MIS) is produced by functioning male testes. Production of MIS is determined by the SRY gene on the Y chromosome in males. In the female fetus, there is no production of MIS, so the Wolffian ducts atrophy while the Mullerian ducts develop into the uterus, cervix, and fallopian tubes.

BASIC SCIENCE PEARL	STEP 1

Remnants of the Wolffian ducts in females can be found in the mesosalpinx (forming paraovarian and paratubal cysts) and as the Gartner's duct (can form cystic lesions within the lateral walls of the vagina).

What if the patient had no pubic hair but a short (2 cm) vagina? What is the most likely diagnosis in this scenario?

A patient without any pubic hair but who does have a vaginal opening with minimal vaginal length most likely has complete androgen insensitivity (CAIS).

What is the pathophysiology of CAIS and the associated karyotype?

CAIS is a condition in which there is a defect in the androgen receptor resulting in the absence of masculinization. The karyotype is 46, XY, and the gonads produce testosterone. However, since there are no functional androgen receptors, the external genitalia are not masculinized and pubic hair is absent or sparse. CAIS patients have high levels of serum testosterone which is peripherally converted to estrogen resulting in normal breast development.

BASIC SCIENCE PEARL	STEP 1

Patients with CAIS do not have internal Mullerian structures (uterus, fallopian tubes, or upper vagina) because MIS is still produced, causing regression of the Mullerian ducts during embryologic development. External genitalia appear female due to the lack of functional androgen receptors preventing masculinization in utero.

CLINICAL PEARL STEPS 2/3

Gonads are typically intra-abdominal in patients with CAIS, but they sometimes can be found within an inguinal hernia (either unilateral or bilateral). An ovary found within an inguinal hernia in a young girl should always raise suspicion for CAIS or Mullerian agenesis.

Your patient and her mother return for a review of all the results, and you explain her diagnosis and treatment options. She says she isn't ready for any treatment yet, but wants to consider dilation starting when she is 16 or 17. During a confidential interview, she asks if she will be able to have a normal sex life when she is older and if she can contract any sexually transmitted infections.

How do you counsel an adolescent with MRKH about sexuality?

You should counsel all adolescent patients about safe sexual practices. Even though a patient with Mullerian agenesis cannot become pregnant, she could still contract sexually transmitted infections such as gonorrhea, *Chlamydia*, herpes simplex virus (HSV), or human immunodeficiency virus (HIV). She is also at risk for exposure to human papilloma virus (HPV) and vaccination should be recommended. Satisfying sexual experiences are possible for women with Mullerian agenesis with or without creation of a neovagina. Her anatomy should be explained to her using diagrams or a mirror if she feels comfortable. Women with a new diagnosis of MRKH should be referred to appropriate support groups, such as the Beautiful You MRKH Foundation (www.beautifulyoumrkh.org).

BEYOND THE PEARLS

- Women with Mullerian agenesis/MRKH may have rudimentary uterine horns (single or bilateral). Generally the horns are not functional, but 2%–7% will have some functional endometrium, which can lead to accumulation of menstrual blood in the horns (hematometrium) and cyclic pain. Retrograde menstruation can occur from the horns and result in endometriosis and pelvic pain. MRI can be useful in identifying small rudimentary horns and assessing for endometrium; laparoscopic resection of the rudimentary horns is recommended when functional endometrium is present.
- Patients with complete CAIS were historically recommended to have a bilateral gonadectomy after puberty in order to prevent possible malignancy of the internal gonads. However, this recommendation is now considered controversial due to the very small risk of malignancy, high cure rates of the rare gonadal malignancies that do occur, and the risks and burden of lifelong estrogen therapy required to maintain hormones in these women following gonadectomy. Bilateral gonadectomy is no longer a universal recommendation, so CAIS should be evaluated and cared for by a knowledgeable multispecialty team.

Case Summary

- A 15-year-old adolescent girl presents with no menses and normal development of secondary sexual characteristics. Her exam is consistent with a lack of uterus and a blind-end vagina, which indicates either Mullerian agenesis or CAIS. Her normal testosterone levels and imaging confirm Mayer-Rokitansky-Kuster-Hauser syndrome (MRKH), or Mullerian agenesis.
- The patient is offered vaginal dilation, which she wants to wait to start until she feels more ready, around age 16–17. She is curious about future sexual activity and sexual infection risk, so you advise her about safe sex practices and future fertility options.

References

ACOG Committee Opinion No. 651: Menstruation in girls and adolescents: using the menstrual cycle as a vital sign. (2015). *Obstetrics and Gynecology 126*(6), e143–e146.

Committee Opinion No. 562: Mullerian agenesis: diagnosis, management, and treatment. (2013). *Obstetrics and Gynecology 121*(5), 1134–1137.

Londra, L., Chuong, F. S., & Kolp, L. (2015). Mayer-Rokitansky-Kuster-Hauser syndrome: a review. *International Journal of Women's Health 7*, 865–870.

Nakhal, R. S., & Creighton, S. M. (2012). Management of vaginal agenesis. *Journal of Pediatric and Adolescent Gynecology 25*(6), 352–357.

Lauren Damle, MD

A 14-Year-Old Girl With Heavy Menstrual Bleeding Since Menarche

A 14-year-old girl with a 1-year history of heavy menstrual bleeding presents to the office with her mother. She reports that she started menses at age 12. She states that she menstruates every 27–29 days (she has been tracking it using her phone), and her menstrual bleeding lasts 6–7 days. During her menstrual period, she passes large clots, has a sensation of flooding, and has episodes where blood overflows her sanitary pad, including such accidents at school. She complains of fatigue and quit the school soccer team as a result.

What additional history would be helpful to assess this patient?

It is important to ask patients with heavy menstrual bleeding, especially adolescents, about history of other types of bleeding such as epistaxis or surgical bleeding. A pictorial bleeding assessment calendar can be very useful in quantifying blood loss (an example is shown in Fig. 50.1). Family history of bleeding disorders and the menstrual history of the patient's mother and sisters are also important. Finally, a confidential interview is essential to determine her level of sexual activity and her risk for sexually transmitted infections (STIs) and to assess possible contraception needs which may influence the diagnosis and treatment.

CLINICAL PEARL   **STEPS 2/3**

The HEADSS acronym can be used to remember the key topics of the social history for an adolescent patient, and these should be asked in a confidential interview with the adolescent.

  Home: living situation, family composition, history of incarceration or running away
  Education/Employment: school attendance, performance, after school jobs, future career plans
  Activities: sports, extracurricular activities, peer group
  Drugs: use by peers, family members and patient including alcohol and tobacco
  Sexuality: sexual orientation, number of partners, contraception, history of STIs, sexual abuse or rape
  Suicide/Depression: depressive symptoms, self-harm such as cutting, suicidal thoughts or plans

---

The patient and her mother report she had a tonsillectomy at age 5 years that was uncomplicated, but she reports a history of frequent nose bleeds and easy bruising. Her mother had a postpartum hemorrhage when she delivered her daughter and has since had an endometrial ablation for heavy menstrual bleeding. During a confidential interview, the patient denies any past sexual activity and does not intend to have sex at any time in the near future.

Pictorial Bleeding Assessment Chart recording document

Day 1 of Menstruation:

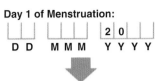

Score	Towels	1	2	3	4	5	6	7
			No bleeding ☐	No bleeding ☐	No bleeding ☐	No bleeding ☐	No bleeding ☐	No bleeding ☐
1								
5								
20								
Tampons								
1								
5								
10								
1	Small Clots / Flooding							
5	Large Clots / Flooding							

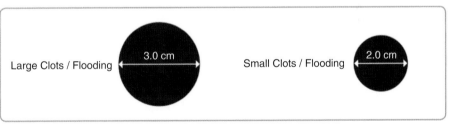

Large Clots / Flooding ←— 3.0 cm —→   Small Clots / Flooding ←— 2.0 cm —→

Fig. 50.1 Pictorial chart that can help to illuminate menstrual patterns in patients who have menstrual abnormalities. Patients tally their menstrual products each day during their menstrual cycle. Lightly soaked product = 1 point, moderately soaked = 5 points, and heavily soaked = 20 points. Small clots receive 1 point and large clots 5 points. A score of 100 or more indicates significant heavy menstrual bleeding. *(From Donnez J et al. Efficacy and safety of repeated use of ulipristal acetate in uterine fibroids. Fertil Steril. 2015 Feb 1;103(2):519–27.e3, suppl. fig. 3.)*

What is in the differential diagnosis of abnormal uterine bleeding in an adolescent?

Abnormal uterine bleeding (AUB) can be the result of heavy menstrual bleeding or intermenstrual bleeding. The mnemonic PALM-COEIN is used to remember the potential etiologies of AUB, just as with adults, but the most common etiologies are different. Structural causes and malignancy (the PALM portion of the PALM-COEIN system) are extremely rare in adolescent females, whereas physiologic causes (the COEIN portion) are more common. Ovulatory dysfunction secondary to immaturity of the hypothalamic-pituitary-ovarian axis is particularly common in adolescence. Pregnancy-related uterine bleeding and STIs (cervicitis or pelvic inflammatory disease) can also cause AUB in this age group. Any adolescent female with history of heavy AUB resulting in anemia, transfusion, or severe symptoms should be evaluated for a bleeding disorder, because 10%–62% of adolescents with heavy menstrual bleeding have an underlying coagulation disorder.

> On physical examination, her temperature is 37°C (98.6°F), blood pressure is 115/64 mm Hg, heart rate is 75/min, respiration rate is 14/min, and oxygen saturation is 99% on room air. Her height is 63 inches and weight is 114 pounds (body mass index of 20.2 kg/m²). She is a well-developed, well-nourished teenager in no apparent distress. Her conjunctiva are pale, but there are no ecchymosis or petechiae noted on her skin, and her cardiac and pulmonary exams are normal. Her abdomen is soft and nontender with no palpable masses. A limited genitourinary exam reveals normal external female genitalia, Tanner 4 development, a patent vaginal opening, and an estrogenized hymen. An internal exam is not performed, given the patient's young age.

What laboratory tests and/or radiology studies should be ordered in the evaluation of this patient?

A female with heavy menstrual bleeding needs to be evaluated for possible anemia with a complete blood count (CBC). Iron studies and ferritin should be added if anemia is found. For the evaluation of heavy AUB since menarche, coagulation studies are recommended. If menstrual bleeding patterns are irregular (cycles lasting less than 21 days or longer than 40 days in an adolescent patient), an endocrine workup may be considered including thyroid-stimulating hormone (TSH), prolactin, follicle-stimulating hormone (FSH), luteinizing hormone (LH), and androgens (testosterone, dehydroepiandrosterone [DHEAS], and 17-hydroxyprogesterone [17-OHP]). For patients who are sexually active, STI screening is indicated, and all menstruating females with AUB, regardless of their report of sexual activity, need a urine pregnancy test. Imaging of the female pelvis is not always indicated as structural abnormalities such as leiomyoma and endometrial polyps are rare in adolescents. An ultrasound may be helpful to evaluate the ovaries in a patient in whom polycystic ovarian syndrome (PCOS) is suspected. Ultrasonography is also indicated in a patient with severe pain or palpable mass on physical examination.

Should this patient be evaluated for a bleeding disorder?

Von Willebrand disease (vWD) is the most common bleeding disorder diagnosed in women and often presents as heavy menstrual bleeding at the time of menarche. Reported prevalence ranges from 1%–2% among African-American girls with heavy AUB to 10%–20% among Caucasian girls with heavy menses. Patients may have a history of recurrent epistaxis or easy bruising, but not necessarily. Platelet function disorders can also present with heavy bleeding at the time of menarche. The laboratory evaluation for vWD is a panel of three tests: von Willebrand factor (vWF) antigen, von Willebrand ristocetin cofactor activity, and factor VIII activity. Platelet function tests, such as bleeding time, prothrombin time (PT), and partial thromboplastin time (PTT), are needed to diagnose a platelet dysfunction disorder.

> The patient's laboratory results are shown in Table 50.1. Ultrasound imaging is not recommended at this time. After the results are received, you meet with the patient and her mother to discuss the diagnosis and treatment plan. You inform the patient that her diagnoses are vWD and iron deficiency anemia. In addition to referring the patient for a hematology consultation, you discuss immediate plans for treatment of anemia and control of heavy menstrual bleeding.

TABLE 50.1 ■ **Laboratory Results in This Adolescent Patient With Heavy Menstrual Bleeding**

Laboratory	Result
Urine β-human chorionic gonadotropin	Negative
Leukocytes	6700/μL
Hemoglobin	9.1 g/dL
Hematocrit	27.3%
Platelets	213,000/μL
Mean corpuscular volume (MCV)	74.8 fL
Prothrombin time (PT)	13.4 seconds
Partial thromboplastin time (PTT)	29.8 seconds
Total iron binding capacity (TIBC)	412 μg/dL
Serum iron	34 μg/dL
Ferritin	5 ng/mL
Von Willebrand factor activity	24 IU/dL
Von Willebrand ristocetin cofactor activity	28 IU/dL
Factor VIII activity	67%

How is iron deficiency anemia treated?

Iron deficiency is treated with iron replacement at a dose of 15–30 mg/kg per day of oral, elemental iron, divided into 2–3 daily doses. Iron supplementation is given in the form of ferrous salt tablets such as ferrous sulfate (325 mg contains 65 mg of elemental iron), ferrous gluconate (325 mg contains 36 mg of elemental iron), or ferrous fumarate (325 mg contains 105 mg of elemental iron). There is also a liquid formulation (15 mg/mL elemental iron). With appropriate replacement and control of blood loss, anemia should resolve within 6–8 weeks.

CLINICAL PEARL   **STEPS 2/3**

Iron supplements should not be taken with calcium-rich foods or within 2 hours of antacid medication. Coadminstration with 250 mg of ascorbic acid or a small glass of orange juice can enhance absorption.

What is the pathophysiology of von Willebrand disease?

vWD is caused by abnormal vWF, a protein that binds platelets and endothelial components at the site of endothelial injury and acts as a carrier protein for factor VIII, therefore contributing to fibrin clot formation. Quantitative and qualitative defects in the vWF lead to impaired hemostasis and are known as type 1 and type 2 vWD, respectively. Type 3 vWD is caused by a complete absence of vWF and is both very severe and extremely rare. vWD is the most common bleeding disorder in the general population, present in 1% of randomly tested patients. To confirm a diagnosis of vWD, levels of less than 30 IU/dL of vWF or ristocetin cofactor activity level must be documented. If levels are low but not diagnostic, the labs can be repeated since there can be variation in the values on different days.

BASIC SCIENCE PEARL   **STEP 1**

Most cases of vWD are autosomal dominant and can affect males and females, although an acquired form of the disease does exist. In contrast, hemophilia A (factor VIII deficiency) and hemophilia B (factor IX deficiency) are X-linked disorders that are only expressed in male offspring of female carriers.

How should the patient's heavy menses be treated?

The management of heavy menstrual bleeding depends on the underlying etiology, meaning infectious causes are treated with antibiotics, endocrine causes with hormone treatment, and so on. Adolescents with a bleeding disorder, as well as those with heavy bleeding without a specific identifiable etiology, should be managed with either progestin or combined progestin and estrogen therapies. First-line therapy is combined oral contraceptive medications containing ethinyl estradiol and progestin given in the form of oral contraceptive pills (OCPs), vaginal ring, or transdermal patch. The progestin-releasing intrauterine device can also be considered first-line, especially in sexually active adolescents or those who have a contraindication to estrogen use. Progestin-only pills (POPs) and depot medroxyprogesterone acetate (DMPA) intramuscular injections are also options.

BASIC SCIENCE PEARL   **STEP 1**

Estradiol is produced through a process of aromatization of androgens, which are produced in the ovary's theca cells. Progesterone is secreted by the corpus luteum, a functional cyst that develops after ovulation during the normal menstrual cycle. Pharmacologic administration of progesterone causes thinning or atrophy of the endometrial lining, while estrogens stabilize the lining.

What are the risks and benefits of combined OCPs?

Combination estrogen and progestin contraception provides the benefit of decreased menstrual bleeding and the possibility of increasing the interval between menstrual bleeding episodes. With use for at least 5 years, there is a significant reduction in the future risk of ovarian cancer and endometrial cancer. However, estrogen-containing therapies increase the risk of venous thromboembolism (VTE). Patients with a family history of VTE, personal known thrombophilia, or personal risk factors such as poorly controlled diabetes mellitus or chronic hypertension should consider progestin-only therapies.

> Once you counsel the patient about her diagnosis and possible treatment options, she and her family express worry about future bleeding episodes. The patient asks, "What if someday I bleed so much that I pass out or have to go to the emergency room?"

How can acute, heavy vaginal bleeding be managed in an adolescent patient?

Part of the treatment of coagulation disorders is to empower the patient and family with education about what levels of bleeding are abnormal, how and why to access emergency care, and what to tell new providers about their history. In emergency settings, higher doses of estrogen and progesterone are needed to stop acute bleeding. Combined OCPs, given in higher doses, are very effective. There are multiple regimens, but one simple strategy is to give four tablets of a combined OCP that contains 30 or 35 mcg of ethinyl estradiol at time of initial presentation. If the patient is stable for discharge home, she can be instructed to take three tablets per day until the bleeding ceases and then take two tablets per day for 14 days, followed by one pill per day until she is seen in the office. It is important to instruct the patient to only take the active pills in the package and discard the placebo pills. Alternative treatments for heavy, emergent bleeding are intravenous estrogen or high-dose progestins. Patients who are also hemodynamically unstable will need admission to the hospital, adequate intravenous access and fluid resuscitation, and transfusion with packed red blood cells.

BASIC SCIENCE PEARL   **STEPS 1/2/3**

In vWD, vWF defects prevent platelet cross-linking, so transfusing more platelets will not allow a patient with vWD to improve their coagulation. For this reason, patients with this disorder will not benefit from other transfusion products, like cryoprecipitate. For episodes of hemorrhage, factor VIII concentrates, which also contain vWF (such as Humate P) can be used.

The patient elects to start therapy using combined OCPs. Due to her diagnosis of vWD and iron deficiency anemia, you recommend continuous OCPs and iron replacement. She returns after 3 months and reports that her menstrual bleeding is significantly decreased, and she has been compliant with her iron supplementation. Repeat laboratory studies reveal a hemoglobin level of 11.1 g/dL and hematocrit level of 32.2%. You advise her to continue her OCPs and take a daily multivitamin containing iron.

BEYOND THE PEARLS

- Tranexamic acid is an antifibrinolytic medication that decreases plasmin formation and fibrinolysis. It was approved by the U.S. Food and Drug Administration (FDA) in 2009 for the treatment of heavy menstrual bleeding in a dose of 1300 mg orally 3 times per day for a maximum of 5 days during bleeding.
- Many factors can spuriously influence the findings of vWF laboratory studies. Exogenous estrogens, such as OCPs, can falsely increase the detected activity and quantity of vWF, as can exercise and stress. Also, patients with type O blood have vWF levels about 25%–30% lower than other blood types.
- Synthetic vasopressin (desmopressin or DDAVP) stimulates the release of vWF into the plasma, so can be used to treat vWD. Patients can receive factor VIII concentrates or DDAVP in emergencies or prior to surgeries to give them 8–10 hours of improved clotting.

Case Summary

- A 14-year-old girl with heavy menstrual bleeding since menarche, a history of easy bruising, and a family history of heavy menstrual bleeding presents to your office and has prolonged bleeding times, decreased factor VIII and von Willebrand factor activity, and iron deficiency anemia. Her findings are consistent with vWD.
- She starts on OCPs and has more regular menses with less heavy bleeding, and she takes oral iron with improvement in her anemia and iron studies.
- You educate the patient and her family on vWD and prepare them with a plan to access medical care and receive treatment in the event of a bleeding emergency.

References

Ahuja, S. P., & Herweck, S. P. (2010). Overview of bleeding disorders in adolescent females with menorrhagia. *Journal of Pediatric and Adolescent Gynecology, 23*, S15–S21.

American College of Obstetrics and Gynecology (2012). Diagnosis of abnormal uterine bleeding in reproductive-aged women. Practice bulletin No. 128. *Obstetrics and Gynecology, 120*, 197–206.

American College of Obstetrics and Gynecology (2015). Menstruation in girls and adolescents: using the menstrual cycle as a vital sign. Committee Opinion No. 651. *Obstetrics and Gynecology, 126*, e143–e146.

Venkateswaran, L., & Dietrich, J. E. (2013). Gynecologic concerns in pubertal females with blood disorders. *Journal of Pediatric and Adolescent Gynecology, 26*, 80–85.

Jason Jarin, MD ■ Lauren Damle, MD

An 11-Year-Old With Gender Identity Concerns

An 11-year-old preteen presents to your office accompanied by her parents. She reports a several-year history of feeling that something "wasn't right" about her body and distress about her female anatomy. Her parents note that she has started to dress in a more masculine manner and has asked them to use male pronouns when referring to her.

What is gender dysphoria?

Gender dysphoria (GD) is defined in the *Diagnostic and Statistical Manual of Mental Disorders* (DSM-5) as significant distress experienced by transgender individuals due to persistent cross-gender identification and discomfort with one's sex or gender role. Transgender individuals have a gender identity that differs from those typically associated with gender assigned at birth. Gender identity is distinct from sexual orientation (which gender[s] one finds sexually attractive) or gender expression (how one chooses to behave in a gender role). Evidence demonstrates improved outcomes with the initiation of gender-affirming interventions, including long-term counseling, cross-sex hormone therapy (CSHT), gender reassignment surgery, and social and legal transition to the desired gender.

What are the initial steps in caring for this patient?

Care for individuals with GD starts with creating a welcoming clinical environment. Changing intake forms to reflect sexual minorities in the gender field and educating clinic staff can promote patient confidence and comfort during the first encounter. Providers should also ask what name and pronoun the patient prefers and take a history of the patient's gender experience using open-ended questions. This includes asking about the age of initial transition and any prior supplement or hormone use. Individual goals should be discussed during the first visit, understanding that not all GD patients choose to undergo medical or surgical transition. Many transgender individuals are very uncomfortable with genital examinations, therefore, a problem-oriented examination is sufficient in most cases, and the genital exam can be deferred until the patient feels comfortable. Regardless of the patient's age or depth of transition, psychotherapy with a qualified mental health provider is recommended. The diagnosis of GD is made only by a mental health provider, and any potential medical or surgical intervention in the future is highly contingent on meeting this diagnosis and continuing mental health care.

CLINICAL PEARL   **STEPS 2/3**

Continuing psychotherapy for gender dysphoria (GD) patients is beneficial after the diagnosis is made, given the increased risk of mental health disorders, depression, substance abuse, and even suicide in individuals affected by GD. The aim of any psychotherapy is *not* to impose a certain gender role or identity on the individual, but to help patients deal with feelings and struggles associated with GD. Individuals should be referred to a therapist who is comfortable treating GD.

TABLE 51.1 ■ Gender Terminology

Gender dysphoria (GD)	Distress that is caused by a discrepancy between a person's gender identity and that person's gender at birth
Gender identity	An individual's sense of being male, female, or an alternative gender
Gender expression	How individuals present themselves socially in their speech, mannerisms, and clothing, independent of their gender identity
Gender variance/gender nonconformity	Gender identity that does not fully fit male or female gender norms
Sexual orientation	An individual's attraction to members of the same sex and/or a different sex (i.e., lesbian, gay, bisexual, heterosexual, or asexual)
Female-to-Male (FTM)	Describes transgender men/boys, or individuals assigned female gender at birth who are changing their body/gender role to a more masculine body/gender role
Male-to-Female (MTF)	Describes transgender women/girls, or individuals assigned male gender at birth who are changing their body/gender role to a more feminine body/gender role

Your patient and his family return 6 months later. He has been seeing a mental health provider who confirmed a diagnosis of GD. The patient has transitioned to a male gender role socially and is consistently using male pronouns. The patient reports feeling well supported by his family and peers and intends to enroll as a boy when he starts junior high next year. He notes worsening distress over some breast development, and his parents express concern that a first menses might be imminent.

How does the onset of puberty affect the management of this patient?

The distress that accompanies GD typically worsens during puberty as adolescents experience unwanted changes in their body. The Endocrine Society clinical practice guidelines support the use of medical suppression of puberty when a child reaches Tanner stage 2, signaled by breast budding in girls and a testicular volume of 4 mL or more in boys. A letter of support from the mental health provider detailing the need for medical intervention is needed before puberty suppression can be initiated. Puberty suppression can prevent the development of secondary sexual characteristics that may later be difficult to alter, such as the Adam's apple, deepened voice, notable breasts, or gender-specific fat distribution. Gonadotropin-releasing hormone (GnRH) agonists can be administered in the form of an implantable rod (histrelin) or intramuscular injections (leuprolide) for puberty suppression. Depo-medroxyprogesterone acetate may also be used in cases in which insurance does not cover the costs of GnRH agonists. Physical and laboratory evaluation (Table 51.2) should be performed every 3 months during puberty suppression.

CLINICAL PEARL   **STEPS 2/3**

The Endocrine Society clinical practice guidelines recommend that bone density be followed annually after initiating puberty suppression therapy as suppression of endogenous testosterone and estrogen contribute to lower bone mineral density. Adult transgender individuals who undergo gonadectomy and then choose to stop hormone therapy are at high risk for osteopenia and osteoporosis and should be monitored.

Is any additional history needed for this patient?

As with any adolescent patient, no visit with a medical provider is complete without a thorough, confidential interview. Sexual minorities, which include gay, lesbian, transgender and gender

TABLE 51.2 ■ Medical Management of Gender Dysphoria

	Puberty Suppression	FTM	MTF
Types of medications	Implantable GnRH analogs (histrelin) Intramuscular GnRH analogs (leuprolide) Depo-medroxyprogesterone	Testosterone (oral, transdermal, intramuscular, subcutaneous)	Estrogen (oral, transdermal, parenteral) Antiandrogens (Spironolactone)
Monitoring	Every 3 months: Height/weight LH, FSH, estradiol, testosterone Every year: LFTs, renal profile, lipids, insulin, HgbA1c BMD, bone age	Every 3 months: Height/weight, CBC LH, FSH, estradiol, testosterone, LFTs, renal profile, lipids, insulin, HgbA1c Every year: BMD, bone age	Every 3 months: Height/weight, LH, FSH, estradiol, testosterone, prolactin, LFTs, renal profile, lipids, insulin, HgbA1c Every year: BMD, bone age
Benefits	Prevention of secondary sexual characteristics of the assigned gender	Deepened voice, facial and body hair growth, increased libido, amenorrhea, clitoral enlargement (variable), and increased muscle mass percentage compared to body fat	Breast growth (variable), decreased testicular size, and increased percentage of body fat compared to muscle mass Antiandrogens may reduce effects of endogenous testosterone (e.g., reduction in new hair growth)

BMD, Bone mineral density; *GnRH,* gonadotropin-releasing hormone; *LH,* luteinizing hormone; *FSH,* follicle-stimulating hormone; *CBC,* complete blood count; *LFT,* liver function test; *HgbA1c,* hemoglobin A1c.

variant youth, are at increased risk of suicide, substance abuse, and high-risk sexual behavior. Salient issues such as substance abuse, bullying, and body image should always be discussed separately from parents. A detailed sexual history should be taken for older adolescents and young adults. It is important to address sexual health, including the risks of sexually transmitted infections and, if the patient is engaging in vaginal-penile sex, the risk of pregnancy. The confidential interview is also an opportunity to determine if there are issues with acceptance of the patient's gender identity among his or her family and friends.

> The patient decides to have a histrelin implant placed. Prior to the end of his visit, he enquires about cross-sex hormone therapy. He has read on the Internet that some kids are using testosterone during their transition, and he would like to know more about this treatment. His parents are unsure about him "using hormones" at such a young age and are concerned that this may affect his ability to have children in the future.

What medical treatment options are available to transgender patients?
Regardless of whether or not puberty was suppressed, the Endocrine Society clinical practice guidelines support initiation of cross-sex hormone therapy (CSHT) around the age of 16. Physicians should extensively counsel adolescents who are considering CSHT regarding the expected results and their possible adverse health effects (Table 51.2). It is appropriate to start to discuss future treatment with this patient while emphasizing that he is still too young to initiate CSHT. At age 16, this patient may be referred for CSHT by his mental health provider. It is important for health care providers to be aware that many transgender youth may purchase medications through the Internet and self-treat to hasten their transition. Emphasizing the

importance of only taking medication prescribed by a physician knowledgeable in transgender care is crucial. Testosterone is used for masculinization in female-to-male transitions and may be administered intramuscularly or subcutaneously to suppress menses and virilize the body, face, and hair. Serum testosterone levels are measured every 2–3 months. For male-to-female transitions, feminizing therapy with estrogen is used. Estrogen can be given orally, as a transdermal patch, or parenterally (intramuscular or subcutaneous injection). Estrogen will promote breast growth, redistribute fat to the hips, and reduce facial hair growth. After starting estrogen therapy, serum testosterone and estradiol levels are measured every 3 months. Spironolactone, which has antiandrogenic properties, is given in addition to estrogen to decrease masculine features such as unwanted hair and acne.

BASIC SCIENCE/CLINICAL PEARL   **STEPS 1/2/3**

Testosterone therapy carries with it risks of polycythemia vera (overabundance of red blood cells), liver inflammation, hyperlipidemia, and diabetes. Individuals on CSHT with testosterone should have evaluation with hemoglobin and hematocrit to evaluate for polycythemia, as well as liver function tests, lipid panels, and hemoglobin A1c to assess for development of diabetes.

Does hormonal treatment have an effect on future fertility? What are this patient's options?
Prolonged use of CSHT may have negative effects on ovarian and testicular function. Providers should engage transgender patients in discussion regarding plans for future childbearing *before* initiating CSHT. Female-to-male transgender individuals may opt for embryo cryopreservation or oocyte cryopreservation to preserve fertility. The success of embryo freezing has been well documented, and oocyte-freezing techniques have improved dramatically in recent years. It is important to note, however, that unintended pregnancies have occurred in trans-men receiving testosterone, so contraceptive needs must be addressed, especially in patients who have maintained their uterus and are engaging in penile-vaginal intercourse. Male-to-female transgender individuals may choose to undergo sperm cryopreservation to preserve fertility. This can be accomplished at sperm banking facilities.

> Your patient and his family also have questions about long-term health issues and recommended screening tests. Specifically, he wants to know if he will need to have Pap tests or mammograms as he gets older. He is also wondering what type of surgery he may want to consider in the future.

What surgical options are available to transgender patients?
Some individuals undergoing transition consider surgery essential to gender affirmation, while other transgender patients are comfortable and satisfied without undergoing any surgery. The Endocrine Society recommends that surgery be deferred until age 16 for breast reduction and 18 for other surgical procedures. For female-to-male transitions, surgical interventions include reduction or removal of breast tissue (often referred to as "top surgery"), hysterectomy with or without bilateral salpingo-oophorectomy, and/or surgical creation of a phallus ("bottom surgery"). For male-to-female transgender patients, breast augmentation can be offered as well as complex genital reconstruction to reduce the phallus and create a functional vagina. Genital reconstruction surgeries are performed by highly specialized surgeons with expertise in these procedures.

What long-term health considerations need to be discussed specific to transgender patients?
Individuals undergoing long-term estrogen supplementation require counseling regarding the increased risks of venous thromboembolism (VTE). Monitoring of weight and blood pressure,

directed physical exams, routine health questions focused on risk factors and medications, and lab tests including complete blood count, renal and liver functions, glucose levels, and lipid profile should be standard care for transgender adults. Estrogen is generally continued until the average age of menopause (51 years). Female-to-male transgender patients who still have a cervix are recommended to have routine cervical cancer screenings starting at age 21, and immunization against human papilloma virus (HPV) is recommended for all transgender patients aged 9–26 just as it is for cis-gender patients. The American Cancer Society (ACS) recommends age-appropriate screening for breast cancer in all transgender patients who have any breast tissue. The risk of endometrial cancer should also be discussed with female-to-male patients who have retained their uterus while receiving long-term testosterone treatment. Though routine endometrial biopsy is discouraged, any abnormal uterine bleeding needs to be evaluated. Transgender male-to-female patients should receive prostate cancer screening according to ACS guidelines. Last, it is crucial to emphasize the importance of long-term mental health follow-up for all transgender patients.

CLINICAL PEARL   **STEPS 2/3**

Transgender patients are at increased risk for sexual abuse, high-risk sexual behavior, and confusion about sexual orientation and relationships. Regular screening for high-risk sexual behavior and abuse should take place at all visits, and transgender individuals who are sexually active in any form should be routinely screened for sexually transmitted infections. A urine specimen can be used for gonorrhea and *Chlamydia* screening if the patient is uncomfortable with a genital exam. As with all young people, they need to be screened for self-destructive behaviors or thoughts of self-harm; concerns should be taken seriously and promptly addressed. Young people with substance abuse disorders, particularly addiction, should be offered information on counseling, rehabilitation, or 12-step programs.

The patient enrolls in middle school as a boy and feels increasingly comfortable in his gender role; continued visits over the ensuing years reveal safe practices. He endures some verbal bullying as a middle school student but continues psychotherapy and learns to manage worries and anxiety about this. The patient opts to undergo cryopreservation of oocytes and, when he turns 16, initiates CSHT with testosterone. The patient is attracted to females and initiates a romantic relationship with a girl at age 17; he reports no abuse in that relationship.

BEYOND THE PEARLS

- Patients who desire male-to-female surgical transition of the genitalia often have formation of a neovagina, a vaginal vault that is made of other autologous tissue (tissue from elsewhere on the patient's body). Neovaginas are created by first dissecting the perineal space, usually after removal or revision of the testicles and formation of the scrotal skin into labia majora, and then placing the patient's skin on a mold (McIndoe procedure). Colonic tissue or other autologous tissue in this space serves as the epithelium of the new vagina. Skin from the penis can also be used to create a neovagina. Successful procedures are marked by patient comfort with the appearance and, usually, the ability to use the vagina for sexual activity.
- Transgender individuals sometimes want to see medical providers in specialties appropriate for the gender with which they identify. For this reason, gynecologists may see patients who are genetically male or even have male or ambiguous genitalia who wish to have pelvic or gynecologic exams to more fully identify with their female gender identity. Modern providers should be aware of this possibility and know their own comfort level, boundaries, and knowledge limitations in caring for these patients. It is vital to create an open and nonjudgmental environment that prioritizes the patient's health needs, with referral to other providers as appropriate.

Case Summary

- An 11-year-old preteen, assigned female gender at birth, presents with feelings of discomfort with her body and the sense that she identifies as a male. Evaluation by a mental health professional confirms a diagnosis of gender dysphoria (GD).

- The patient lives as a boy socially for 6 months, feels comfortable with the new identity, and enrolls in middle school as a boy. Puberty is suppressed using a gonadotropin-releasing hormone agonist implant (histrelin) until the age of 16, when he starts testosterone therapy. Prior to initiation of testosterone therapy, the patient opts for cryopreservation of oocytes to preserve future fertility options.

- Going forward, the patient feels increasingly confident in his male gender identity. He continues counseling therapy, and, as he identifies as being attracted to women, forms a safe, romantic relationship with a female partner when he is in high school.

References

American Psychiatric Association (2013). *Diagnostic and Statistical Manual of Mental Disorders* (5th ed.). Arlington VA: American Psychiatric Association.

Hembree, W. C., Cohen-Kettenis, P., Delemarre-van de Waal, H. A., et al. (2009). Endocrine Society. Endocrine treatment of transsexual persons: an Endocrine Society clinical practice guideline. *The Journal of Clinical Endocrinology and Metabolism*, *94*(9), 3132–3154.

World Professional Association for Transgender Health (WPATH) (2012). *Standards of care for the health of transsexual, transgender, and gender-nonconforming people.* 7th Version. World Professional Association for Transgender Health.

Amanika Kumar, MD

A 65-Year-Old Postmenopausal Woman With Abdominal Distension

A 65-year-old postmenopausal woman presents to her general practitioner with 6 months of progressively worsening abdominal pain, early satiety, and abdominal distension. The pain is dull, achy, and constant; does not change with oral intake; and is accompanied by a decrease in appetite. She says her clothes "haven't been fitting" her, but she thought she "was just gaining weight." Her medical history is significant for hypertension, which is well-controlled, and class I obesity with a body mass index of 31 kg/m².

What are the next steps in the evaluation of this patient?
The differential diagnosis of abdominal pain is wide. It includes pathology involving any system in the abdomen: gastrointestinal, genitourinary, vascular, or musculoskeletal, and, less frequently, referred pain from the pulmonary or cardiac system. The complaints of weight and appetite change in the postmenopausal patient increase the suspicion for more serious pathology. The next best step for this patient is a full physical exam, which should include a pelvic exam in any woman with these complaints.

Physical exam confirms a temperature of 37°C (98.7°F), blood pressure of 118/76 mm Hg, heart rate of 95/min, respiratory rate of 20/min, and an oxygen saturation of 96% on room air. Her exam is significant for a nontender, distended abdomen with a fluid wave, and pelvic exam reveals a palpable pelvic mass that is fixed to the rectovaginal septum. You order a CA 125 and computerized tomography (CT) scan of the chest, abdomen, and pelvis. Her CA 125 is elevated to 1365 U/mL (Table 52.1). Her CT scan is significant for peritoneal carcinomatosis with omental cake, ascites, and a left ovarian mass.

CLINICAL PEARL   **STEPS 2/3**

Tumor markers obtained in the setting of suspected intraabdominal malignancy in a postmenopausal woman include carcinoembryonic antigen (CEA), CA 125, CA 19-9, and CA 27-29. CEA is a marker for colorectal cancer, CA 19-9 is a marker for pancreatic cancer, and CA 27-29 is a marker for breast cancer. CA 125 is the most nonspecific of the tumor markers, but is more specific in postmenopausal women and is used in diagnosis and to monitor treatment of epithelial ovarian cancer.

The patient is taken to the operating room of gynecologic oncology. There she is diagnosed with high-grade serous carcinoma of the ovary.

BASIC SCIENCE PEARL	STEPS 2/3

There are five histologic subtypes of epithelial ovarian cancer: serous, mucinous, endometrioid, transitional cell, and clear cell. The most common subtype is high-grade serous carcinoma.

TABLE 52.1 ■ Causes of Elevated CA 125

Epithelial ovarian, fallopian tube, and primary peritoneal carcinoma
Endometrial carcinoma
Benign ovarian neoplasms
Endometriosis
Pregnancy
Ovarian hyperstimulation
Pelvic inflammatory disease
Menstruation
Cirrhosis
Ascites of any etiology
Colitis
Intraabdominal abscess or infection
Pancreatitis
Pleural effusion
Pericardial disease
Heart failure
Recent abdominal surgery
Sarcoidosis
Lupus
Malignancy of other etiology including breast, colon, hematologic

How is epithelial ovarian cancer staged?

At the time of diagnosis, the first step for management of any malignancy is determining the stage of the cancer. For ovarian cancer, this is done surgically. The staging procedure includes total hysterectomy, bilateral salpingo-oophorectomy, pelvic and paraaortic lymphadenectomy, omentectomy, and peritoneal washing.

BASIC SCIENCE/CLINICAL PEARL	STEPS 1/2/3

Cancers can spread lymphatically, hematogenously (by the blood stream), and by direct extension. Ovarian cancer can spread in all of these manners but is most commonly spread by direct extension to peritoneal surfaces and other intraabdominal organs at the time of diagnosis.

What are the goals of surgery for ovarian cancer?

The goals of surgery for epithelial ovarian cancer are twofold: (1) to surgically stage a cancer to determine the extent of spread, and (2) to "cytoreduce" tumor to no visible disease. Tumor debulking, sometimes called surgical cytoreduction, is a procedure in which each visible area of tumor in the abdomen is removed. Optimal cytoreduction is defined as all tumor greater than 1 cm being removed (so no single site of tumor left is greater than 1 cm), as studies have shown improved survival in patients with this surgical outcome. More recent studies have shown that leaving *no* residual disease (no tumor palpable or visible) improves overall and progression-free survival.

The gynecologic oncology service performs an exploratory laparotomy, drainage of 3 L of ascites, total abdominal hysterectomy, bilateral salpingo-oophorectomy with en bloc resection of the distal sigmoid/proximal rectum, stapled reanastomosis of bowel, omentectomy, diaphragm stripping, and pelvic and paraaortic lymphadenectomy. At the end of the procedure, there is no visible tumor in the abdomen. She has a stage IIIC, high-grade, serous carcinoma of the ovary. She would like to know her future options for treatment (Fig. 52.1).

BASIC SCIENCE PEARL   **STEP 1**

The log kill hypothesis provides the theoretical underpinnings for why cytoreductive surgery leads to better outcomes in ovarian cancer. It states that chemotherapy kills the same proportion of tumor cells (as opposed to the same absolute number of cells) regardless of the size of the tumor at chemotherapy initiation.

CLINICAL PEARL   **STEPS 2/3**

When diagnosed with epithelial ovarian cancer, 60%–70% of patients are diagnosed with stage III or IV cancer. This is due to the lack of symptoms and reliable screening tests for this cancer.

Is there an alternative treatment to primary debulking surgery for advanced epithelial ovarian carcinoma?

The first step to management of a patient with advanced ovarian cancer is to determine whether a neoadjuvant chemotherapy or a primary debulking surgery approach is most appropriate, and this must be individualized to the patient and the center at which the patient is being seen. Some factors used to decide on approach include the extent of tumor as seen on CT scan, evidence of disease outside the abdomen, evidence of comorbidities, functional status, age, and evidence of venous thromboembolism at the time of diagnosis. At the time of primary debulking surgery, the first step of the surgery is to determine whether or not an optimal or complete cytoreduction is feasible. This can be done laparoscopically or through a mini-laparotomy; the approach is determined by surgeon and center preference.

CLINICAL PEARL   **STEPS 2/3**

Primary debulking surgery is when a patient's first treatment is surgery, meaning it is done before the administration of chemotherapy. Chemotherapy given after surgery is termed adjuvant chemotherapy. Neoadjuvant chemotherapy is chemotherapy given *before* surgery. Surgery performed *after* chemotherapy for ovarian cancer is called interval debulking surgery.

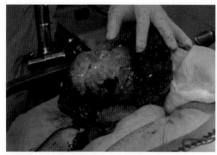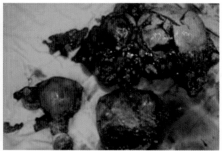

Fig. 52.1 Abdomen in surgery and pelvic organs after removal showing a large amount of abdominal carcinomatosis and a large omental "cake" of tumor. *(From Chia CC, Huang SC. Rapid progression of synchronous ovarian and endometrial cancers with massive omental carcinomatosis. Taiwan J Obstet Gynecol. 2012 Sep 1;51(3):452–4, fig. 2.)*

The patient is hospitalized for 5 days after her complete cytoreduction and discharged home. She follows up 3 weeks after surgery with gynecologic oncology to discuss chemotherapy.

What are chemotherapy options for patients with advanced high-grade serous carcinoma of the ovary?

Adjuvant chemotherapy is recommend for patients following primary debulking surgery for epithelial ovarian cancer. Chemotherapy consists of a platinum-containing regimen, most commonly carboplatin and paclitaxel. In general, six cycles of chemotherapy are given, and each cycle is 21 days. A gynecologic oncology group (GOG) study demonstrated progression-free survival and overall survival benefit to intraperitoneal (IP) chemotherapy of 15.9 months and a Japanese GOG study of dose-dense chemotherapy demonstrated improved survival of 38.3 months, both being compared to standard chemotherapy. IP chemotherapy and dose-dense chemotherapy are currently being compared to each other in a GOG study.

BASIC SCIENCE PEARL	STEP 1

Carboplatin is a DNA adducting agent. It intercalates into replicating DNA, specifically in the S-phase of the cell cycle, and causes DNA double strand breaks. Paclitaxel is a taxane derivative and is a topoisomerase II inhibitor, which means that it inhibits the enzyme that recoils the DNA strands during the M-phase of the cell cycle (Table 52.2).

The patient goes on to receive chemotherapy in a dose-dense fashion for six cycles. During her chemotherapy, her CA 125 drops to normal (<35 U/mL) after three cycles and remains normal through the completion of chemotherapy.

What does the patient do next?

After completion of chemotherapy and with normalization of the tumor marker of her cancer (in this case, CA 125), the patient is considered in a state of no evidence of disease (NED). She will now undergo surveillance for recurrence. Surveillance is done with a clinical history and exam every 3 months for the first 2 years. Following CA 125 every 3 months is optional and warrants discussion between the patient and the provider. Routine imaging is not recommended and should be performed only when prompted by clinical symptoms, clinical exam, or change in CA 125.

TABLE 52.2 ■ Side Effects of Chemotherapy

Chemotherapy	Common Side Effects	Less Common Side Effects
Carboplatin	Bone marrow suppression Fatigue Nausea/emesis	Skin rash Kidney dysfunction Changes in hearing Hair loss Changes in vision Changes in taste
Paclitaxel	Bone marrow suppression Hair loss Myalgias Peripheral neuropathy	Allergic reaction Nausea/emesis Diarrhea Palpitations Finger/toenail changes

BEYOND THE PEARLS

- In a patient with a clinically apparent stage I ovarian cancer, paraaortic lymphadenectomy will find metastases and upstage the patient to stage IIIA in 30% of cases.
- The origin of high-grade serous carcinoma of the ovary is now established to be the fallopian tube, most commonly the fimbriated end. Precursor lesions to high-grade serous carcinomas can be found in the fallopian tube and are called serous tubal intraepithelial carcinomas (STICs).
- Several centers use a laparoscopic approach to evaluate the ability to debulk at the time of primary surgery. One such scoring tool, the Fagotti score, looks at the presence or absence of peritoneal carcinomatosis, omental cake, mesenteric retraction, diaphragmatic carcinomatosis, bowel infiltration, stomach infiltration, and liver metastasis to predict the ability to completely cytoreduce ovarian cancer.
- Paclitaxel is derived from the yew tree and is given in a diluent called cremophor. This cremophor, rather than the drug itself, is often the cause of hypersensitivity reactions during infusion. Preventing these reactions is important, so patients are pretreated with corticosteroids and histamine blockers before paclitaxel infusion.
- Randomized controlled trials demonstrated equivalent oncologic outcomes between primary surgery and neoadjuvant chemotherapy, but these trials had low rates of optimal and complete cytoreduction.
- A study performed in England demonstrated that early identification of elevated CA 125 (as opposed to diagnosing recurrence by identification of suspicious symptoms) showed no difference in overall survival, and early identification with CA 125 was associated with longer chemotherapy and a worsened quality of life.

Case Summary

- A postmenopausal woman presents with symptoms of abdominal pain, early satiety, and abdominal distension.
- A history and physical exam is concerning for malignancy, and an elevated CA 125 biomarker and computed tomography (CT) scan confirm this suspicion.
- The patient undergoes surgery to stage the ovarian cancer and to cytoreduce (debulk) the cancer to no gross residual disease.
- After surgery she is given carboplatin and paclitaxel chemotherapy for six cycles, during which time her CA 125 returns to normal.
- Following completion of surgery and chemotherapy she is free of disease and undergoes surveillance for recurrence.

References

Armstrong, D., Bundy, B., Wenzel, L., et al. (2006). Intraperitoneal cisplatin and paclitaxel in ovarian cancer. *The New England Journal of Medicine, 354*(1), 34–43.

Barakat, R. (2013). *Principles and practice of gynecologic oncology* (6th ed.). Philadelphia: Wolters Kluwer.

Berek, J. S., & Hacker, N. F. (2006). *Berek and Hacker's gynecologic oncology* (6th ed.). Philadelphia: Wolters Elsevier.

Katsumata, N., Yasuda, M., Isonishi, S., et al. (2013). Long-term results of dose-dense paclitaxel and carboplatin versus conventional paclitaxel and carboplatin for treatment of advanced epithelial ovarian, fallopian tube, and primary peritoneal cancer (JGOG 3016): a randomized, controlled open-label trial. *Lancet Oncology, 14*, 1020–1026.

Levine, D. A., De Los Santos, J., Fleming, G., et al. (2015). *Handbook for principles and practice of gynecologic oncology* (2nd ed.). Philadelphia: Wolters Kluwer.

Alexis Hokenstad, MD

CASE 53

A 52-Year-Old Perimenopausal Woman With Irregular Bleeding

A 52-year-old G0 woman presents with irregular vaginal bleeding and bleeding following inter-course. Her last cervical cytology test was 8 years ago and was abnormal, requiring cervical biop-sies. Speculum exam reveals a large (3.5-cm) ulcerated lesion on the cervix that does not appear to extend to the vagina. Bimanual exam reveals a firm lesion with a small and mobile uterus. Recto-vaginal exam does not reveal any nodules in the parametrial areas. The remainder of the physical exam, including supraclavicular node assessment, is normal.

What are your next steps?

You have assessed the cervix and uterus, which was an important first step. Because a lesion is visualized on the cervix, it is very important to get a biopsy. A cervical cytology alone, commonly known as a Pap smear, is not adequate here. Consideration should also be given to obtaining endocervical curettings and an endometrial biopsy.

What is the likely diagnosis?

At this time, your exam is concerning for invasive cervical cancer. Uterine cancer protruding through the cervix, a metastasis to the cervix, cervical or endometrial polyp, and myometrial leio-myoma are also on the differential diagnosis.

CLINICAL PEARL	**STEPS 2/3**

A very common clinical presentation of cervical cancer is bleeding after intercourse.

You inform the patient that your exam is concerning for cervical cancer and perform a cervical biopsy, endocervical curettage, and endometrial biopsy in the office.

What is the incidence of cervical cancer?

Cervical cancer is the third most common cancer in women worldwide and the 12th most common cancer among women in the United States. More than 80% of all cervical cancer cases are from less developed countries due to limited access to cervical cancer screening and prevention programs.

What are some risk factors for the development of cervical cancer?

Risk factors for cervical cancer are associated with an increased risk of acquiring human papilloma virus (HPV), such as early age at first intercourse, multiple sexual partners, and a history of sexu-ally transmitted infections (STIs). Immunocompromise due to human immunodeficiency virus (HIV) infection or immunosuppressive drugs, smoking, low socioeconomic status, and African-American race are also risk factors.

What are the main histologic subtypes of cervical cancer?

Squamous cell carcinoma (SCC) is the most common histologic type and accounts for 80% of invasive cervical cancers with the vast majority associated with HPV infection. Adenocarcinomas account for approximately 20% of invasive cervical cancers and are associated primarily with HPV 18. Other histologic subtypes include neuroendocrine carcinoma, adenoid cystic carcinoma, glassy cell carcinoma, and cervical lymphomas.

CLINICAL PEARL   STEPS 2/3

Adenocarcinoma of the cervix is commonly multifocal (occurring in multiple sites or "foci") and is associated with "skip lesions." Up to 15% of the lesions are located within the endocervical canal, as opposed to on the surface of the cervix where routine Pap specimens are taken, so adenocarcinoma can be missed with routine screening.

CLINICAL PEARL   STEPS 2/3

The average age of diagnosis for cervical cancer is 40–59 years, with a bimodal distribution with peaks at 35–39 years and 60–64 years. This correlates with the HPV peak prevalence between ages 25 and 35 years.

What is the pathogenesis for cervical cancer?

Cervical SCCs arise at the squamocolumnar junction from preexisting dysplastic lesions, usually following high-risk HPV (HR-HPV) infection. HR-HPV can be detected in 99.7% of cervical cancers. Most women clear HPV infection, but persistent infections may lead to preinvasive dysplastic disease. Progression from dysplasia to cancer generally takes several years, although this can vary. HPV is a double-stranded DNA virus. More than 40 HPV types infect the anogenital tract, with approximately 15 known to be oncogenic, or high-risk, types (HR-HPV). HPV 16 and 18 are associated with more than 70% of cervical cancers. HR-HPV serotypes make viral oncoproteins E6 and E7, which bind to tumor suppressor genes p53 and RB, respectively, and inhibit their function.

BASIC SCIENCE PEARL   STEP 1

Retinoblastoma (Rb) protein inhibits cell growth or induces cell apoptosis in response to DNA damage. When E7 binds to Rb, Rb is inactivated, allowing damaged cells to progress through the cell cycle. P53 is a tumor suppressor gene, which negatively regulates cell growth by stopping the progression of a cell through the cell cycle when DNA damage occurs and allows time for DNA repair. P53 protein is degraded following the binding of the E6 protein from the high-risk HPV virus, resulting in unregulated cellular cycling and accumulation of chromosomal mutations without DNA repair.

How is cervical cancer staged?

Cervical cancer is staged clinically, not surgically, in contrast to other gynecologic cancers. The International Federation of Gynecology and Obstetrics (FIGO) guidelines allow the following examinations in determining the staging of cervical cancer: physical exam, cervical biopsies with endocervical curettage and conization, endoscopy with hysteroscopy, cystoscopy, and proctoscopy, and imaging studies including intravenous pyelogram to assess for urinary tract obstruction and plain radiographs to assess for metastases. Computed tomography (CT) scans, magnetic resonance imaging (MRI), and positron emission tomography (PET) scanning may be useful for treatment planning but are not considered part of staging.

BASIC SCIENCE/CLINICAL PEARL	STEPS 1/2/3

PET scan is a nuclear medicine study that uses radioisotope-tagged glucose substrates (2-[18F]-fluoro-2-deoxy-D glucose) to create images based on substrate metabolism in the body. Cancer cells have increased metabolic activity, and therefore areas of metastasis will light up on imaging.

TABLE 53.1 ■ Clinical Staging of Cervical Cancer

Stage	Description
I	Tumor confined to cervix
IA	Invasive carcinoma diagnosed only by microscopy
IA1	Stromal invasion of <3.0 mm in depth and extension of <7.0 mm
IA2	Stromal invasion of >3.0 mm and not >5.0 mm in depth with extension of <7.0 mm
IB	Clinically visible lesions limited to the cervix or preclinical cancers greater than stage IA
IB1	Clinically visible lesion <4.0 cm
IB2	Clinically visible lesion >4.0 cm
II	Extension beyond cervix but not to pelvic side wall or lower one-third vagina
IIA	Without parametrial involvement
IIA1	Clinically visible lesion <4.0 cm
IIA2	Clinically visible lesion >4.0 cm
IIB	Parametrial involvement
III	Extended to pelvic side wall and/or lower one-third of vagina
IIIA	Lower one-third of vagina
IIIB	Extension to pelvic side wall or hydronephrosis
IV	Beyond pelvis
IVA	Spread to adjacent pelvic organs, bladder, or bowel
IVB	Spread to distant organs

How is cervical cancer treated?

The management of cervical cancer is determined by stage. In general, early-stage disease (stage IA–IB1, IIA) is treated surgically, and locally advanced disease (stage IB2, IIB–IVA) is treated with chemoradiation. Stage IVB cervical cancer is treated with palliative chemotherapy.

The patient returns to clinic to discuss her biopsy results. Pathology shows invasive squamous cell carcinoma. You inform the patient that she has Stage IB1 cervical cancer. Her imaging (PET/CT) does not show any spread of disease.

What is the recommended treatment of early-stage cervical cancer?

Early-stage cervical cancer can be surgically managed. Alternatively, chemoradiation is curative and can also be offered, particularly in the patient who is not a surgical candidate.

CLINICAL PEARL	STEPS 2/3

Pelvic lymphadenectomy, or removal of lymph nodes from the distal half of the common iliac vessels, internal and external iliac vessels, and obturator space, is done prior to the hysterectomy for cervical cancer. If the pelvic lymph nodes are positive, the hysterectomy is usually abandoned to minimize surgical complications and to avoid delaying adjuvant radiation therapy.

CLINICAL PEARL   STEPS 2/3

Simple or radical trachelectomy, or removal of the entire cervix with or without paracervical tissue, can be offered to select patients who desire to retain fertility. Candidates for trachelectomy must be of childbearing age, have tumor diameter of less than 2 cm without lymph vascular space invasion, and have no high-risk features such as positive pelvic lymph nodes or unusual histology.

What is chemoradiation for cervical cancer?

Locally advanced cervical cancer (Stage IB2–Stage IVA) is treated with primary chemoradiation with combination external beam radiation therapy (radiation from outside the body) and brachytherapy (radiation administered locally within certain sites of the body). Outcomes are improved when chemotherapy is used to sensitize tumor cells to the radiation, most commonly with the drug cisplatin.

What is a radical hysterectomy?

Radical hysterectomy refers to the excision of the uterus en bloc with the parametrium (the round, broad, cardinal, and uterosacral ligaments) and the upper one-third to one-half of the vagina. The degree of radicality (extent of dissection) is determined by the size of the tumor and clinical stage.

The patient undergoes modified radical hysterectomy with pelvic lymph node dissection. The final pathology shows a 3.0-cm squamous cell carcinoma with stromal invasion of 8 mm. Twenty five lymph nodes are removed, and all are negative for cancer. Her postoperative course is complicated by urinary retention, for which the patient learns self-catheterization. She recovers normal bladder function by postoperative day 30.

BASIC SCIENCE/CLINICAL PEARL   STEPS 1/2/3

A common complication of radical hysterectomy is bladder dysfunction and urinary retention. This results from the disruption of the pelvic splanchnic nerve, which supplies parasympathetic activity to the detrusor muscle of the bladder. The splanchnic nerves travel through the parametria, and disruption during dissection leads to detrusor hypotonicity. Nerve-sparing radical hysterectomy procedures have been proposed to limit the dorsal extent of parametrial resection to avoid these complications.

BEYOND THE PEARLS

- Patients with coitarche (initiation of vaginal sexual intercourse) and menarche within the same year have an increased risk of cervical dysplasia and cancer due to possible exposure to HPV at a time of metaplasia in the transformation zone.
- Depth of stromal invasion of greater than 10 mm, tumor size of greater than 3 cm, and lymph vascular space invasion are tumor characteristics that predict decreased survival and poor overall prognosis in cervical cancer.
- Cisplatin makes cells more sensitive to radiation by forming adducts with guanine bases and causes DNA kinks that cannot be easily repaired.
- Bevacizumab is an antiangiogenesis agent that inhibits vascular endothelial growth factor (VEGF); it was recently approved by the U.S. Food and Drug Administration (FDA) for use in advanced, recurrent, and progressive cervical cancer.
- In 2006, a quadrivalent HPV vaccine (Gardasil) became commercially available. It targets HR HPV serotypes 16 and 18, as well as low-risk (papilloma-causing) serotypes 6 and 11. The vaccine is more than 99% effective for the prevention of low- and high-grade cervical dysplasia. The 9-valent (HPV 6, 11, 16, 18, 31, 33, 45, 52, and 58) vaccine, Gardisil-9, became available in 2014. Vaccination is recommended for both males and females aged 9 through 26.

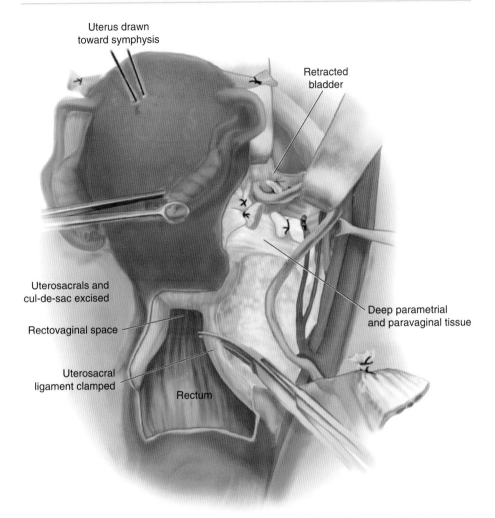

Fig. 53.1 Radical hysterectomy parametrial resection, demonstrated that all the parametrial and paravaginal tissues are dissected out laterally and divided near the origin of the uterine artery, superior to the ureter passing under the uterine artery's origin. *(From Schellhas HF, Baggish MS. Atlas of pelvic anatomy and gynecologic surgery, Elsevier Philadelphia (PA); 2016: 247–62, fig. 13.22.)*

Case Summary

- A 52-year-old woman presents with abnormal menstrual bleeding and bleeding after intercourse; she is found on exam to have a 3.5-cm cervical lesion.
- Biopsy of this cervical lesion is consistent with invasive squamous cell cervical cancer (SCC), and, based on the size and physical findings, she is diagnosed with stage IB1 cervical cancer.
- Based on the patient's stage, which is determined clinically (not surgically, as in other types of gynecologic cancer), she is a candidate for surgical management as opposed to chemoradiation.
- The patient undergoes surgical management with a modified radical hysterectomy and pelvic lymphadenectomy.
- After the surgery, the patient experiences postoperative urinary retention that requires intermittent self-catheterization. Her retention resolves after 30 days.

References

Delgado, G., Bundy, B., Zaino, R., Sevin, B. U., Creasman, W. T., & Major, F. (1990). Prospective surgico-pathological study of disease-free interval in patients with stage IB squamous cell carcinoma of the cervix: A Gynecology Oncology Group study. *Gynecology Oncology, 38,* 352–357.

Frumovitz M. *Invasive cervical cancer: epidemiology, risk factors, clinical manifestations and diagnosis.* In B Goff, DS Dizon, editors. *UpToDate.* Waltham, MA: UpToDate.

Palefsky JM, Cranston RD. *Virology of human papillomavirus infections and the link to cancer.* In BJ Dezube, DS Dizon, editors. *UpToDate.* Waltham, MA: UpToDate.

Tewari, K. S., Sill, M. W., et al. (2014). Improved survival with bevacizumab in advanced cervical cancer. *The New England Journal of Medicine, 370,* 734–743.

Sumer Wallace

A 58-Year-Old Woman With Postmenopausal Bleeding

A 58-year-old woman presents to your gynecologic clinic for evaluation of vaginal spotting. She first noticed blood on her tissue 4 months ago, with at least one episode of spotting each month since that time. She reports that her last menstrual period was approximately 5 years ago.

CLINICAL PEARL	**STEPS 2/3**

A woman is defined as menopausal after 12 months without menses. The average age of menopause in the United States is 51.

What can cause postmenopausal bleeding?
The differential diagnosis for postmenopausal bleeding includes atrophic endometrium, cervical or endometrial polyp, endometrial hyperplasia, endometrial cancer, and vaginal atrophy. The source of bleeding must be identified and distinguished from a urinary tract or rectal/gastrointestinal source. Although the most common cause of vaginal bleeding in postmenopausal women is genital atrophy (vaginal and/or endometrial) from lack of estrogen hormones, these patients must have endometrial cancer ruled out.

With what symptoms does a patient with endometrial cancer usually present?
The most common presenting sign of endometrial hyperplasia or cancer is vaginal bleeding. In the premenopausal woman, this may present as heavy and/or irregular menstrual bleeding, and the differential diagnosis of abnormal uterine bleeding in these women is broad. In the postmenopausal women, vaginal bleeding is the most common symptom. Any type of vaginal bleeding in this population should raise suspicion of endometrial cancer.

What are risk factors for endometrial cancer?
Risk factors for endometrial cancer include age, obesity, unopposed estrogen, early menarche, late menopause, nulliparity, hypertension, diabetes, history of abnormal bleeding or anovulation, polycystic ovarian syndrome, family history of uterine or colon cancer including hereditary syndromes, or a former diagnosis of endometrial hyperplasia. Endometrial hyperplasia is an abnormal overgrowth of the glands of the endometrium that is a precursor to endometrial cancer. Hyperplasia is categorized as simple hyperplasia, simple hyperplasia with atypia, complex hyperplasia, and complex hyperplasia with atypia, with hysterectomy recommended as the preferred treatment for complex hyperplasia with atypia due to the high risk for malignancy. When evaluating a patient with postmenopausal bleeding, like this patient, it is important to ask them about these risk factors.

BASIC SCIENCE/CLINICAL PEARL	STEPS 1/2/3

Lynch syndrome is a hereditary syndrome that increases the risk of endometrial cancer, as well as other cancers such as colon, urinary tract, and ovary, among others. Lynch syndrome is an autosomal-dominant mutation of mismatch repair genes MSH2, MSH6, MLH1, and PMS2.

You investigate the patient's risk factors associated with endometrial cancer. She does not have any pain associated with the bleeding or other symptoms. She has a history of hypertension, hyperlipidemia, and type 2 diabetes. There is no history of cancer in the patient's family. On physical exam, her body mass index (BMI) is 34.5 kg/m².

How do you classify endometrial cancer?

There are two types of endometrial cancer, type I and type II. Type I cancers are often diagnosed in an earlier stage (when they are less advanced) and have endometrioid histology. These cancers are associated with unopposed exposure to estrogen, meaning that the patient has a higher level than normal of circulating estrogens without a corresponding elevation in serum progestins. Women with obesity, such as this patient, are at increased risk for type I endometrial cancer. Type II cancers are not related to estrogen exposure and typically are higher-risk histologies, such as serous, carcinosarcoma, or clear cell carcinoma.

BASIC SCIENCE PEARL	STEP 1

Obese women are at higher risk for endometrial cancer because adipose contains aromatase, which converts androstenedione to estrone, creating an environment of unopposed estrogen that promotes endometrial proliferation.

BASIC SCIENCE PEARL	STEP 1

Endometrioid histology in endometrial cancer indicates that the malignant cells are formed from endometrial glands, with overgrowth and "crowding" of the glands on microscopy. Endometriod histology is graded according to the ratio of glands to solid components (Grade 1 ≤5%, Grade 2 5%–50%, Grade 3 >50%). Cellular and nuclear atypia such as enlarged nuclei, increasing mitotic figures, and prominent nucleoli also play a role in grading, and abnormal features can "upgrade" a cancer. Grade 1 and grade 2 endometriod endometrial cancers are considered low grade, whereas grade 3 endometriod cancer and all nonendometrioid histologies are considered high grade.

Physical exam is notable for her elevated BMI, and her vital signs are normal. On pelvic exam, there is a small amount of blood on vaginal speculum exam, and the remainder of the pelvic exam is unremarkable. The patient consents to an in-office endometrial biopsy, which reveals endometrial carcinoma of the endometrioid type.

What is the initial evaluation of endometrial cancer?

Initial evaluation of the endometrium can be performed via pelvic ultrasound, endometrial biopsy, or dilation and curettage. The endometrial thickness of a postmenopausal woman should be 4 mm or less. Biopsy should be performed for any woman with the following characteristics: persistent abnormal uterine bleeding with unopposed uterine estrogen, age older than 45, abnormal uterine bleeding, or postmenopausal bleeding.

CLINICAL PEARL	STEPS 2/3

Note that endometrial cancer, like other types of gynecologic cancer, is staged after the patient has had removal of relevant tissues in a surgery. This, however, is unlike cervical cancer, where the cancer is staged by clinical exam only.

What tests should be ordered for evaluation of endometrial cancer and presurgical planning?
Prior to surgery, basic lab values are obtained. These labs include a complete blood count and electrolyte panel with creatinine. In addition, in patients with diabetes, glucose and hemoglobin A1C should be recorded. Further medical evaluation of patient comorbidities can be performed if needed, such as an electrocardiogram in patients with a cardiac history. A chest X-ray is performed to investigate for pulmonary pathology or metastatic disease. Further imaging, such as a computed tomography (CT) scan, may be performed in patients with high-risk endometrial cancer or with concerning symptoms or physical exam findings but is not routine.

What is the treatment for endometrial cancer?
The definitive treatment for endometrial cancer is surgery, which includes total hysterectomy, bilateral salpingo-oophorectomy, and possible lymph node evaluation. Pelvic lymphadenectomy may be performed depending on characteristics of the patient's tumor, such as size, depth of invasion, histology, and grade. In high-risk cancers, paraaortic lymphadenectomy may need to be performed. This type of surgery can be performed using a minimally invasive technique, such as a laparoscopic or robotic-assisted laparoscopic approach. Final stage is determined based on the surgical pathology (Table 54.1).

Alternatively, if the patient has too many medical morbidities to undergo surgery or wishes to preserve her childbearing ability, medical management of endometrial cancer is an option. Hyperplasia and grade 1 endometrial cancer can be treated with progestin therapy administered orally, by injection, or with an intrauterine device (IUD). Prior to committing to medical management of endometrial cancer, deeply invasive disease must be ruled out with imaging such as pelvic magnetic resonance imaging (MRI). After progestin therapy is started, an endometrial biopsy should be performed every 3 months to assess for response to treatment.

TABLE 54.1 ■ **Endometrial Cancer Staging**

Stage I:	Confined to uterus
IA	Tumor invades <50% into myometrium
IB	Tumor invades ≥50% into myometrium
Stage II:	Tumor invades cervical stroma
Stage III:	Tumor involves regional structures
IIIA	Tumor involves of uterine serosa or adnexa
IIIB	Tumor involves vagina or parametrium
IIIC1	Tumor involves pelvic lymph nodes
IIIC2	Tumor involves para aortic lymph nodes
Stage IV:	Tumor involves distant structures
IVA	Tumor involves bladder and/or rectal mucosa
IVB	Distant disease, including inguinal lymph nodes and abdominal spread (including abdominal/pelvic metastases)

The patient undergoes a robotic-assisted laparoscopic hysterectomy with bilateral salpingo-oophorectomy and bilateral pelvic lymphadenectomy. Her uterus demonstrates endometrioid carcinoma invading less than half of the thickness of the myometrium, and the fallopian tubes, ovaries, cervix, and bilateral pelvic nodes, which were sampled in this case, were negative for carcinoma. Based on this, she is diagnosed with stage IA endometrioid endometrial carcinoma.

Does the patient need additional treatment?

Adjuvant chemotherapy and radiation is recommended in more advanced stages and with more concerning histology, such as clear cell or serous endometrial cancer. Risk factors for recurrence include lympho-vascular space invasion (LVSI), myometrial invasion, and higher tumor grade. Therefore, patients with these risk factors often receive additional postoperative treatment with adjuvant chemotherapy and/or radiation. Radiation is most often given as vaginal brachytherapy alone, but some cases will also require external pelvic radiation. Chemotherapy is reserved for patients with high-grade histology or metastatic disease. This patient has a low-grade, low-risk carcinoma, the most common presentation of endometrial cancer, and does not require additional treatment.

CLINICAL PEARL   **STEPS 2/3**

The two most commonly used chemotherapy medications for endometrial cancer are paclitaxel and carboplatin.

You counsel your patient that she does not require any more treatment at this time, and she is quite relieved to hear this. However, she is worried about the cancer "coming back again" and wants to know what she can do to prevent this.

How common is recurrence, and what could be done if the cancer returns?

Although endometrial cancer recurrence is rare, it most commonly occurs at the vaginal cuff and is usually detected within the first 3 years following diagnosis. Recurrent endometrial cancer can be treated with radiation, both vaginal brachytherapy and pelvic external beam, or surgery followed by adjuvant radiation and/or chemotherapy. In addition to surgery and radiation, hormonal therapy such as progestins or selective estrogen response modulators (SERM) can be considered.

What does the patient do next?

The patient should undergo surveillance. Surveillance includes monitoring for recurrence with symptoms and physical exam with pelvic exam every 3–6 months for 2 years and then approximately every 6 months for the following 3 years.

BEYOND THE PEARLS

- A rare tumor of the uterus, carcinosarcoma (sometimes called malignant mixed mullerian tumor or MMMT), is considered one of the most aggressive and dangerous cancer types of the uterus. The 5-year survival rate, even for stage I tumors, is as low as 50%. Carcinosarcoma is so named because the cancer includes both cancerous epithelial cells (carcinoma) and cancerous connective tissue cells (sarcoma); however, it is now known that these are epithelial in origin. Women with carcinosarcoma often present with large, necrotic, and friable tumors, and this nonviable tissue may cause a severe pelvic infection. Treatment is surgical resection, staging, and possibly treatment with a chemotherapy regimen.

BEYOND THE PEARLS—cont'd

- Emerging studies for evaluation of lymph nodes in endometrial cancer have led to the idea of performing sentinel lymph node excision. This is done by injecting fluorescent dye into the cervix and following the lymph channels to the sentinel lymph node, or the first lymph nodes that would be reached by the cancer, in the pelvic lymph node group on each side of the body.
- Endometrial cancer patients benefit from risk stratification, meaning that the clinician uses certain characteristics of the patient and the cancer to determine what treatment and/or surveillance they need based on their risk of the cancer advancing or returning after treatment. These studies use age and tumor characteristics such as depth of invasion, cervical stromal invasion, tumor grade, tumor histology, and presence of lymphovascular space invasion. Stratification is into three categories: low-risk, intermediate-risk (which also includes high-intermediate risk), or high-risk.

Case Summary

- A 58-year-old woman who has been menopausal for 5 years presents with new onset of vaginal bleeding. She has a normal physical exam except for an elevated BMI consistent with obesity and a slight amount of blood in the vaginal vault.
- Concerned with this patient's risk for endometrial cancer, you perform an office biopsy of her endometrium and the pathology confirms the diagnosis of endometrial cancer, specifically endometrioid type.
- The patient undergoes robotic hysterectomy, bilateral salpingo-oophorectomy, and sampling of pelvic lymph nodes. Her final diagnosis based on pathology is IA endometrioid endometrial cancer.
- After the surgery, the patient does not have risk factors that qualify her for further treatment, but she is advised to continue surveillance with gynecologic exams every 3–6 months for 2 years and then every 6 months for the following 3 years.

References

Cosin, J. A., Kesterson, J. P., & Olawaiye, A. B. (2014). *Staging of gynecologic malignancies handbook* (4th ed.). Society of Gynecologic Oncology.

Dowdy, S. C., Mariani, A., & Lurain, J. R. (2012). Uterine cancer. In J. S. Berek (Ed.), *Berek & Novak's gynecology* (15th ed). Philadelphia, PA: Lippincott, Williams, & Wilkins.

Hoffman, B. L., Schorge, J. O., Bradshaw, K. D., Halvorson, L. M., Schaffer, J. I., & Corton, M. M. (2016). Endometrial cancer. In B. L. Hoffman, J. O. Schorge, K. D. Bradshaw, L. M. Halvorson, J. I. Schaffer, & M. M. Corton (Eds.), *Williams gynecology* (3rd ed). New York: McGraw-Hill.

McMeekin, D. S., Yashar, C., Campos, S., & Zaino, R. J. (2013). Corpus: epithelial tumors. In R. R. Barakat, A. Berchuck, M. Markman, & M. E. Randall (Eds.), *Principles and practice of gynecologic oncology* (6th ed). Philadelphia, PA: Lippincott, Williams, & Wilkins.

Alexis Hokenstad, MD

A 35-Year-Old Woman With a Family History of Ovarian Cancer

A 35-year-old G3P3 presents to her gynecologist for a routine health maintenance exam. She is feeling well and is healthy. She becomes tearful when she discloses that her mother recently was diagnosed with ovarian cancer. Her mother's testing for genetic mutations associated with ovarian cancer is pending.

Which inherited genetic disorders carry an increased risk of ovarian cancer?
Hereditary ovarian cancer represents 15%–25% of all ovarian cancers. More than 90% of inherited ovarian cancer is caused by germline mutations in the breast cancer 1 and 2 (BRCA) genes. Hereditary nonpolyposis colon cancer syndrome (HPNCC), also known as Lynch syndrome, and Peutz-Jeghers syndrome are also associated with an increased risk of ovarian cancer.

BASIC SCIENCE/CLINICAL PEARL	STEPS 1/2/3
Lynch syndrome, or HNPCC, is caused by a defect in mismatch repair genes and is associated with an increased risk of colon, endometrial, and ovarian cancers.	

BASIC SCIENCE/CLINICAL PEARL	STEPS 1/2/3
Peutz-Jeghers syndrome is associated with a mutation of the serine/threonine kinase 11 (STK11) gene. Hallmark features include pigmented mucocutaneous lesions and hamartomatous polyps in the gastrointestinal (GI) tract, as well as increased risk of GI, breast, and nonepithelial ovarian cancers.	

Who should be offered hereditary cancer risk assessment for hereditary breast and ovarian cancers?
A thorough evaluation of a patient's risk for hereditary breast and ovarian cancer should be a routine portion of obstetric and gynecology practice, with focus on personal and family history of cancer. Patients with a 20%–25% chance of having an inherited mutation, as well as those with a personal history of ovarian, fallopian tube, or primary peritoneal cancer, should be referred for genetic counseling and possible genetic testing (Table 55.1).

What genetic testing should be offered to women with or at increased risk of ovarian/fallopian tube/primary peritoneal cancer?
Genetic testing should begin with the individual who has ovarian or breast cancer, termed the proband. As there are more than 1000 known mutations of BRCA1 and BRCA2 genes, full sequencing of both genes is performed. If a specific mutation is detected in the proband, testing for that specific mutation in blood relatives should be performed, called *predictive testing*. If no affected individual is available for testing, then patients at increased risk due to family history may still undergo testing.

TABLE 55.1 ■ Society of Gynecology Oncology Criteria for BRCA Mutation Testing

Women affected with:
- Epithelial ovarian, tubal, or peritoneal cancer diagnosed at any age
- Breast cancer ≤45 years
- Breast cancer plus a close relative with breast cancer ≤50 years or close relative with epithelial ovarian, tubal, or peritoneal cancer at any age
- Breast cancer ≤50 years with limited family history
- Breast cancer plus ≥2 close relatives with breast cancer at any age
- Breast cancer plus ≥2 relatives with pancreatic cancer or aggressive prostate cancer
- Two primary cancers of the breast (i.e. one in each breast or two different breast cancer cell types) with the first diagnosed prior to age 50
- Triple-negative breast cancer ≤60 years
- Breast cancer and Ashkenazi Jewish ancestry
- Pancreatic cancer at any age plus ≥2 close relatives with breast, ovarian, tubal, primary peritoneal, pancreatic, or aggressive prostate cancer

Women unaffected with cancer, but with:
- A first-degree relative or several close relatives who meet one of the above criteria
- A close relative carrying a known BRCA1 or BRCA2 mutation
- A close relative with male breast cancer

The patient returns to your office 3 months later. She states that her mother was positive for a BRCA1 mutation. The patient was subsequently tested and found to also carry the BRCA1 mutation.

What is the BRCA gene, and how common are mutations?

The BRCA genes are inherited in an autosomal dominant fashion. BRCA1 is located on chromosome 17, and BRCA2 is on chromosome 13. BRCA1 and BRCA2 are tumor suppressor genes that encode proteins that function in the repair of double-stranded DNA breaks, a process called homologous recombination. The BRCA genes function like most tumor suppressors in that two defective copies of the allele are required for cancer formation. Individuals inherit one defective allele from their mother or father, but most patients have a second functional allele. If this second allele becomes nonfunctional, cancer can develop. This is called the "two-hit hypothesis." The prevalence of BRCA mutations ranges from 1:300 to 1:800 in the general population, but certain ethnic groups such as Ashkenazi Jews, French Canadians, and Icelanders have a higher prevalence due to founder mutations.

BASIC SCIENCE PEARL   **STEP 1**

A variety of DNA repair mechanisms are available, and the type employed at a given time in the body depends on the type of DNA damage present. Single-strand breaks are repaired with base excision repair, nucleotide excision repair, and mismatch repair. Double-strand breaks may be repaired with homologous recombination, which has high fidelity with minimal mistakes, or nonhomologous end joining, which is more prone to mistakes. The BRCA genes are involved with homologous recombination.

BASIC SCIENCE PEARL   **STEP 1**

Tumor suppressor genes are involved with cell cycle regulation, which promotes repair of cell damage prior to entering the cell cycle or apoptosis. Mutation of these genes results in inactivation and unregulated progression of damaged cells through the cell cycle, thus promoting cancer. Examples of tumor suppressors include BRCA, p53, and Retinoblastoma (Rb).

TABLE 55.2 ■ Estimated Risks for Cancer With BRCA Mutation

Cancer Type	Risk for Carriers to Age 70 Years		
	BRCA1 mutation	BRCA2 mutation	General population
Breast	55%–70%	45%–70%	12%
Ovarian	39%–46%	12%–20%	1.3%
Male breast	1%	8%	0.1%
Pancreatic	Unclear	5%	1.5%

What is the lifetime risk of ovarian and breast cancer in a patient with BRCA mutation?
In the general population, the lifetime risk for development of breast cancer is approximately
12%, and the ovarian cancer risk is approximately 1.3%. The risk for breast cancer increases to
65%–74% in women with a BRCA1 or BRCA2 mutation. The ovarian cancer risk increases to
39%–46% in women with a BRCA1 mutation and 12%–20% in women with a BRCA2 mutation. Fallopian tube and primary peritoneal cancers also are included in the spectrum of diseases
associated with a BRCA mutation.

CLINICAL PEARL   **STEPS 2/3**

In addition to breast and ovarian cancers, patients with a BRCA mutation are at increased
risk for development of other cancers including pancreatic cancer, male breast cancer, and
prostate cancer. Because male breast cancer is quite rare outside of BRCA mutations, a family history of male breast cancer should arouse a high suspicion of a familial BRCA mutation
(Table 55.2).

Your patient is very worried to hear about her increased risk for these cancers, and she urgently
wants to "do everything possible" to prevent these cancers.

**What are the recommendations for surveillance and risk reduction for breast cancer in
BRCA-positive women?**
Specific recommendations for screening in women with BRCA mutation include self-breast
examinations starting at age 18, clinical breast examinations every 6–12 months starting at
age 25, annual breast magnetic resonance imaging (MRI) starting at age 25, and annual mammogram and breast MRI at age 30. The age at screening initiation can be altered depending on
the specific family history. A prophylactic bilateral mastectomy can reduce breast cancer risk by
90%. Oophorectomy reduces the risk of breast cancer by 50% due to the decrease in systemic
estrogen.

**How should women with BRCA mutations be counseled regarding surveillance for ovarian
cancer?**
Current recommendations for screening include pelvic exam, transvaginal ultrasonography, and
serum testing for cancer antigen 125 (CA 125) every 6 months beginning at age 30 or 5–10 years
prior to the earliest age of diagnosis of ovarian cancer in the family.

BASIC SCIENCE PEARL   **STEP 1**

CA 125 is a large transmembrane glycoprotein derived from both coelomic (pericardium, pleura,
peritoneum) and Müllerian (fallopian tubal, endometrial, endocervical) epithelia.

CA 125 testing has low sensitivity and specificity for ovarian cancer, especially in premeno-pausal women, as increased cellular turnover or inflammation in the pelvis, whether normal or pathologic, can cause increased CA 125, and such issues (fibroids, endometriosis, inflamma-tory bowel disease, ruptured ovarian cysts) are more common in premenopausal women. This serum biomarker is primarily used as part of an evaluation for malignancy in women with an adnexal mass or for monitoring women with ovarian cancer during and after treatment.

What options are available for ovarian cancer risk reduction in women with BRCA mutations?

Combined oral contraceptives have been shown to reduce the risk of ovarian cancer by approximately 50%; however, a slight increase in breast cancer risk has been shown. Due to limitations in screening, risk-reducing bilateral salpingo-oophorectomy (BSO) is recommended in patients with BRCA muta-tions and reduces the risk of ovarian/fallopian tube/primary peritoneal cancer by 90%. For most women, risk-reducing surgery should occur at age 35–40 or when the patient is finished with childbearing.

The patient proceeds with the recommended screening and returns to your office to discuss the results. Upon review, she had a normal mammogram, normal pelvic ultrasound, and a CA 125 level within the normal range (<35 U/mL). She has completed childbearing and desires to proceed with a risk-reducing BSO.

How should a risk-reducing BSO be performed?

The procedure should be performed laparoscopically with a thorough inspection of the peritoneal cavity, pelvic washings, and biopsy of any abnormal tissue. All ovarian and fallopian tube tissue should be removed, and the ovarian vessels should be ligated at the pelvic brim with at least 2 cm of the gonadal vessels removed.

Occult microscopic cancer has been identified in 5%–12% of patients with BRCA mutations undergoing risk-reducing surgery. Therefore thorough pathology review with serially section-ing every 2–3 mm of the entire ovary and fallopian tube is recommended, with particular attention to the fimbriated end.

The patient undergoes an uncomplicated laparoscopic risk-reducing BSO. Pathology with appro-priate serial sectioning shows normal bilateral ovaries and fallopian tubes and negative pelvic washings. She continues to follow recommended screening for breast cancer and is considering a risk-reducing mastectomy.

- Patients who have received an allogenic bone marrow transplant should not have molecu-lar genetic testing via blood or buccal sample due to unreliable test results from contami-nation by donor DNA.
- A variant of unknown significance (VUS) is a variation in the normal sequence of a gene whose association with disease is unknown. At this time, VUSs should be considered normal variants and should not be pursued with additional testing.

BEYOND THE PEARLS—cont'd

- It is important to be aware of legislation that addresses issues of discrimination and privacy raised by increasingly comprehensive genetic information. The Genetic Information Nondiscrimination Act (GINA), passed in 2008, prohibits health insurers and employers from discriminating on the basis of genetic information.
- In women with ovarian cancer, those with BRCA mutations have a significantly longer survival compared to those without a BRCA mutation. The loss of function of the BRCA protein may result in a more favorable response to platinum-based chemotherapy.
- Poly-ADP ribose polymerase (PARP) is an enzyme involved with repair of single-strand DNA breaks. Olaparib is the first of the PARP inhibitor drugs to be approved in the United States for treatment of recurrent ovarian cancer in patients with BRCA mutations.
- Current guidelines recommend prophylactic BSO in patients with BRCA1 and BRCA2 mutations by age 35–40; however, surgery may be delayed in patients with a BRCA2 mutation only as their ovarian cancer risk does not increase until age 50–55.
- Prophylactic salpingectomy at the time of pelvic surgery (i.e., hysterectomy or permanent sterilization) may provide an opportunity to reduce risk of ovarian cancer in the general population. Further studies are ongoing to assess the total impact of salpingectomy at the time of benign pelvic surgery.

Case Summary

- A 35-year-old woman without complaints reveals in a routine gynecologic visit that her mother was recently diagnosed with ovarian cancer at age 60.
- Based on the patient's risk of a genetic cancer syndrome, she is tested and found to carry the breast cancer (BRCA) 1 mutation.
- The patient is counseled about her elevated breast and ovarian cancer risk and is informed of recommended breast and ovarian cancer screening.
- The patient is informed that prophylactic bilateral mastectomy would reduce her risk of breast cancer. She is also informed that prophylactic bilateral salpingo-oophorectomy (BSO), which would be appropriate when finished with childbearing or by age 35–40 years, would reduce her risk of gynecologic cancers and breast cancer associated with the BRCA mutation.
- The patient is finished with childbearing and opts for risk-reducing BSO and is considering a future bilateral mastectomy.

References

American College of Obstetricians and Gynecologists (2008). Elective and risk-reducing salpingo-oophorectomy. ACOG Practice Bulletin No. 89. *Obstetrics and Gynecology, 111*, 231–241.

American College of Obstetricians and Gynecologists (2009). Hereditary breast and ovarian cancer syndrome. ACOG Practice Bulletin No. 103. *Obstetrics and Gynecology, 113*, 957–966.

NCCN Clinical Practice Guidelines. BRCA-related breast and ovarian cancer syndromes. Version 2.2016. Available at: http://www.nccn.org.

Peshkin, B. N., & Isaacs, C. (2008). BRCA1 and BRCA2-associated hereditary breast and ovarian cancer. In A. B. Chagpar, B. Goff, & D. S. Dizon (Eds.), *UpToDate*. Waltham, MA: UpToDate.

Beverly Long

A 29-Year-Old Woman With Vaginal Bleeding

A 29-year-old G2P1011 presents to the emergency department with 2 days of heavy vaginal bleeding. She is unsure of her last menstrual period, but reports intermittent spotting since a miscarriage 3 months ago. She believes she was "two and a half months pregnant" but did not receive medical care. She reports abdominal cramping. Her past medical history is unremarkable, and she had an uncomplicated, term vaginal delivery 2 years ago.

What is the differential diagnosis of vaginal bleeding?

There are many problems that can cause this pattern of vaginal bleeding. However, in a reproductive-age woman, it is important to promptly evaluate pregnancy status, since pregnancy-related complications can be emergencies. History and physical exam will also narrow the differential diagnosis.

On physical exam, blood pressure is 114/72 mm Hg, heart rate is 96/min, respiration rate is 16/min, and oxygen saturation in 100% on room air. Her abdomen is minimally tender with no rebound or guarding. On bimanual exam, the uterus is 12 weeks in size, and the cervix is closed without bleeding. Urine pregnancy test is positive, and serum β-human chorionic gonadotropin (β-hCG) is 138,000 mIU/mL. Ultrasound shows a 5-cm hypervascular intrauterine mass.

What is the most likely diagnosis?

This patient's presentation is most consistent with gestational trophoblastic neoplasia (GTN), a class of malignant neoplasms that arise from placental trophoblastic tissue. Gestational trophoblastic disease (GTD) encompasses all abnormal trophoblastic proliferation, including both benign and malignant conditions (Table 56.1). Complete and partial molar pregnancies are types of benign GTD. GTN includes invasive mole, choriocarcinoma, placental site trophoblastic tumor (PSTT), and epithelioid trophoblastic tumor (ETT).

BASIC SCIENCE PEARL   **STEPS 1/2**

Partial molar pregnancy occurs when a normal ovum is fertilized by two sperm, resulting in a triploid karyotype (XXY, XYY) made up of both maternal and paternal chromosomes. In a complete mole, an empty ovum is fertilized by a normal sperm. Complete moles have diploid karyotypes (XX) and are usually composed entirely of paternal genetic material.

TABLE 56.1 ■ Classification of Gestational Trophoblastic Disease

Benign	Malignant
Benign nonneoplastic trophoblastic lesions (incidental histologic findings)	Invasive mole
• Exaggerated placental site	Choriocarcinoma
• Placental site nodule	Placental site trophoblastic tumor
Hydatiform mole	Epithelioid trophoblastic tumor
• Complete mole (46,XX; 46,XY)	
• Partial mole (69,XXX; 69XXY; 69XYY)	

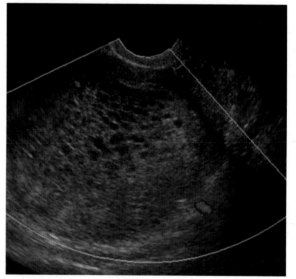

Fig. 56.1 Snowstorm appearance of a complete molar pregnancy on ultrasound view of the uterus. *(From Kopp P. Endocrinology: adult and pediatric. 2016: 1500–14.e5, fig. 85-3.)*

Molar pregnancy typically presents with vaginal bleeding, elevated β-hCG, and abnormal ultrasound findings. A complete molar pregnancy is more likely to present with the classic "snowstorm" appearance of hydropic, swollen chorionic villi on ultrasound with no fetal parts (Fig. 56.1). Hyperemesis, hyperthyroidism, or preeclampsia may be present due to hyperstimulation by β-hCG. A partial molar pregnancy may mimic an incomplete or missed abortion and can coexist with a fetus, although β-hCG elevation is usually less extreme.

CLINICAL PEARL   **STEPS 2/3**

High levels of β-hCG can cause hyperthyroidism due to the homology between thyroid-stimulating hormone (TSH) and the β-subunits of hCG.

Invasive mole or choriocarcinoma is usually recognized months after a pregnancy event due to elevated β-hCG during postmolar surveillance, vaginal bleeding, or metastatic symptoms. Our patient's GTN probably developed after her miscarriage, although antecedent partial mole is possible as the aborted tissue was not examined.

Who is at risk for developing GTN?

The risk is highest after a complete (15%–20%) or partial mole (1%–5%). GTN is rare following nonmolar pregnancy (<1 in 15,000). Risk factors for postmolar GTN include uterine size greater than dates, β-hCG levels of greater than 100,000 mIU/mL, or theca lutein cysts. Many women, like our patient, will have no risk factors.

What are the next steps for diagnosis in our patient?

Final diagnosis is based on pathologic examination after suction dilation and curettage (D&C). D&C is both diagnostic and therapeutic for hydatiform mole. Following D&C, β-hCG levels are monitored weekly until they are negative for 3 weeks. In contrast, GTN is a clinical diagnosis. During surveillance following hydatiform mole, diagnosis is made based on increasing or persistently elevated β-hCG. After nonmolar pregnancy, diagnosis is based on elevated β-hCG and ultrasound findings.

Where is GTN most likely to metastasize?

Approximately 5% of GTN patients present with distant metastases. The most common sites are lung (80%), vagina (30%), central nervous system (CNS) (10%), and liver (10%). Metastatic sites are highly vascular, and signs of bleeding from a lesion may be the initial presentation of metastatic GTN. Biopsy of suspected metastatic lesions is not recommended due to risk of hemorrhage.

> You tell the patient she has GTN and explain the risks. She wants to know what additional testing and treatment is needed.

What laboratory or imaging studies should be ordered?

Pretreatment evaluation should include complete blood count (CBC), liver and renal function tests, and a chest radiograph (CXR). If CXR reveals lung metastases or specific symptoms are present, computed tomography scan (CT) or magnetic resonance imaging (MRI) of the brain, abdomen, or pelvis should be performed to rule out other sites of metastasis.

> The patient's labs are within normal limits. CXR shows three distinct densities consistent with metastatic disease, but CT scans of the head, abdomen, and pelvis show no additional lesions.

How is GTN staged?

Staging is based on the FIGO staging system (Table 56.2) and the World Health Organization (WHO) Prognostic Scoring System (Table 56.3). Patients with WHO scores of less than 7 have "low-risk" disease and are expected to respond favorably to monotherapy. Patients with scores of 7 or higher have "high-risk" disease and must be treated with multiagent chemotherapy regimens. Our patient has stage III disease and a WHO score of 8.

How is GTN treated?

Because most GTN is extremely chemosensitive, the primary treatment is chemotherapy, and surgery is usually unnecessary. Patients are treated with single or multiagent chemotherapy

TABLE 56.2 ▨ **International Federation of Gynecology and Obstetrics (FIGO) Staging System for Gestational Trophoblastic Neoplasia (GTN)**

Stage I	Disease localized to the uterus
Stage II	Disease extends to the adnexa and/or pelvis
Stage III	Pulmonary metastases
Stage IV	Metastases to any distant organ (not including pulmonary)

TABLE 56.3 ▨ **World Health Organization (WHO) Prognostic Scoring System for Gestational Trophoblastic Neoplasia (GTN)**

Risk Factor	Points			
	0	1	2	4
Age (years)	<40	≥40	-	-
Antecedent pregnancy type	Mole	Abortion	Term	-
Months from antecedent pregnancy	<4	4–6	7–12	>12
Pretreatment serum β-hCG (mIU/mL)	<10^3	10^3–10^4	10^4–10^5	>10^5
Size of largest tumor (cm)	<3	3–<5	≥5	
Metastatic site(s)	Lung	Spleen, kidney	GI tract	Brain, liver
Number of metastases	0	1–4	5–8	>8
Prior failed chemotherapy	–	–	Single-drug	2+ drugs

based on their WHO score. Patients in the low-risk category are treated with single-agent methotrexate or actinomycin-D. Patients with high-risk disease receive multiagent therapy with etoposide, methotrexate, actinomycin-D, cyclophosphamide, and vincristine (EMA-CO) with leucovorin support. PSTT and ETT are less chemosensitive, so prognosis for metastatic disease is poor.

BASIC SCIENCE PEARL   **STEP 1**

Methotrexate is a folate antagonist; it competitively inhibits dihydrofolate reductase (DHFR), which converts oxidized folate to the reduced form used in DNA, RNA, and protein synthesis. Leucovorin (folinic acid) is a reduced form of folate, which normal cells can use for biosynthesis to bypass DHFR and continue normal proliferation.

This patient undergoes chemotherapy with EMA-CO. After six cycles, her weekly β-hCG levels normalize and remain negative over 3 consecutive weeks.

How should this patient be monitored?

Serum β-hCG is very sensitive for recurrence, so imaging is not recommended if β-hCG levels are consistently declining. Monthly β-hCG levels should be followed until negative for 12 months. Repeat imaging should be performed if persistent or recurrent disease is suspected. Reliable contraception is necessary during posttreatment surveillance.

BEYOND THE PEARLS

- Persistent elevation of serum β-hCG is not always due to GTN. False-positive results can occur due to heterophilic antibodies. Heterophilic antibodies are more common in veterinary or farm workers because these patients develop antibodies against animal-derived antigens used in commercial immunoassays. False-positive β-hCG values are typically less than 1000 mIU/mL. Heterophilic antibodies are not present in urine, so check a urine pregnancy test to verify the serum result.
- Patients with a large amount of disease from GTN are at risk for death from pulmonary or brain hemorrhage due to rapid tumor breakdown in response to full-dose chemotherapy. Slow induction of chemotherapy with low-dose cisplatin and etoposide prior to full-dose EMA-CO chemotherapy has been shown to reduce the risk of early death in high-risk patients.
- Following treatment for GTD, fibrotic lesions may remain visible at previous sites of disease. Positron emission tomography (PET) scan imaging, is able to distinguish between metabolically active and inactive lesions, of which neoplasia is the former and fibrotic lesions are the latter, and may be necessary to characterize these lesions and guide further management.

Case Summary

- A 29-year-old woman presents with vaginal bleeding and markedly elevated serum β-hCG several months after reported spontaneous abortion, and her laboratory work and imaging are consistent with GTN.
- Our patient is found to have metastatic lung lesions, consistent with stage III GTN. A WHO prognostic score of 8 necessitated multiagent chemotherapy.
- After multiagent chemotherapy with EMA-CO, β-hCG remains negative.

References

Berkowitz RS, Goldstein DP, Horowitz NS. Gestational trophoblastic neoplasia: Epidemiology, clinical features, diagnosis, staging, and risk stratification. In: Goff B, Dizon DS, editors. *UpToDate*. Waltham, MA: UpToDate.

Berkowitz RS, Goldstein DP, Horowitz NS. Initial management of high-risk gestational trophoblastic neoplasia. In: Goff B, Dizon DS, editors. *UpToDate*. Waltham, MA: UpToDate.

Berkowitz RS, Goldstein DP, Horowitz NS. Initial management of low-risk gestational trophoblastic neoplasia. In: Goff B, Dizon DS, editors. *UpToDate*. Waltham, MA: UpToDate.

Amanika Kumar, MD

A 63-Year-Old With Known Ovarian Cancer and New-Onset Abdominal Symptoms

A 63-year-old woman with a history of high-grade serous ovarian cancer, treated formerly with primary debulking surgery followed by six cycles of carboplatin and paclitaxel, presents for a routine surveillance visit to her gynecologic oncologist. She has been cancer free for 18 months. Upon her visit, you elicit a recent history of bloating and abdominal pain for a "few weeks." A proton pump inhibitor that she started taking with her dinner has not improved her abdominal symptoms. She denies chest pain, shortness of breath, fatigue, nausea, changes in bowel or bladder habits, or vaginal bleeding.

What are the next steps in this patient's care?

In cancer surveillance, a full history and physical, including a pelvic exam, should be performed every 3 months for the first 2 years. If abnormalities are found, this should prompt laboratory testing with a relevant cancer marker (in this case: Ca 125) and imaging studies, most commonly a computed tomography (CT) scan.

You perform a physical exam, and vital signs are normal. No abdominal masses are palpated and no tenderness is elicited on abdominal or pelvic exam. Given her new symptoms, you order a Ca 125 and a CT scan of the chest, abdomen, and pelvis. On CT scan, there is a 4-cm mass located at the hilum of the spleen, a 2-cm nodule in the pelvic peritoneum, and moderate ascites. Ca 125 returns elevated at 400 U/mL, confirming recurrent serous epithelial ovarian cancer.

What are options for treatment for recurrent epithelial ovarian cancer?

Advanced epithelial ovarian cancer recurs in 75%–80% of patients. The majority of recurrences are found in the peritoneal cavity, but they can also occur in the chest, bones, and, more rarely, the central nervous system (CNS). Recurrence can be diagnosed by clinical symptoms, physical exam findings, Ca 125 elevation, or imaging findings. The first determinant of management for recurrent ovarian cancer is whether the disease is platinum sensitive or resistant. Options for management at the time of recurrence include surgery, chemotherapy, radiation, a combination of the former, and hospice. In the setting of platinum-sensitive disease, when disease is isolated to a few sites of recurrent cancer than can be safely removed, a removal or "debulking" of all recognizable recurrent tumor can be offered. This procedure is called secondary cytoreduction or secondary debulking. Several studies have demonstrated that overall survival is correlated with ability to achieve a complete cytoreduction at the time of secondary debulking. If complete cytoreduction is not achievable, chemotherapy is a better choice of treatment.

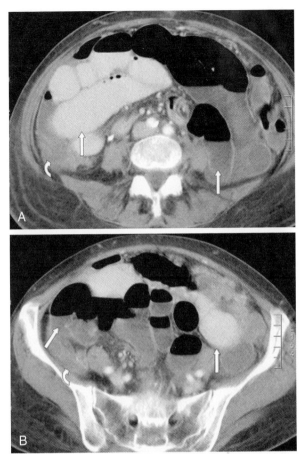

Fig. 57.1 Computed tomography (CT) scan of recurrence of ovarian cancer and small bowel obstruction in a patient formerly undergoing chemotherapy. Panel A shows the lumbar region and Panel B displays the pelvic level. The CT scan shows loops of dilated, fluid-filled bowel *(white arrows)* and an abdomen with a large burden of ascites *(curved arrow)* and carcinomatosis. *(From Cronin CG, O'Connor M, Lohan DG et al. Imaging of the gastrointestinal complications of systemic chemotherapy. Clin Radiol. 2009; 64(7):724–33, fig. 10.)*

CLINICAL PEARL   **STEPS 2/3**

Cancer stage never changes for a patient. When a cancer is diagnosed, it is staged at initial presentation. If a cancer recurs, regardless of location, the original stage does not change.

CLINICAL PEARL   **STEPS 2/3**

Platinum sensitivity in epithelial ovarian cancer is defined as a disease-free interval (time from the completion of platinum-based chemotherapy to the recurrence) of greater than 6 months. If cancer has recurred in 6 months or less from completion of chemotherapy, it is considered platinum-resistant.

Given the patient's ascites and after discussion between the patient and her family, she wishes to pursue chemotherapy rather than surgery. She had significant neuropathy following her first line of chemotherapy and one of her hobbies is knitting, so she is concerned that although she can now knit again, this problem may occur in the future.

What chemotherapy is given at the time of recurrent ovarian cancer?

Chemotherapy in recurrent ovarian cancer depends on prior chemotherapies, disease-free interval, platinum sensitivity, and side-effect profiles. In patients with platinum-sensitive disease, a platinum doublet (a combination of two chemotherapy agents that include carboplatinum) is preferred to single-agent therapy, but with consideration of side-effect profile and potential hypersensitivity reaction to platinum. A large multicenter study has shown noninferiority between platinum-based doublet chemotherapy options, and patients with platinum-resistant disease receive single-agent nonplatinum therapy.

The patient begins chemotherapy with carboplatin and liposomal doxorubicin. However, after 3 cycles of chemotherapy, her Ca 125 has risen to 800 U/mL. On history, the patient has had progressive abdominal distension and nausea with difficulty eating. A CT scan shows increased tumor consistent with progression of disease, a large amount of ascites, and mildly dilated loops of small bowel without a clear transition point.

What options does the patient have now?

The patient's options at this point are third-line chemotherapy either on or off a clinical trial. The patient would also have the options of palliative care, which may include hospice.

What is palliative care?

Palliative care is medical care aimed at relieving the symptoms of serious illnesses. This kind of care can and should be provided by any number of medical specialists with special training. Ideally, palliative care begins with the diagnosis of an advanced ovarian cancer and can be provided in parallel with disease-directed therapy. As disease progresses, disease-directed therapy decreases and palliative care increases (Fig. 57.2). Palliative care should be ruled by the concept

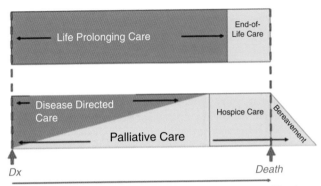

Fig. 57.2 Palliative care/cancer care paradigms, illustrating the former, more traditional paradigm with palliative care ensuing only after medical care is exhausted *(top diagram)* and the newer, more veritable paradigm with palliative care integrated into medical oncological care throughout the course of the disease from diagnosis to death. *(From Epstein AS, Goldberg GR, Meier DE. Palliative care and hematologic oncology: the promise of collaboration. Blood Rev. 2012 Nov 1;26(6):233–9, fig. 1.)*

of person-centered medicine, which addresses the values and wishes for a patient and symptom impact on her quality of life.

> The patient now is considered to have platinum-resistant disease and starts on gemcitabine 1000 mg/m^2 every 4 weeks. Three months into treatment, the patient comes to the emergency room with emesis for 48 hours and an inability to tolerate oral intake. An abdominal X-ray shows air–fluid levels, a distended stomach, and dilated loops of small bowel.

What is the patient's diagnosis at this time?
Sadly, patients with progressing ovarian cancer frequently develop small bowel obstruction (SBO) from the malignancy at some point. Malignant SBO is the final common pathway of ovarian disease and the way the majority of patients die. This patient's diagnosis is malignant SBO.

CLINICAL PEARL **STEPS 2/3**

SBO and ileus can be difficult to distinguish, as both disorders present with abdominal distension and vomiting. In general, physical exam findings on ileus include a lack of bowel sounds with a distended abdomen, while small bowel obstruction produces hyperactive, high-pitched bowel sounds. Radiologic findings in ileus generally present with gaseous distension of large and small bowel, whereas SBO displays distended loops of bowels with air–fluid levels and minimal or absent colonic gas.

What is the management of SBO in this patient?
Patients with a new malignant SBO should be evaluated immediately, so the patient should be urgently brought to a hospital or emergency room setting if not already in this environment. Workup includes a physical exam, abdominal radiograph, electrolyte panel, complete blood count, serum lactate, and usually but not necessarily a CT scan. If the patient is stable, conservative management can be pursued. A nasogastric (NG) tube should be placed at bedside with low, intermittent wall suction. Intravenous (IV) fluids and pain medicine should be given, and electrolytes should be evaluated. NG tube decompression should provide immediate relief of obstruction symptoms, but does not address the underlying malignancy. If this management does not relieve the SBO in 5–7 days, small bowel diversion is pursued. The two most commonly used options are loop ileostomy or percutaneous endoscopic gastrostomy (PEG) tube placement. It is important that a decision for operative management is taken in light of overall goals of care.

The patient decides to stop tumor-directed therapy and gets a venting PEG tube placed, which immediately relieves her symptoms. She then enrolls in hospice.

What is hospice?

Hospice is a subset of palliative care in which all disease-directed therapy is stopped; treatments are now completely aimed at symptom relief. Hospice enrollees must have a life expectancy 6 months or less, and enrollment requires a paradigm shift for patients, families, and providers. Hospice care requires an understanding that disease is not curable and that death is inevitable. The Institute of Medicine wrote a groundbreaking report on the end of life:

"*A decent or good death* is one that is: free from avoidable distress and suffering for patients, families, and caregivers; in general accord with patients' and families' wishes; and reasonably consistent with clinical, cultural, and ethical standards. A *bad death*, in turn, is characterized by needless suffering, dishonoring of patient or family wishes or values, and a sense among participants or observers that norms of decency have been offended. Bad deaths include those resulting from or accompanied by neglect, violence, or unwanted and senseless medical treatments."

The goal of hospice is to help patients and their families at the end of life and through the bereavement process.

MEMBERS OF THE HOSPICE TEAM   **BOX 57.1**

- Physicians—gynecologic oncology, medical oncology, radiation oncology, palliative care
- Social work
- Nursing, especially hospice nursing
- Physical therapy/occupational therapy
- Pharmacists
- Chaplains
- Psychologists/psychiatrist
- Dieticians
- Family

The patient enrolls in hospice, and she dies 1 month later at home with her family.

BEYOND THE PEARLS

- Bevacizumab is a vascular endothelial growth factor (VEGF) inhibitor that has been studied in both the upfront and recurrent ovarian cancer setting. The addition of bevacizumab in recurrent, platinum-resistant disease treatment improves progression-free and overall survival, so it is improved only in this instance.
- Double-strand DNA breaks are repaired in two ways: homologous recombination, which is a more "faithful" error-free process, or nonhomologous end joining, which is a more error-prone process. Patients with breast cancer gene mutations (BRCA) have impaired homologous recombination. Poly ADP ribose polymerase (PARP) is an enzyme involved in single-strand DNA break repairs, and PARP inhibitors increase cell death associated with single-strand breaks. PARP inhibitors can be used in patients with BRCA mutations to prevent the "cell immortality" that leads to cancer formation. Olaparib, a PARP inhibitor, is approved by the U.S. Food and Drug Administration (FDA) for recurrent epithelial ovarian cancer in BRCA mutation patients.
- Studies in palliative care in advanced cancer have shown improved quality of life, fewer emergency room visits, decreased hospitalization, lower costs, increased patient and family satisfaction, and even prolonged survival in patients with advanced cancer who receive palliative care simultaneous to tumor-directed therapy.

Case Summary
- A patient with a history of ovarian cancer presents with abdominal symptoms at her routine surveillance visit 18 months after completion of her primary treatment, prompting an evaluation with a CT scan. This confirms the presence of recurrent ovarian cancer.
- As the patient has a platinum-sensitive recurrence, she undergoes surgery followed by chemotherapy. However, she has progression of her disease despite chemotherapy, so the platinum-based chemotherapy regimen is changed to an alternative agent.
- The patient continues to have progressive cancer and presents with malignant SBO. She is treated initially with NG tube decompression and then with a palliative PEG tube. She enrolls in hospice, dying at home shortly thereafter.

References

Field, M. J., & Cassel, C. K. (Eds.), (1997). *Approaching death: improving care at the end of life committee on care at the end of life*. Washington DC: Institute of Medicine.

NCCN Clinical Practice Guidelines. Ovarian cancer including fallopian tube cancer and primary peritoneal cancer. Version 2.2015. Nccn.org

Temel, J., Greer, J., Muzikansky, A., et al. (2010). Early palliative care for patients with metastatic non-small-cell lung cancer. *The New England Journal of Medicine, 363*(8), 733–742.

Kate V. Meriwether, MD ■ Rebecca G. Rogers, MD

A 57-Year-Old Woman With Pain on Sexual Intercourse

A 57-year-old woman presents complaining of pain with sexual intercourse for 8 months that is severe enough that she avoids intercourse with her husband. She has seen three physicians and has been told that it is "in her head." She is desperate to find a solution.

Why is it important to ask about and address sexual concerns among women?

Sexual problems are very common, with as many as 40% or more of U.S. women having a sexual problem and more than 10% having a very distressing sexual problem; it is even more common in middle-aged women (aged 45–64). Sexual problems are associated with poor health, low education, and depression, so gynecologists must ask about and know how to treat these issues.

When a woman has pain with intercourse, what do you need to know about her history?

Any organ system in the pelvis can lead to pain with intercourse: reproductive, gastrointestinal (GI), urinary, integumentary, musculoskeletal. First, ask the patient about the pain using the PPQRST format (palliation, provocation, quality, radiation, severity, timing), and ask if this type of pain has happened before. If this is the woman's first episode of pain, it makes the case for a new, inflammatory problem (such as infection or trauma). If the pain is long term, the patient may have changes in nerve response that characterize chronic pain, or pain existing for 6 months or longer. The clinician must ask the patient about her sexual practices (type and frequency of intercourse, partners, sexual abuse, sexually transmitted infections [STIs]), if the pain occurs in all sexual situations, and any past injuries or surgeries in the pelvic area. Establish the patient's menopausal status, if she is using any hormonal medications, and if she has vaginal dryness. As the mean age of menopause is 51 in the United States, this woman is likely to be postmenopausal. Ask the patient about vaginal symptoms such as itching or discharge that would indicate vaginitis and any bleeding from the vagina around sexual intercourse (Table 58.1).

TABLE 58.1 ■ **Types of Female Sexual Dysfunction Included in the Current** *Diagnostic and Statistical Manual of Mental Disorders* **(DSM-5)**

Type of Sexual Dysfunction (DSM-5)	Definition (Required for at Least 6 Months Causing Significant Distress)
Female sexual interest/arousal disorder	Difficulty with interest in or desire to engage in sexual activity and/or difficulty obtaining physical arousal
Female orgasmic disorder	Difficulty with achieving orgasm with adequate sexual stimulation
Genito-pelvic pain/penetration disorder	Pain in a genital or pelvic location caused or exacerbated by sexual activity that inhibits or prevents comfortable sexual activity

The patient tells you her pain is sharp, 7/10 in severity, worsened by vaginal intercourse, alleviated 20–30 minutes after stopping intercourse, centered in the vagina, and radiating to the bilateral pelvis. The patient has one male partner with whom she has vaginal-penile intercourse about once a week, without any history of STI. She has been menopausal since age 52 and has had vaginal dryness for 10 years for which she uses a lubricant for sex. She notes a malodorous, clear discharge from the vagina for the last 3–4 months, and spotting of blood for 1–2 days after the last two times she attempted intercourse. Two years ago, she a hysterectomy and an anterior repair for pelvic organ prolapse which included the placement of vaginal polypropylene mesh.

What clues in the history might point toward vaginal atrophy?

In postmenopausal women, estrogen decline in the vaginal tissues causes a decrease in cellular turnover, increase in basal cells, increase in the vaginal pH from 4.7 (premenopausal level) to approximately 5.7, and a decrease in the population of *Lactobacilli*. For many women, these changes result in lack of lubrication, bleeding and/or odor after vaginal intercourse, and an increased risk of bacterial vaginosis (BV). On exam, women with vaginal atrophy have thin, pale, and dry mucosa that lacks some of the typical vaginal folds (rugae). This woman has experienced vaginal dryness for the past 10 years, which could be explained by atrophy, but her pain with intercourse started more recently.

What clues in the history might point toward a musculoskeletal origin of the pain?

If the woman has a history of pain or injury in the back or hip region (like a recent car accident or fall), musculoskeletal upset may have caused the pelvic muscles to spasm. Pain with intercourse can arise due to irritation of the levator ani or obturator muscle groups when joints in the area are compromised by injury. On vaginal exam, one can palpate the levator muscle group at 4 o'clock and 7 o'clock, 1–2 cm inside the hymen as a slight band of muscle. The obturator internus lies laterally on the internal pelvic side wall, and having the patient try to externally rotate the hip while palpating this muscle may elicit pain.

BASIC SCIENCE PEARL   **STEP 1**

The levator ani group consists of three paired muscles (puborectalis, pubococcygeus, and iliococcygeus) around the levator hiatus, the space through which the vagina and rectum pass.

In addition to evaluating the vaginal mucosa for atrophy and the pelvic muscles for pain, what other information should be gathered from this patient on pelvic exam?

Any patient with sexual pain should have an abdominal and pelvic exam. Her external genitalia should be inspected for lesions, which might indicate vaginal infections, chronic irritation (chronic scratching or allergic reactions to clothing or detergents), or even skin diseases or cancers. Any suspicious changes should have a biopsy to rule out malignancy. If the patient has pain upon entry during intercourse (insertive dyspareunia), a moistened Q-tip should be used to palpate the external genitalia. Pain out of proportion to the stimulation (hyperalgesia) or the sensation of pain with a nonpainful stimulation (allodynia), particularly in the vestibule area, increases suspicion for vulvodynia or vulvar vestibulitis. A speculum exam should be performed to look for vaginal discharge, lesions, foreign objects, or masses. The uterus, adnexa, and pelvic muscles should be palpated to determine if pain is reproduced. It is important to help coach the woman through the exam as you are trying to find the site of the pain.

The patient has a temperature of 36.5°C (97.8°F), a heart rate of 95/min, a blood pressure of 135/80 mm Hg, and a soft, nontender abdomen. On pelvic exam, she has no external genital lesions or pain on Q-tip exam. A speculum exam reveals thin, pale, smooth vaginal mucosa. There is a 1 cm area of "plastic-like" material protruding out of the anterior vaginal wall; the tissue around this is erythematous and bleeds easily. Her levator muscles are tender and tense.

What is the foreign body in this woman's vagina, and how does that relate to her pain?

The differential diagnosis on a vaginal foreign body in an adult includes a retained hygiene device (such as a tampon), a retained contraceptive device (such as a condom or diaphragm), a bezoar formed from hair, objects inserted by the patient, or objects inserted for medical use (such as an intrauterine device or a pessary). This woman has erosion of the vaginal mesh material that was used to support her vaginal walls in her recent vaginal prolapse surgery. Vaginal grafts of many types are implanted in the vaginal walls by gynecologic surgeons to treat pelvic organ prolapse or incontinence. These graft materials can be biologic or synthetic, and synthetic materials can be absorbable or permanent. The most common type of implanted permanent vaginal graft is polypropylene mesh. Up to 10% of women who have vaginal mesh implanted experience vaginal erosion, which can result in pain with intercourse, vaginal bleeding or discharge, or pelvic infection (Fig. 58.1).

CLINICAL PEARL   **STEPS 2/3**

Permanent suture or mesh material in medical use includes polypropylene and silk. Absorbable suture and mesh materials used in medicine include polydioxanone (PDS) suture, a monofilament suture which is at half-strength 8 weeks after placement, and polyglactin 910 (Vicryl), a multifilament suture with half-strength at about 3 weeks. The quickest absorbing suture is "catgut," a multifilament collagen suture that retains strength for only 1–2 weeks.

What treatment options exist for this woman's vaginal mesh erosion?

If a woman is not sexually active or has no symptoms (not the case with this patient), it is an option to observe the erosion. In the case of a small erosion (<5 mm mesh), treatment for 3 months with vaginal medications (such as 0.5 g of conjugated equine vaginal estrogen cream, 0.625 mg/g, applied every other night and alternating with metronidazole gel) is an option. If the erosion is large (>5 mm), the patient quite bothered, or treatment with medication is not successful for 3 months, surgical excision of the eroded area should be offered.

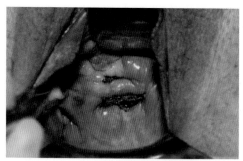

Fig. 58.1 A vaginal mesh erosion in a patient who had former implantation of permanent polypropylene mesh in the anterior vaginal wall for pelvic organ prolapse correction. *(From Karram MM. Atlas of pelvic anatomy and gynecologic surgery. 2016: 739–48, fig. 59-1B.)*

The woman is distressed by this problem and wants to proceed with excision of the vaginal mesh in the operating room.

What does the patient need to know prior to having the mesh removed?

Very small vaginal mesh erosions (<3 mm) can sometimes be excised under local anesthesia in the clinic. Be aware that the vagina is highly vascular and sensitive, and the surgeon must be prepared for bleeding and pain. The woman should also be counseled that, if the entire mesh is not excised, the erosion may occur again. In many cases, excision of the mesh requires the expertise of a female pelvic reconstructive surgeon. She should know that removing the mesh carries surgical risks, such as entry into nearby organs (bladder or urethra), return of the problem the mesh was placed to treat (like prolapse or leakage of urine), bleeding, infection of the area, or more mesh erosions in the future. The patient should also be counseled that not all pain may resolve immediately following surgery. In this case, the woman's vaginal atrophy and levator spasm will likely need treatment as well.

The patient undergoes excision of the anterior mesh with minimal bleeding and no complications. The patient returns for a visit 6 months after vaginal mesh excision and states that while her partner no longer feels a "scratching," she still feels pain on vaginal entry. The patient is faithfully using the vaginal estrogen. Repeat exam reveals well-estrogenized tissue, no mesh erosion, and pain over bilateral levator muscle groups. The patient is "disappointed" because she thought "the surgery would get rid of all the pain."

What treatments can you offer the patient at this point?

You cannot blame a patient for being discouraged; only 51% of women with excision of mesh erosion have resolution of all symptoms. This establishes the importance of setting expectations before the surgery. This woman can be offered pelvic floor physical therapy or injections of local anesthesia into "trigger points" or the pudendal nerve. The pudendal nerve supplies somatic innervation to the vulva and distal vagina, and blocks can break the pain cycle. The injection site for the pudendal nerve is through the vagina, 2 cm medial, posterior, and superior to the ischial spine. These injections are done weekly for 6–8 weeks, and it is prudent to engage in a long-term treatment like physical therapy.

BASIC SCIENCE PEARL   **STEP 1**

Local anesthetics, all of which have names ending in "-caine," come from two groups—amines and esters—based on their chemical makeup. Esters are more prone to cause allergic reactions because of hypersensitivity to the ester metabolite para-aminobenzoic acid (PABA), so most clinically used local anesthetics, like lidocaine and bupivacaine, are amines. Local anesthetics work by blocking sodium-gated ion channels that allow the nerve cell to depolarize and transmit pain signals. Side effects of intravascular local anesthetics include periorbital numbness or ringing in the ears. If a patient experiences these side effects with injection, the injection should be immediately stopped to avoid cardiac complications (like arrhythmias) from toxicity.

The patient is not interested in pudendal nerve blocks as she "lives too far away," but she is able to see a physical therapist in her area. She returns to your office 3 months later with minimal tenderness of the levator group and has been able to have comfortable intercourse.

BEYOND THE PEARLS

- Women with sexual dysfunction and pain are often discouraged, shuffled from physician to physician, and feel that nobody understands their problem. Always be thorough and set aside time to listen; it may take several visits to gather information and find solutions.
- The most common type of implanted, synthetic vaginal mesh for pelvic support procedures is polypropylene "Type I" mesh, which is knitted monofilament mesh with large pores (>75 μm) that allow immune cells to circulate around the mesh and prevent formation of bacterial films.
- Ospemifene, a selective estrogen receptor modulator that acts as an estrogen agonist in the vagina and increases vaginal lubrication and epithelial thickness, has recently been approved for the treatment of sexual pain in postmenopausal women.
- If less invasive treatments of chronic musculoskeletal pain in the pelvis, such as physical therapy, are not successful, emerging evidence suggests that injections of botulinum toxin into the muscle of pain origin may be helpful.

Case Summary

- A 57-year-old postmenopausal woman presents with pain with vaginal intercourse and a past history of vaginal mesh insertion. Physical exam reveals that patient has a vaginal mesh erosion, vaginal atrophy, and levator muscle pain and spasm.
- The patient opts for surgical excision of the mesh and begins vaginal estrogen treatment for her vaginal atrophy.
- After the surgery, the patient still has residual pain attributed to her levator muscle group and is offered treatment with physical therapy and bilateral pudendal nerve block injections. She does physical therapy with biofeedback and experiences improvement.

References

Abed, H., Rahn, D. D., Lowenstein, L., et al. (2011). Systematic Review Group of the Society of Gynecologic Surgeons. Incidence and management of graft erosion, wound granulation, and dyspareunia following vaginal prolapse repair with graft materials: a systematic review. *International Urogynecology Journal, 22*(7), 789–798.

Crosby, E. C., Abernethy, M., Berger, M. B., et al. (2014). Symptom resolution after operative management of complications from vaginal mesh. *Obstetrics and Gynecology, 123*(1), 134–139.

Hokenstad, E. D., El-Nashar, S. A., Blandon, R. E., et al. (2015). Health-related quality of life and outcomes after surgical treatment of complications from vaginally placed mesh. *Female Pelvic Medicine and Reconstructive Surgery, 21*(3), 176–180.

Lev-Sagie, A. (2015). Vulvar and vaginal atrophy: physiology, clinical presentation, and treatment considerations. *Clinical Obstetrics and Gynecology, 58*(3), 476–491.

Lucas, M., Pickersgill, A., & Smith, A. R. B. (2006). Chronic pelvic pain: diagnosis and management. In C. R. Chapple, et al. (Ed.), *Multidisciplinary management of pelvic floor disorders* (pp. 319–334). Philadelphia: Elsevier.

Muffley, T. M., & Barber, M. D. (2010). Insertion and removal of vaginal mesh for pelvic organ prolapse. *Clinical Obstetrics and Gynecology, 53*(1), 99–114.

Portman, D., Palacios, S., Nappi, R. E., & Mueck, A. O. (2014). Ospemifene, a non-oestrogen selective oestrogen receptor modulator for the treatment of vaginal dryness associated with postmenopausal vulvar and vaginal atrophy: a randomised, placebo-controlled, phase III trial. *Maturitas, 78*(2), 91–98.

Shifren, J. L., Monz, B. U., Russo, P. A., et al. (2008). Sexual problems and distress in United States women. *Obstetrics and Gynecology, 112*(5), 970–978.

Vaccaro, C. M., & Pauls, R. N. (2013). Female sexual dysfunction. In R. G. Rogers, C. B. Iglesia, & V. Sung (Eds.), *Female pelvic medicine and reconstructive surgery* (pp. 315–338). New York: McGraw Hill.

Casey Kinman, MD

A 62-Year-Old Woman With Urinary Urgency and Incontinence

A 62-year-old G3P3 Caucasian female presents to your office reporting a 6-month history of having to urinate every 30 minutes. On her way to the restroom, she feels that she must "rush to get there." If she is unable to get there quickly, she will usually have leakage for which she wears 1–2 sanitary pads per day. This affects her performance at her job as a warehouse supervisor. She denies any pain with urination or blood in her urine. She has smoked 1 pack of cigarettes per day for the past 25 years and has a history of hypertension.

What are some causes of urinary frequency and urgency?

Urinary urgency is the sudden, compelling desire to pass urine which is difficult to defer. Urinary frequency is defined as eight or more voids during waking hours. There are many conditions that can result in the symptoms of urinary frequency and urgency, and a careful history and physical will help determine the etiology of the patient's symptoms. Specific attention should be paid to history of pelvic surgeries or radiation, neurological disorders, and medications the patient is taking that might cause or worsen urinary urgency and frequency.

TABLE 59.1 ■ **Causes of Urinary Urgency and/or Frequency or Overactive Bladder (OAB)**

Category	Disease Process
Neurogenic	• Multiple sclerosis • Stroke • Parkinson's disease • Spinal cord injury • Dementia
Idiopathic	• Most common (~90%)
Myogenic	• Muscular disorders • Outflow obstruction (commonly from prior antiincontinence surgery or severe pelvic organ prolapse)
Inflammatory	• Interstitial cystitis • Bladder tumor/foreign body

What initial workup should be performed at her first visit?

Urinalysis should always be performed in patients who present with urinary urgency and frequency. The presence of bacteria, leukocytes, nitrites, or leukocyte esterase is indicative of a urinary tract infection (UTI), in which case urine culture should be sent and possible antibiotics prescribed. Postvoid residual (PVR) should be checked using either a bladder scanner or catheter to ensure that the patient's symptoms are not due to incomplete bladder emptying; a PVR of less than 100–150 mL is considered normal.

When should you consider cystoscopy in the evaluation of a patient with lower urinary tract symptoms?

Cystoscopy should be considered for women with hematuria or whose urinary symptoms do not improve with behavioral and first-line medical therapies. Cystoscopy can detect pathology that could be causing her symptoms: intravesical polyp or mass, foreign body such as a stone, stricture, diverticulum, chronic cystitis, or even bladder cancer. This patient, with her history of smoking, is at increased risk for bladder malignancy, so should be evaluated by cystoscopy if first-line treatment fails.

> The patient denies any prior abdominal or pelvic surgeries and experienced menopause 9 years ago. She is on three different medications for her blood pressure, including a "water pill," but admits to noncompliance with her medications. Physical exam reveals an obese female in no apparent distress with a height of 1.5 m (5'3"), weight of 102 kg (225 lbs), and a blood pressure of 155/85 mm Hg. Pelvic exam reveals mild vaginal atrophy but no masses or pelvic organ prolapse. Her urinalysis is negative for leukocytes, nitrites, and bacteria, and PVR by bladder scanner is 45 mL.

What is the patient's likely diagnosis?

Overactive bladder (OAB) is defined by the International Continence Society as "urinary urgency, usually accompanied by frequency and nocturia, with or without urgency urinary incontinence, in the absence of urinary tract infection or other obvious pathology." OAB is a common condition that affects 8%–29% of the U.S. population and over half of women older the age of 60; one-third of women with OAB have incontinence associated with this. Understandably, OAB causes significant socioeconomic and quality-of-life impact. Older age, higher body mass index (BMI), parity, smoking, menopause, and pelvic organ prolapse are all risk factors for OAB. This patient has no other clues in her history or exam findings that would indicate another etiology. OAB is a diagnosis of exclusion, and the majority of cases are idiopathic; so only patients like this one without evidence of organic pathology can have a diagnosis of OAB.

> The patient wants to try and "do something about this problem" as soon as possible and would like to start with "easy" treatments first.

What are some first-line therapies to treat OAB?

This patient should first be counseled on lifestyle modifications for OAB: avoidance of dietary irritants, decreasing caffeine and tobacco use, weight loss, fluid management, and timed voiding. Weight loss of as little as 5%–10% of body weight, which would have additional health benefits in this obese patient, has been shown to decrease urinary incontinence significantly. Additionally, pelvic floor exercises are a low-risk, minimally invasive therapy which are effective in decreasing OAB symptoms. Behavioral treatments are generally either equivalent to or superior to medications for the treatment of OAB. If conservative therapies do not control the patient's symptoms, she should be offered medical therapy.

> The patient returns to your office 2 months later. She has decreased her tobacco and caffeine intake by half, lost about 3 kg (7 lbs) with diet and exercise, and eliminated acidic foods from her diet. However, she still has 3–4 episodes of incontinence per day associated with an urge to void and remains frustrated.

What medical treatment can you offer the patient, and what is the mechanism of action?

Anticholinergics are the most common medical therapy for OAB and should be offered to patients whose symptoms are not sufficiently improved with behavioral therapy. Antimuscarinics are the specific type of anticholinergic medication utilized for OAB treatment; they block muscarinic receptors that normally respond to acetylcholine from postsynaptic parasympathetic neurons in the pelvic nerve. Muscarinic receptors are present throughout the body, so these medications have commonly reported side effects such as primarily dry mouth, dry eyes, constipation, and blurry vision. Antimuscarinics are contraindicated in patients with narrow-angle glaucoma due to their potential to precipitate an attack, and they should be avoided in patients with gastric retention or urinary retention. Furthermore, they should be used with caution in elderly populations due to their potential central nervous system (CNS) effects.

A newer medication that acts as a β_3-adrenoceptor agonist, mirabegron, was approved by the U.S. Food and Drug Administration (FDA) for OAB in 2012. This is a good option for patients who are unable to tolerate the side effects of or have contraindications to anticholinergic medications. However, mirabegron is contraindicated in patients with poorly controlled hypertension or tachycardic arrhythmias, so would not be a good option for this patient.

Long-term adherence to medications for OAB is low, with more than half of patients stopping medications within 6 months of initiation. Therefore, patients should have appropriate counseling about side effects and the plan for indefinite use (if the medication is effective) before starting these medications.

BASIC SCIENCE/CLINICAL PEARL   **STEPS 1/2/3**

There are five known subtypes of muscarinic receptors (M1–M5) with M2 and M3 being the predominate subtypes in the bladder. Some newer antimuscarinics have selectivity for M3 receptors and subsequently have less peripheral side effects.

BASIC SCIENCE/CLINICAL PEARL   **STEPS 1/2/3**

Narrow-angle glaucoma involves increased pressure in the compartment of the eye enclosed by the cornea and the iris. When the lens of the eye and the iris change shape due to relaxation of the ciliary muscles (accommodation), pressure increases in this compartment. Antimuscarinic medications inhibit the parasympathetic reflex that allows the ciliary muscles to contract, increasing pressure in the eye, so these medications are contraindicated in narrow-angle glaucoma.

You discuss these medication options with the patient and decide to start her on oxybutynin extended-release tablets 5 mg once daily. When she returns 12 weeks later, she has noted only slight improvement in her symptoms and has developed bothersome dry mouth. She still has 1–2 episodes of urinary leakage and nocturia 3 times per night. Due to her smoking history and failure of first-line therapy, she has a cystoscopy in your office and it is normal. She would like to explore other therapy options.

What third-line treatments exist for the treatment of OAB?

Third-line treatments for patients unable to tolerate, comply, or succeed with lifestyle changes and medications include intradetrusor onabotulinum toxin A (BTX-A) injection, sacral neuromodulation (SNM), and percutaneous tibial nerve stimulation (PTNS). Intradetrusor BTX-A, administered through cystoscopic injection, is approved for both refractory idiopathic OAB and neurogenic

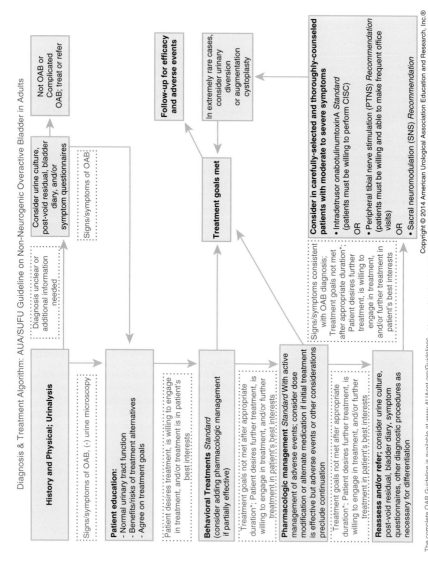

Fig. 59.1 Treatment algorithm for overactive bladder (OAB), with or without urinary urgency incontinence. *(From Gormley EA, Lightner DJ, Faraday M, et al. Diagnosis and treatment of overactive bladder (non-neurogenic) in adults: AUA/SUFU guideline amendment. J Urol. 2015 May 1;193(5):1572–80.)*

detrusor overactivity. BTX-A, which is produced by the bacteria *Clostridium botulinum*, has an 80%–90% efficacy rate for OAB, but patients usually require reinjection every 6–12 months for symptom control. Patients opting for BTX-A treatment need to be aware of the risk of incomplete bladder emptying (4%–43%) and be willing to self-catheterize should they need it. SNM involves the placement of a wire through the S3 sacral foramen which delivers nonpainful, mild electrical pulses to the sacral nerve roots that control the bladder and pelvic floor. Patients wear an external battery for 1–2 weeks, and women with 50% improvement in symptoms are candidates for a permanent lead wire and battery. SNM is currently FDA approved for refractory OAB, nonobstructive urinary retention, and fecal incontinence. Success rates with the permanent implant are approximately 85%. PTNS is another form of neuromodulation that avoids the permanent implantation of any foreign material. The tibial nerve is a mixed nerve, containing both sensory and motor fibers from the L4–S3 levels of the spinal cord. Patients undergoing PTNS have 10–12 weekly office sessions where low-voltage stimulation is applied to a 34-gauge needle placed 3–5 cm cephalad to the medial malleolus. Success rates are around 60%–70%.

BASIC SCIENCE PEARL   **STEP 1**

BTX-A acts by inhibiting calcium-mediated release of acetylcholine vesicles at the presynaptic neuromuscular junction in peripheral nerve endings, decreasing the muscle's ability to contract.

BASIC SCIENCE PEARL   **STEPS 2/3**

Metal implants, such as the implant used in SNM, are contraindicated in the case of patients who need body magnetic resonance imaging (MRI) on a regular basis, such as patients with certain types of neurological disease like multiple sclerosis. The magnetic field used in MRI may heat or move metal implants, such as the lead wires in a sacral neuromodulator, and this could damage surrounding tissue or move the device.

The patient opts to undergo intradetrusor BTX-A injection and experiences good symptom control following the procedure. She is only getting up to the restroom one time at night and is sleeping better "than she has in years." She is emptying her bladder well, and only has 1 leakage episode per month. You advise her to follow-up in 6 months to discuss her symptoms, with a plan for reinjection if her symptoms return sooner.

BEYOND THE PEARLS

- Some patients with urinary incontinence may not clearly have leakage due to urgency or may not feel the detrusor contraction that causes their leakage. In other words, particularly in patients with neurological disease (such as patients with diabetes), OAB may not present in a classic way.
- Urodynamic testing should be considered for patients with refractory incontinence, prior anti-incontinence surgery, pelvic radiation, or voiding difficulty to help determine the underlying pathology and best treatment strategies.
- A recent randomized trial showed that BTX-A may have a slightly better improvement in leakage per day than sacral neuromodulation, but the difference between them was small and both led to greater than 60% treatment satisfaction.
- Recent studies have found that vaginal estrogen cream has similar efficacy to antimuscarinic medications for the treatment of OAB symptoms.

Case Summary

- A 62-year-old woman presents with urinary urgency, frequency, and urinary incontinence. History and physical exam reveal that the patient has no infection, normal emptying, and is likely to have idiopathic overactive bladder.
- The patient first tries conservative therapies but her symptoms are still bothersome. She begins an antimuscarinic medication, but this does not provide adequate symptom control.
- She undergoes a cystoscopy due to her history of smoking, and this is normal.
- The patient decides to try a third-line treatment, intradetrusor BTX-A injection, which results in good symptom control.

References

Abrams, P., Cardozo, L., Fall, M., Standardisation Sub-committee of the International Continence Society, et al. (2002). The standardisation of terminology of lower urinary tract function: report from the Standardisation Sub-committee of the International Continence Society. *Neurourology and Urodynamics, 21*, 167–178.

American Urological Association 2014 (2016). *Diagnosis and Treatment of Overactive Bladder (Non-Neurogenic) in Adults: AUA/SUFU Guideline (PDF)*. Retrieved June 1, 2016.

Amundsen, C. L., Richter, H. E., Menefee, S. A., et al. (2016). Onabotulinumtoxin A vs sacral neuromodulation on refractory urgency urinary incontinence in women: a randomized clinical trial. *JAMA, 316*(13), 1366–1374.

De Boer, T. A., Salvatore, S., Cardozo, L., et al. (2010). Pelvic organ prolapse and overactive bladder. *Neurourology and Urodynamics, 29*, 30–39.

Stewart, W. F., Van Rooyen, J. B., Cundiff, G. W., et al. (2003). Prevalence and burden of overactive bladder in the United States. *World Journal of Urology, 20*, 327–336.

Temml, C., Heidler, S., Ponholzer, A., & Madersbacher, S. (2005). Prevalence of the overactive bladder syndrome by applying the International Continence Society definition. *European Urology, 48*(4), 622–627.

Visco, A. G., Brubaker, L., Richter, H. E., et al. (2012). Pelvic Floor Disorders Network. Anticholinergic versus botulinum toxin A comparison trial for the treatment of bothersome urge urinary incontinence: ABC trial. *Contemporary Clinical Trials, 33*(1), 184–196.

Deslyn T. G. Hobson, MD

A 51-Year-Old With Frequent Urinary Tract Infections and Vaginal Dryness and Burning

A 51-year-old G6P6 postmenopausal woman presents to your office with three urinary tract infections (UTIs) over the past year. For 6 months, she has also noticed vaginal dryness, itching, burning, and discomfort during intercourse. She is sexually active with one male partner that she has had for the past 7 months.

What type of history is important to discuss with this patient and why?
Genitourinary syndrome of menopause (GSM), former known as "vulvovaginal atrophy," is defined as symptoms and signs associated with a decrease in estrogen in the genital tract and can appear in early menopause years or long after cessation of menses. GSM symptoms include vaginal dryness and burning, lack of lubrication, sexual pain, urinary urgency or frequency, dysuria, and recurrent UTIs. Symptoms of GSM are experienced by 50% of postmenopausal U.S. women, but only 25% seek medical help. Therefore, physician–patient dialogue about these symptoms is key. The physician should take a thorough history involving the symptoms experienced, the timing of symptom onset and menopause, the use of hormone therapy, a sexual history including partners and sexually transmitted infections (STIs), vaginal discharge or postmenopausal bleeding, and the use of any vaginal products or douches. Important urinary symptoms to ask about include urinary urgency, frequency, incontinence, and UTIs.

The patient reports urinary frequency and dysuria when she has UTIs, and these resolve with antibiotic treatment. She experiences symptoms of vaginal burning and itching "all the time," but vaginal pain and dryness is "terrible when I have sex." She denies any bleeding or discharge. She has vaginal intercourse with her male partner once a week.

What are physical signs of GSM? What physical exam is indicated to evaluate this patient?
Estrogen maintains vaginal blood flow and vaginal elasticity, so physical signs of GSM include vaginal redness, pallor, and petechiae; loss of vaginal caliber; a small, atrophic cervix; lack of moisture; attenuated labia minora; and loss of rugae (Fig. 60.1). The vulva should be checked for lesions which may indicate skin disease, and vulvar lesions should be biopsied to exclude malignancy. Women with postmenopausal bleeding need cervical cancer screening and an endometrial biopsy. Because of this patient's sexual activity, she should be tested for STIs and common causes of vulvovaginitis with appropriate polymerase chain reaction (PCR) tests, saline and 10% potassium hydroxide (KOH) microscopy, and litmus paper pH. Vaginal secretions for microscopy and pH should be taken from the mid-vagina as cervical secretions are more acidic. GSM, *Trichomonas* infection, and bacterial vaginosis all elevate vaginal pH, so pH should be done in concert with microscopy.

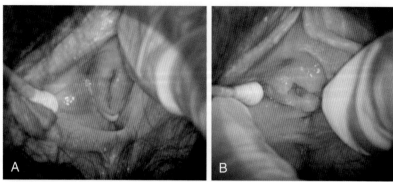

Fig. 60.1 A: External genitalia in a menopausal woman demonstrates scarce pubic hair, diminished elasticity and turgor of the vulvar skin and periurethral tissue, increased erythema around the urethra, decreased introital moisture, and fusion of the labia minora anteriorly and posteriorly. In contrast (B), a premenopausal female has more vaginal color, moisture, and tissue flexibility around the introitus. *(From Shindel AW, Goldstein I.* Campbell-Walsh urology. *Philadelphia: Elsevier: 2016:749–64.e9, fig. 32-5A.)*

On pelvic exam, the patient has attenuated labia minora and a narrowed introitus without lesions. A speculum exam reveals a pale, smooth vagina and a small cervix. Saline microscopy shows increased parabasal cells (Fig. 60.2), lack of *Lactobacilli*, less than 20% clue cells, and a pH of 5.5. KOH microscopy reveals no spores or hyphae, and gonorrhea/chlamydia testing is negative. Given these findings, you tell her that GSM is the most likely diagnosis.

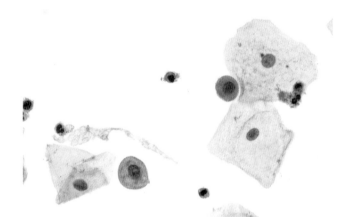

Fig. 60.2 Photomicrograph of parabasal cell on Papanicolaou smear. Parabasal cells are immature squamous epithelial cells that are rounded and have a large nucleus-to-cytoplasm ratio. In contrast, mature squamous epithelial cells (also seen in this photograph) are larger, cuboidal, with a smaller nucleus-to-cytoplasm ratio. *(From Nephron, Own work, CC BY-SA 3.0,* https://commons.wikimedia.org/w/index.php?cur id=42760076)

How do you establish a diagnosis of recurrent UTI in this patient?

Of all women, 3%–5% will have recurrent UTI, so it is important to understand the definition of recurrent UTI: three or more laboratory-confirmed UTIs in 12 months or two or more infections in 6 months. It is important to distinguish recurrent UTIs from urinary symptoms associated with overactive bladder or interstitial cystitis/bladder pain syndrome. This patient meets criteria for recurrent UTIs based on her history.

> To evaluate this patient's UTI history and assess for current infection, you do a urine culture. The culture reveals more than 100,000 colony-forming units per milliliter (10^5 CFU/mL) of *Escherichia coli* that is sensitive to nitrofurantoin.

CLINICAL PEARL   **STEPS 2/3**

Urine dipstick, 75% sensitive and 82% specific for a UTI if positive for leukocyte esterase or nitrates, adds little clinically in acutely symptomatic patients but can guide therapy "in the moment" for patients with an uncertain diagnosis. Urine microscopy detects bacteria, leukocytes, and red blood cells, but only 50% of UTIs demonstrate microscopic hematuria. Urine culture showing more than 10^5 CFU/mL of a single uropathogenic organism (or 10^2 CFU/mL in a catheter specimen) is considered the gold standard in diagnosis but is not mandatory to make a diagnosis in straightforward, uncomplicated UTI.

What are the common organisms isolated in recurrent UTIs?

Escherichia coli (*E. coli*, O, K, and H antigen serotypes) causes 80%–90% of all UTIs. *Staphylococcus saprophyticus*, detected in 3% of all UTIs, is rare in postmenopausal patients. UTIs of other Enterobacteriaceae (such as *Proteus, Pseudomonas, Klebsiella, Serratia, Morganella*) are frequently associated with an abnormal urinary tract, catheters, and calculi.

What are the risk factors for recurrent UTIs in postmenopausal women?

Menopause is a major risk factor for recurrent UTIs as lack of estrogen decreases *Lactobacilli*, increases genital pH, and predisposes the patient to pathologic bacterial growth. Factors that worsen bladder emptying, such as vaginal prolapse and neurogenic diseases, and factors that alter vaginal microbes and pH, such as spermicides, anal intercourse, and diabetes mellitus, are also risk factors. Some women may have a genetic predisposition due to enhanced adherence of uropathogenic *E. coli* to their urinary tract, such as nonsecretors of ABH blood group antigens.

How would you manage recurrent UTIs in the postmenopausal woman?

Management of recurrent UTIs should start with addressing risk factors, including treatment of GSM with vaginal estrogen therapy in this patient. Her current infection should be treated with therapeutic antibiotics for 3–7 days, and she should also be offered a 6-month course of continuous prophylaxis for suppression (Table 60.1). Although suppression reduces risk of recurrence up to 95%, up to 50% of women will have a recurrence of UTI when the suppression is stopped. Most women with recurrent UTIs, especially if they recur despite therapy or have risk factors for urinary tract abnormalities (such as former bladder surgery or a history of stones) or malignancy (such as smoking), should have cystoscopy and appropriate upper tract imaging.

TABLE 60.1 ■ Prophylaxis Regimens for Recurrent Urinary Tract Infections

Antibiotic	Dose	Frequency
Trimethoprim-Sulfamethoxazole	40/200 mg or 80/400 mg	Daily
Nitrofurantoin	50 mg or 100 mg	Nightly
Cephalexin	125 mg or 250 mg	Nightly
Trimethoprim alone (useful if sulfa allergy)	100 mg	Nightly
Fosfomycin	3 g powder suspended in water	Every 7–10 days

CLINICAL PEARL   STEPS 2/3

In settings with a 10%–15% prevalence of resistance to trimethoprim-sulfamethoxazole (TMP-SMX), the cure rate with this antibiotic is equivalent to ciprofloxacin or nitrofurantoin. TMP-SMX should not be used for initial UTI treatment if local resistance rates of uropathogens exceed 20%.

The patient has a normal renal ultrasound and a normal cystoscopy in the office. Her urinalysis is negative for hematuria after her current UTI is treated, and no other red flags exist in her history.

CLINICAL PEARL   STEPS 2/3

Noncontrast computed tomography (CT) is the current gold standard for radiographic diagnosis of calculi as it is more likely than ultrasound and plain-film radiography of kidneys, ureters, and bladder (KUB) to identify small or radiolucent stones. Contrast CT is best to detect upper urinary tract malignancy.

What measures can be taken to prevent recurrent UTIs?

The treatments best supported by evidence for UTI prevention are vaginal estrogen (for postmenopausal women) and prophylactic antibiotics. Vaginal estrogen treatment normalizes the vaginal microbiome and reduces UTI frequency in postmenopausal women by an average of 1.1 UTIs/year. Commonly discussed behavioral changes (e.g., front-to-back wiping, urinating after sex) have not been demonstrated to be effective. Adhesion blockers such as D-mannose and bacteriostatic methenamine salts are mildly effective, and vaginal probiotics (such as active *Lactobacillus* cultures) have some benefit. Cranberry products, sadly, have not clearly demonstrated efficacy in prevention of UTIs in systematic reviews, but some individual studies have shown a mild benefit.

The patient returns for a visit 6 months later. She has taken daily prophylaxis with nitrofurantoin for 6 months and is happy to report that she has not had any UTI symptoms. She avoided vaginal estrogen due to concern "about hormones," and she is still experiencing vaginal dryness and pain with sex.

What treatments can you offer the patient for her GSM?

Topical, vaginal estrogen is the most commonly used treatment for GSM (Table 60.2). Contraindications to vaginal estrogen include a personal history of estrogen-positive breast cancer, endometrial cancer, personal predisposition to these cancers (such as BRCA mutation), or venous thrombosis. For women who want to avoid vaginal estrogen, vaginal moisturizer three times a week at night or vaginal lubricants used prior to sexual activity are viable options. If the patient has two or more symptoms of GSM, such as burning and dryness, evidence shows benefit to vaginal estrogen over these alternatives. As there is minimal serum absorption from vaginal treatment alone, no progesterone therapy is needed in women with an intact uterus.

TABLE 60.2 ■ **Examples of Vaginal Estrogen Products for Treatment of Genitourinary Syndrome of Menopause (GSM)**

Composition	Form and Trade Name	Dosage (µg)	Regimen (All Administered to Vagina)	Serum Estradiol Level (pg/mL)
Estradiol hemihydrate	Estradiol tablet (Vagifem)	10	Initial: 1 tablet/day for 14 days Maintenance: 1 tablet twice a week	3–11
17β-estradiol	Estradiol ring (Estring)	7.5	Device (2 mg total) releases 7.5 µg/day for 90 days	5–10
17β-estradiol	Estradiol cream (Estrace)	200	Initial: 2–4 g/day for 1–2 weeks Maintenance: 1 g, 1–3 times/week	40–80
Conjugated equine estrogen	CEE cream (Premarin)	300	0.5–2 g/day for 14–21 days, then 2–3 times a week	No change

The patient is prescribed conjugated equine estrogen and is able to have comfortable sexual intercourse 3 months later. She denies any new UTIs. You instruct her to continue the vaginal estrogen three times a week indefinitely.

BEYOND THE PEARLS

- Selective estrogen-receptor modulators (SERMs) that are inhibitory for genital tract estrogen receptors (such as tamoxifen) can aggravate GSM. Ospemifene, a SERM that stimulates estrogen receptors in the genital tract, was recently approved for GSM-associated sexual pain.
- The vaginal maturation index (VMI), a method for examining the menopausal status of the vagina, reports percentages of cell types in vaginal secretions. In estrogenized women, the typical VMI is 40%–70% intermediate, 30%–60% superficial, and 0% parabasal cells. In typical postmenopausal women, the VMI is 65% parabasal, 30% intermediate, and 5% superficial cells.
- Nitrofurantoin can induce hemolytic anemia in patients with glucose-6-phosphate dehydrogenase deficiency. Also, long-term exposure to nitrofurantoin (>12 months) has been associated with pulmonary reactions, chronic hepatitis, and neuropathy.
- Fluoroquinolones (e.g., ciprofloxacin) should not be used as first-line agents in treating uncomplicated urinary tract infections, as these broad-spectrum medications have more risk for resistance, gastrointestinal complications (like *C. difficile* diarrhea), can prolong the cardiac QTc interval, and rarely can cause Achilles tendon rupture.
- Bioidentical hormones, nonestrogen products of isoflavones or soy derivatives, are considered by the U.S. Food and Drug Administration (FDA) to be supplements and are not regulated for purity or dosing or required to undergo rigorous testing for efficacy. They should be avoided in symptomatic patients who want safe, evidence-based, effective treatment.
- Compounded vaginal estrogens, which are mixed in a licensed compounding pharmacy using dosing and concentrations that are proved efficacious for GSM, can be a lower cost alternative for patients who cannot afford brand-name formulations of vaginal estrogens.

Case Summary

- A 51-year-old woman presents with three urinary tract infections (UTIs) per year, vaginal dryness and burning, and painful sexual intercourse. History and physical confirms that the patient has genitourinary syndrome of menopause (GSM) and meets criteria for recurrent UTIs.
- Patient is treated for a current UTI based on urine culture and placed on continuous antimicrobial prophylaxis with nitrofurantoin for 6 months, and she has improvement in her UTI symptoms.
- The patient hesitates on vaginal estrogen treatment for her GSM; symptoms of pain with intercourse and vaginal burning and dryness persist despite moisturizer use. Once she utilizes vaginal estrogen, she gets relief of her symptoms.

References

American College of Obstetricians and Gynecologists (2014). ACOG practice bulletin no. 141: management of menopausal symptoms. *Obstetrics and Gynecology*, *123*(1), 201–216.

American College of Obstetricians and Gynecologists' Committee on Gynecologic Practice & Farrell, R. (2015). ACOG committee opinion no. 659 summary: the use of vaginal estrogen in women with a history of estrogen-dependent breast cancer. *Obstetrics and Gynecology*, *127*(3), 618–619.

Eriksen, B. (1999). A randomized, open, parallel-group study on the preventive effect of an estradiol-releasing vaginal ring (Estring) on recurrent urinary tract infections in postmenopausal women. *American Journal of Obstetrics and Gynecology*, *180*(5), 1072–1079.

Gupta, K., Horton, T. M., Naber, K. G., et al. (2011 March 1). International clinical practice guidelines for the treatment of acute uncomplicated cystitis and pyelonephritis in women: a 2010 update by the infectious diseases society of america and the european society for microbiology and infectious diseases. *Clinical Infectious Diseases*, *52*(5), e103–e120.

North American Menopause Society (2013). Management of symptomatic vulvovaginal atrophy: 2013 position statement of the North American Menopause Society. *Menopause*, *20*, 888–902.

Portman, D. J., & Gass, M. L. (2014). Vulvovaginal Atrophy Terminology Consensus Conference Panel. Genitourinary syndrome of menopause: new terminology for vulvovaginal atrophy from the international society for the study of women's sexual health and the North American Menopause Society. *Menopause*, *21*, 1063–1068.

Rahn, D. D., Carberry, C., Sanses, T. V., et al. (2014). Society of Gynecologic Surgeons Systemic Review Group. Vaginal estrogen for genitourinary syndrome of menopause: a systematic review. *Obstetrics and Gynecology*, *124*(6), 1147–1156.

Simon, J. A., & Maamari, R. V. (2013). Ultra-low-dose vaginal estrogen tablets for the treatment of postmenopausal vaginal atrophy. *Climacteric*, *16*(Suppl), 37–43.

Stapleton, A. E., Au-Yeung, M., Hooton, T. M., et al. (2011). Randomized, placebo-controlled phase 2 trial of a lactobacillus crispatus probiotic given intravaginally for prevention of recurrent urinary tract infection. *Clinical Infectious Diseases*, *52*(10), 1212–1217.

Sara Cichowski, MD

A 32-Year-Old Woman With Urinary Leakage on Exercise

A 32-year-old G2P2 woman presents for evaluation of leakage of urine while jogging. She reports this problem has been present since the birth of her first child 5 years ago and is getting progressively worse.

What are risks factors for stress incontinence?

Stress urinary incontinence (SUI) is defined as involuntary leakage of urine with physical activity or strain on the abdominal wall. Common activities that cause leakage include sneezing, laughing, coughing, or exercise. SUI affects more than 20% of the nation's female population. Many women are embarrassed to discuss SUI or may think it is a normal part of aging, so asking open-ended questions to start a conversation about these symptoms is important. As age increases, so does the prevalence of SUI, making it an important risk factor. Pregnancy and childbirth are the most established risk factors, but SUI is also associated with pelvic organ prolapse, higher body mass index, genetics and family history, caffeine, smoking, depression, constipation, and urinary tract infections (UTIs).

Why does SUI occur?

The mechanisms of SUI are complex and still being researched. The urethra is supported by connective tissues and the levator ani muscles. The urethra itself is a multilayered structure, with striated and smooth muscles and a mucosal lining, and these structures create pressure inward that keeps the urethra closed and the patient continent. Loss of any of these structures, leading to decreased urethral closure pressures, may result in SUI. Urethral hypermobility, when the urethra drops below the pelvic floor, also factors into the pathophysiology of stress incontinence.

BASIC SCIENCE PEARL   **STEP 1**

The female urethra is about 4 cm long. The urethra contains multiple layers that help maintain continence. The longitudinal and circular muscular fibers contribute to the sphincter mechanism.

The patient reports needing to wear a pad constantly and is embarrassed when going to the gym. She is uncertain of future childbearing.

Is there any additional workup needed to make the diagnosis of SUI?

History alone is sufficient to make the diagnosis of SUI. However, the patient should also be asked about other urinary symptoms such as urgency, dysuria, recurrent UTIs, pad usage, and vaginal bulging. On pelvic exam, the vagina should be examined for prolapse (descent of the vaginal walls) and any urethral abnormalities such as urethral diverticulum. Pelvic floor assessment should include evaluation of the woman's ability to contract her pelvic floor. A cough stress test (CST) may also be useful, and the bladder should be checked for complete emptying (post-void residual [PVR]).

BASIC SCIENCE PEARL   **STEPS 2/3**

When intraabdominal pressure, such as with a cough, exceeds urethral closure pressure, there may be leakage of urine and this is called *stress incontinence*.

The patient denies that she has any issues with urgency or dysuria, and she has normal frequency of urination and no nighttime urinary symptoms. Leakage only occurs during physical activity such as jogging and occasionally with a cough, laugh, or sneeze. On physical exam, the woman has normal external genitalia and no evidence of pelvic organ prolapse with straining. She can contract her pelvic floor strongly and hold this around the physician's fingers. When she coughs or strains, she loses drops of urine out of the urethra.

What treatment options are available to her?

Most experts recommend waiting until childbearing is complete before providing surgical intervention. Nonsurgical options for the treatment of SUI include pessaries, pelvic floor exercises, vaginal SUI tampons, vaginal estrogen cream, and weight loss. Presently, there are no oral medications approved for the treatment of SUI in the United States. Self-directed pelvic floor exercises ("Kegels") can be helpful to women for SUI and are described as contracting the muscles in a manner similar to preventing gas passing in a public situation or as if squeezing around a tampon in side the vagina. If a woman is unable to contract her pelvic floor during physical exam, consideration should be given to guidance from a physical therapist. While not available in all areas, there are physical therapists who have additional training and certification in pelvic floor rehabilitation. Performing regular pelvic floor exercises decreases the rate of SUI by 35%–80%. Guidelines recommend performing 8 contractions 3 times a day for 3 months to treat SUI.

Another option for stress incontinence is a vaginal pessary. Pessaries are soft devices made of flexible materials like silicone, and they come in many shapes and sizes. The most common type of pessary used for the treatment of SUI is a ring with knob. The knob provides support to the urethra (Fig. 61.1). Some women only use the pessary during those activities that cause urine leakage. Over-the-counter SUI tampons such as the brand "Impressa" also offer the same type of support. When comparing pelvic floor exercises to pessary, the improvement in symptom bother is similar between groups. Individual preference should be taken into consideration. Vaginal estrogen cream also reduces SUI in postmenopausal woman. However, in premenopausal women like this patient, it would not have benefit as her natural hormone levels are probably still adequate. Also, both surgical and nonsurgical weight loss studies show women have a significant improvement in symptoms with moderate loss of body mass, so weight loss should be recommended as first-line therapy in overweight or obese patients.

CLINICAL PEARL   **STEPS 2/3**

The CST is performed by asking the women with a comfortably full bladder to cough in a supine position. If there is leakage of urine, then the test is positive for SUI. If there is no leakage, the test can be repeated in the standing position.

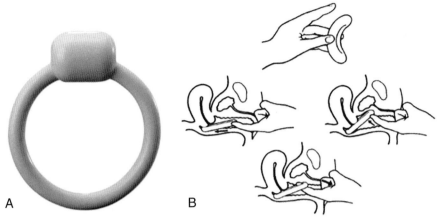

A   B

Fig. 61.1 Pessaries come in many sizes and shapes. The ring with knob pictured here is most commonly used for stress incontinence (A). The pessary is inserted into the vagina and provides support under the urethra, as demonstrated in this view of the woman shown from the side (B). *(From Magali R., et al. Technical update on pessary use. J Obstet Gynaecol Can. 2013 Jul 1;35(7):664–74, fig. 8 and unnamed figure.)*

After discussing the options, the patient is interested in using a pessary and performing Kegel exercises at home, and she is fitted with a ring pessary with knob. She returns 1 year after performing her exercises faithfully and attempting to use the pessary. She found the pessary uncomfortable and did not use it routinely. She and her partner have decided not to attempt further pregnancies. She requests surgical management.

Do you need to perform urodynamic testing prior to antiincontinence surgery?

Multichannel urodynamic studies (UDS), or studies that investigate bladder and abdominal pressures during bladder filling and emptying, are often used to evaluate urinary incontinence. However, UDS are not necessary in uncomplicated SUI. Uncomplicated SUI is defined as stress-predominant symptoms by patient report with observed urinary incontinence during a provocative measure (such as during a CST) in the absence of other pathology. Complicated SUI, or stress incontinence with other possible pathology or factors that would make treatment less straightforward, often requires UDS. Examples of complicated SUI, which would merit UDS, are listed in Box 61.1.

Because this patient demonstrates objective stress incontinence in her initial exam and denies any complicated factors, such as urgency or dysuria, she can be considered to be uncomplicated stress incontinent. She does not have UDS, and she is offered surgical options.

REASONS FOR URODYNAMIC TESTING IN WORKUP OF STRESS URINARY INCONTINENCE   **BOX 61.1**

Reasons to consider multichannel urodynamic testing

Elevated postvoid residual
Mixed incontinence symptoms (leakage of urine both with urgency and physical strain)
Neurologic disorder
Prior history of mid-urethral sling or antiincontinence surgery
Unclear history or patient/family unable to give history

What surgical options are available to treat stress incontinence?

Mesh mid-urethral slings are currently the standard of care for SUI (Fig. 61.2). Other treatment options include retropubic urethropexy (Burch procedure), urethral bulking agents, autologous fascial slings, and artificial sphincters. Mesh is typically avoided in women who have previously had mesh complications or who are undergoing simultaneous urethral diverticulectomy or urethral fistula repair.

> The patient is interested in a mid-urethral sling operation to treat her stress incontinence because this is less invasive than other options available to her. She asks how likely this operation is to "fix" her incontinence and what potential risks there are to undergoing this surgery.

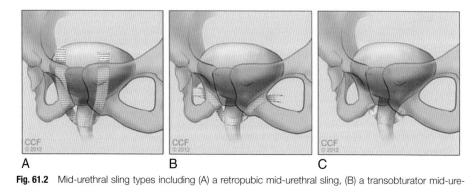

A   B   C

Fig. 61.2 Mid-urethral sling types including (A) a retropubic mid-urethral sling, (B) a transobturator mid-ure-thral sling, and (C) a mini-sling. *(From Ridgeway B, Barber MD. Midurethral slings for stress urinary incon tinence: a urogynecology perspective.* Urol Clin N Am. *2012 Aug 1;39(3):289–97, fig. 1.)*

CLINICAL PEARL   **STEPS 1/2/3**

Retropubic urethropexy (the Burch procedure) attaches the pubocervical fascia at the level of the mid-urethra and urethrovesical junction to Cooper's ligaments using permanent sutures. In order to perform this procedure, the retropubic space (also called the space of Retzius) is accessed.

What are the potential risks to mid-urethral slings?

During the procedure, there are risks of significant bleeding or organ perforation, particularly bladder injury with trocars. Postoperative risks to mid-urethral slings include voiding dysfunction (both temporary and permanent), new-onset or worsening urge incontinence, recurrent UTIs, pain or neuromuscular problems, dyspareunia, and recurrent incontinence. Mesh-specific risks include vaginal mesh exposure and mesh erosion into the urinary tract.

What is the success rate of the operations to treat stress incontinence?

Most mid-urethral sling operations are 80%–85% effective in treating stress incontinence, and more than 90% of women are satisfied with the procedure or would opt to have the operation again if given the opportunity. Of note, these success rates pertain to treatment of SUI and not to other forms of incontinence, such as incontinence with urgency, which may or may not be improved by this operation. As the patient has uncomplicated stress incontinence, she is a good candidate for this operation.

After counseling, the patient opts to undergo a mid-urethral sling, and the procedure occurs without complication. She has resolution of her stress incontinence after the operation, and 3 months after the surgery is happy with her outcome and has no bothersome urinary symptoms.

BEYOND THE PEARLS

- Mid-urethral slings are most commonly placed with two different approaches: retropubic (behind the pubic bone to the anterior abdominal wall) or transobturator (through the obturator foramen) (Fig. 61.2). Retropubic slings carry a higher risk of bladder perforation during the procedure and a higher chance of postoperative voiding dysfunction. Transobturator slings carry a greater risk of leg or groin pain.
- Transobturator slings may be passed from the thigh through the obturator externus muscle, membrane, and obturator internus muscle and come out through a vaginal incision. They can also be placed starting from the vagina, going through the obturator foramen and exiting out the thigh, in reverse order of the course noted above.
- Fascial slings are often made by harvesting the rectus fascia, the thick connective tissue covering on the anterior surface of the rectus abdominis.

Case Summary

- A 32-year-old woman presents with stress urinary incontinence (SUI), wants therapy and possibly more desires more children in the future.
- History and physical reveal that the patient has stress incontinence with a positive empty supine cough stress test (CST).
- The patient opts for nonsurgical management initially with pessary and pelvic floor exercises, but later requests surgical management when her family is complete.
- After the surgery, the patient has resolution of her SUI symptoms.

References

Adams-Piper, E., Buono, K., Whitcomb, E., Mallipeddi, P., Castillo, P., & Guaderrama, N. (2016). A large retrospective series of pregnancy and delivery after midurethral sling for stress urinary incontinence. *Female Pelvic Medicine Reconstructive Surgery* [Epub ahead of print].

Bø, K. (2012). Pelvic floor muscle training in treatment of female stress urinary incontinence, pelvic organ prolapse and sexual dysfunction. *World Journal of Urology, 30*(4), 437–443.

Garely, A. D., & Noor, N. (2014). Diagnosis and surgical treatment of stress urinary incontinence. *Obstetrics and Gynecology, 124*(5), 1011–1027.

Kenton, K., Barber, M., Wang, L., et al. (2012). Pelvic Floor Disorders Network. Pelvic floor symptoms improve similarly after pessary and behavioral treatment for stress incontinence. *Female Pelvic Medicine Reconstructive Surgery, 18*(2), 118–121.

Nager, C. W., Brubaker, L., Litman, H. J., et al. (2012). Urinary Incontinence Treatment Network. A randomized trial of urodynamic testing before stress-incontinence surgery. *The New England Journal of Medicine, 366*(21), 1987–1997.

Rahn, D. D., Carberry, C., Sanses, T. V., et al. (2014). Society of Gynecologic Surgeons Systematic Review Group. Vaginal estrogen for genitourinary syndrome of menopause: a systematic review. *Obstetrics and Gynecology, 124*(6), 1147–1156.

Whitcomb, E. L., & Subak, L. L. (2011). Effect of weight loss on urinary incontinence in women. *Open Access J Urol, 3*, 123–132.

Gregory Kanter, MD, MS

A 43-Year-Old Woman With Pelvic Pain, Symptoms of Bladder Infections Despite Negative Urine Cultures

A 43-year-old G1P0 woman presents to your clinic with 2 years of frequent voiding and pain in her pelvis. Since 2 years ago, she has seen her primary care doctor five times for a "urinary tract infection", with symptoms of dysuria and frequent voiding every 45–60 minutes during the day to avoid pain in the bladder, but her doctor is puzzled because urine cultures results are consistently negative.

Why is it important to differentiate urinary frequency with pain from urinary urgency?
Both interstitial cystitis/bladder pain syndrome (IC/BPS) and overactive bladder (OAB) may be associated with urinary frequency. A hallmark symptom of IC/BPS is pain that is worse with bladder filling and better with emptying, and pain tends to be the sensation that drives patients to void frequently. In OAB, the need to urinate frequently is motivated by urinary urgency as opposed to pain. Treatment of these two conditions is very different, and distinguishing them from the onset is crucial to treatment success. IC/BPS is a diagnosis of exclusion defined by the Society for Urodynamics and Female Urology (SUFU) as "an unpleasant sensation (pain, pressure, discomfort) perceive to be related to the urinary bladder, associated with lower urinary tract symptoms of more than six weeks duration, in the absence of infection or other identifiable causes." In OAB, only urinary urgency must be present. Pain in IC/BPS is often exacerbated by certain foods or drinks that irritate the bladder (such as acidic foods, alcohol, or caffeine), sexual intercourse or pelvic exams, or life stressors. Care should be taken to obtain urine cultures to distinguish an IC/BPS flare from a urinary tract infection (UTI), as symptoms of IC/BPS and UTI can be similar or identical.

What types of questions are important to ask in women with a history of frequent or irritative voiding, as is seen in this patient?
With irritative voiding symptoms, one must consider benign and malignant causes. Benign causes include UTIs genitourinary tract stones, urethral diverticula, and even endometriosis, while malignant causes include tumors of the urinary tract. A thorough history is helpful in setting the level of suspicion for malignancy. IC/BPS often presents in "flares" lasting days or weeks, whereas malignancy usually presents with constant or worsening symptoms. The presence of blood in the urine (either gross or microscopic) may indicate the presence of a stone or malignancy within the urinary tract and requires additional workup. Cyclic blood in the urine that corresponds with the menstrual cycle may indicate endometriosis. A history of smoking or chemical exposure would raise suspicion for cancer.

What is the relationship between IC/BPS and other pain disorders?

Differentiating IC/BPS from other causes of pelvic pain may be difficult because they often co-exist, and there is overlap between etiologies. Fibromyalgia, irritable bowel syndrome, and vulvo-dynia are more common in patients with IC/BPS than in patient without this disorder. Screening for these coexisting disorders is important in the treatment of any of these syndromes, and a higher index of suspicion for IC/BPS is warranted in patients with one of these other issues.

What are important elements of the physical exam if IC/BPS is suspected?

Patients with chronic pain from any origin have an increased risk of having a history of physical or sexual abuse or having had a traumatic experience with pelvic exams in the past. For this reason, the examiner must be particularly gentle during the exam and work on gaining the trust of the patient prior to the examination. The pelvic examination starts externally, inspecting the skin, screening for Bartholin's or Skene's gland cysts or urethral diverticula, and using a moistened cotton swab to map pain if present. A small speculum may then be used to examine for any abnormalities of the vaginal walls or cervix. Discharge may indicate vaginitis or upper genital tract infection, and discharge can be tested for infection if suspected. Using a single digit, the examiner may palpate the anterior vaginal wall beneath the urethra and bladder. Pain in the urethra and the bladder is often present in patients with IC/BPS, whereas the uterus and adnexa would not be expected to be particularly tender unless other disorders that affect these organs (like endometriosis) co-exist. However, the abdominal hand for the bimanual exam may elicit suprapubic tenderness as the bladder is compressed. The muscles of the pelvis (levator ani and obturator internus) should be assessed for pain and spasm and are frequenty also tender in patients with IC/BPS.

> On physical exam, the patient has a temperature of 36.8°C (98.3° F), a heart rate of 84/min, and a blood pressure of 122/78 mm Hg. Her abdomen is soft and without masses, but she experiences mild suprapubic tenderness on palpation. On pelvic exam, the patient has normal external female genitalia with no lesions. Touch with a moistened cotton swab does not elicit pain over the external genitalia. The patient winces with insertion of a small speculum, but the vaginal walls and cervix appear normal. Bimanual exam elicits tenderness over the anterior vaginal wall proximal to the urethral meatus, corresponding to the area of the bladder. The levator muscles are tight and tender.

Are there any diagnostic tests to solidify the IC/BPS diagnosis?

IC/BPS is defined primarily by history and physical, so no diagnostic tests rule in the diagnosis of IC/BPS. However, because this is a diagnosis of exclusion, initial workup should focus on excluding other possible etiologies. A urinalysis and urine culture is necessary to rule out UTI. If blood is noted in the urine, further workup (such as cystoscopy or upper urinary tract imaging) may be necessary to rule out genitourinary malignancy or urinary stones. A bladder diary that includes food and drink may help to establish the diagnosis and guide the patient's treatment. A cystoscopy, which may be performed in the office or operating room, is not necessary for diagnosis, but certain findings may support a diagnosis of IC/BPS. Characteristic lesions include Hunner's lesions and glomerulations (Fig. 62.1), which are only present in a small subset of patients.

> The patient is given a diagnosis of IC/BPS based on a urinalysis that reveals slight leukocyte esterase, no evidence of microscopic hematuria, a negative urine culture, and your history and physical findings. She is very worried and asks, "How did I get this problem?"

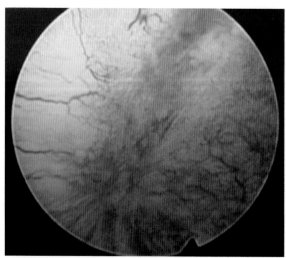

Fig. 62.1 Cystoscopic view of a Hunner's lesion, a characteristic lesion seen in interstitial cystitis/bladder pain syndrome (IC/BPS). *(From Chennamsetty A, Khourdaji I, Goike J, et al. Electrosurgical Management of Hunner Ulcers in a Referral Center's Interstitial Cystitis Population. Urology. 2015 Jan 1;85(1):74–8, fig. 1.)*

What is important for the patient to know about IC/BPS?

The pathophysiology of IC/BPS is poorly understood, and it is impossible to tell this patient what caused her disorder in the first place. Often, it helps patients to understand the disorder as an abnormal reaction by their own body, such as an autoimmune disorder or an allergic reaction, and that it is not malignant or dangerous. The patient should also be informed that IC/BPS can be managed effectively, although it is chronic and may remit and relapse over the patient's life.

BASIC SCIENCE PEARL   **STEP 1**

We do not know for certain what causes IC/BPS, but there are several theories. It is believed that the disease process may be initiated by an insult to the bladder lining, either from trauma or infection. Defects have been found in the glycosaminoglycan (GAG) layer in IC/BPS patients and in animal models, that may make the bladder more permeable and sensitive to irritating substances. As urine is both acidic and contains waste products, it irritates compromised bladder lining. In addition, there appears to be an inflammatory response involving mast cells in IC/BPS patients, and neurological sensitization, either locally within the bladder or in the central nervous system (CNS) plays an important role. This theory may also explain the overlap between IC/BPS and other pain disorders, which all involve increased pain sensitivity.

The patient is willing to "do anything" to help "make this problem go away" as it is affecting her ability to work, function, and have sexual relations with her partner. She wants immediate options for treatment.

Which treatments are most effective for IC/BPS?

No single treatment is useful in every patient, so treatment should be multimodal and individualized to the patient. In general, treatment should begin with conservative measures and progress as needed to medical therapies and more invasive modalities. Treatment can be based on the guidelines from the American Urological Association (AUA), which has devised a useful algorithm. Initially, dietary modifications and other lifestyle changes, such as stress reduction, should be employed.

TABLE 62.1 ■ **Common Dietary Triggers for Interstitial Cystitis/Bladder Pain Syndrome Patients**

Food Group	Examples
Carbonated beverages	Seltzer water, tonic water, sodas, colas
Caffeinated beverages	Energy drinks, coffee, nonherbal tea, colas
Acidic foods	Citrus fruits (lemon/lime/orange), tomatoes, peppers, strawberries, sodas with citric acid
Alcoholic beverages	Beer, wine, dark liquors, vodka, gin, tequila
Artificial sweeteners	Diet drinks, diet shakes

Physicians should recommend that patients be aware of and experiment with decreasing or avoiding these foods and drinks.

If coexisting muscles spasm or tenderness is noted, physical therapy by therapists who specialize in treating pelvic floor disorders is an important modality for IC/BPS treatment. Local anesthetic injection, either in trigger points or directed toward the pudendal nerve, may help with associated musculoskeletal symptoms.

Our patient elects to take a meditation class to aid in stress reduction, and she also keeps a diary of "triggers" for her pain. She notes that her pain seems to be particularly bad after coffee and alcoholic beverages, as well as after spicy foods, so she limits these in her diet. She attends six weekly physical therapy sessions, and she is able to resume intercourse with her husband. She does still have bladder pain that occurs after times of stress and lasts about 1 week. She is interested in further treatments.

What other therapies can be offered to this patient?
After these initial measures, oral and intravesical medications (instilled into the bladder using a catheter) are considered second-line therapy. The effect of all oral medications is modest. The only medication approved for IC/BPS by the U.S. Food and Drug Administration (FDA) is oral pentosan polysulfate, which is thought to adhere to the bladder lining to decrease permeability to irritating solutes. Other oral medications include antihistamines and tricyclic antidepressants. If symptoms are not responsive to one or more oral or intravesical medications, singly or in combination, patients have the option of more invasive therapies. Cystoscopy with hydrodistention and treatment of Hunner's ulcers, if found, may be the next course of action. Intravesical injection of onabotulinum toxin and sacral neuromodulation are further treatment options. In highly refractory cases, augmentation cystoplasty or urinary diversion are options to prevent bladder filling, but these treatments are highly invasive and come with significant risks.

CLINICAL PEARL STEPS 2/3

It is believed that hydrodistention is effective for IC/BPS because these patients have overgrowth and/or hypersensitivity of nerves within the bladder to stimuli. This includes an overgrowth of C fibers, unmyelinated fibers that sense noxious stimuli. Hydrodistention causes bladder stretch, which is believed to decrease the depolarization threshold of such C fibers and prevent them from sending pain signals to the CNS. Unfortunately, this treatment is only effective in 30%–40% of patients, and the duration of relief is highly variable. However, at the time of cystoscopy and hydrodistention, Hunner's lesions may be fulgurated (cauterized with an energy source) or injected with corticosteroid, and the rate of improvement after the treatment of a recognized Hunner's ulcer is up to 86%.

The patient adds pentosan polysulfate to her regimen, but she does not want to take antihistamines because she works as an Uber driver during the weekends and wants to avoid sleepiness. She also starts a weekly course of bladder instillations for 6 weeks and has notable improvement. She continues dietary monitoring and stress reduction with the pentosan polysulfate, and, when you see her 6 months later, she states she has had only two more episodes of symptoms, each lasting about a week. She states that she "handles things better in general" than when the problem started.

BEYOND THE PEARLS

- Tracking patient symptoms in IC/BPS can be done using the O'Leary-Sant Symptom Problem Index, a validated questionnaire and scale for measuring change in disease status. Of note, however, it is not a tool that is ideal for diagnosis.
- Stress reduction therapies that can be employed by IC/BPS patients include meditation-based stress reduction (MBSR), practices such as yoga, and physical exercise.
- High-pressure, long-duration hydrodistention is no longer recommended. After short-duration filling, the bladder is emptied and characteristic Hunner's lesions may be visible on the bladder wall.
- Sacral neuromodulation is a treatment technique that has been used to treat OAB, among other things. For IC/BPS, it is most effective in alleviating frequency symptoms, though not as helpful at treating associated pain.

Case Summary

- A 43-year-old woman presents with long-standing pain that appears to be related to filling of her bladder and that improves after emptying.
- On physical examination, she is found to have pain corresponding to the area of the vagina underlying the bladder. She also is noted to have tenderness to palpation over the muscles of her pelvic floor (the levator ani muscles).
- She has improvement after learning more about her dietary triggers and by using physical therapy to target the muscles of her pelvic floor.
- She adds the oral medication pentosan polysulfate for daily treatment, and this helps to resolve her symptoms, though she still has an occasional flare. Although she does not experience complete cure, she has learned effective strategies to manage them so that they do not dramatically impact her quality of life.

References

Bogart, L. M., Berry, S. H., & Clemens, J. Q. (2007). Symptoms of interstitial cystitis, painful bladder syndrome and similar diseases in women: a systematic review. *Journal of Urology, 177*, 450.

Hanno, P., & Dmochowski, R. (2009). Status of international consensus on interstitial cystitis/bladder pain syndrome/painful bladder syndrome: 2008 snapshot. *Neurourology and Urodynamics, 28*(4), 274–286.

Hanno, P. M., Erickson, D., Moldwin, R., & Faraday, M. M. (2015). Diagnosis and treatment of interstitial cystitis/bladder pain syndrome: AUA guideline amendment. *Journal of Urology, 193*(5), 1545–1553.

Lai, H. H., Vetter, J., Jain, S., et al. (2014). The overlap and distinction of self-reported symptoms between interstitial cystitis/bladder pain syndrome and overactive bladder: a questionnaire based analysis. *Journal of Urology, 192*, 1679.

Rothrock, N. E., Lutgendorf, S. K., Kreder, K. J., et al. (2001). Stress and symptoms in patients with interstitial cystitis: a life stress model. *Urology, 57*, 422.

Sant, G. R., Kempuraj, D., Marchand, J. E., & Theoharides, T. C. (2007). The mast cell in interstitial cystitis: role in pathophysiology and pathogenesis. *Urology, 69*, 34.

Anubhav Agrawal, MD

A 65-Year-Old With Vaginal Bulge and Pelvic Pressure

A 65-year-old woman presents to the clinic with complaints of feeling like she is "sitting on a ball." This problem has bothered her for about 4 years. She reports feeling a constant pressure, relieved by reclining at night but worse as the day progresses. The patient reports embarrassment about this issue, and she is afraid to have sexual intercourse due to this problem.

What questions should you ask when obtaining the patient's history?

The physician has a responsibility to screen for pelvic floor disorders, such as pelvic organ prolapse (POP). POP is a disorder in which the vaginal walls have lost their internal supports and therefore bulge downward toward or through the vaginal opening. The physician can begin by asking, "Have you seen or felt a bulge in your vagina or felt something is falling out of your vagina?" Questions about bowel and bladder habits, sexual complaints, and vaginal symptoms like pressure and heaviness are also helpful. Often patients feel embarrassed about discussing these symptoms, so open-ended questions or written, validated questionnaires may be helpful.

The patient reports that she also feels that it is difficult to start urination or bowel movements. At times, she has to place her fingers in the vagina and lift upward on the bulge to help start urination or a bowel movement.

CLINICAL PEARL   **STEPS 2/3**

POP may include apical prolapse (uterine prolapse or, in women with a prior hysterectomy, prolapse of the top of the vagina), anterior vaginal wall prolapse (formerly known as cystocele), posterior vaginal wall prolapse (formerly known as rectocele), and even prolapse of the vaginal opening or perineum. Surgical repair must address all vaginal compartments, particularly the vaginal apex.

What are some risks factors for POP?

Any prior trauma or injury to the pelvic floor musculature can contribute to POP: pregnancy, childbirth, hysterectomy, pelvic surgery, previous prolapse repair, connective tissue disorders, and congenital abnormalities. In addition, activities that increase abdominal pressure such as chronic constipation, chronic obstructive pulmonary disease, obesity, and heavy lifting may contribute to POP, as does age and lack of hormones from menopause.

What are key physical findings that you should look for?

The physical examination is generally conducted with a speculum and a cotton swab with centimeter markings to allow for measurements. Each compartment of the vagina is individually measured using a standardized POP quantification (POP-Q) examination method, which involves the patient "bearing down" or performing the Valsalva maneuver to exemplify protrusion of the vaginal walls in some measurements (Fig. 63.1). A POP-Q score is assigned to each measurement, and the patient is assigned a prolapse stage (Table 63.1). An evaluation of the S2–S4 nerves and pelvic floor muscle strength is also conducted.

On physical exam, the patient has a temperature of 37°C (98.7° F), a heart rate of 93min, and a blood pressure of 130/80 mm Hg. Her abdomen is soft and nontender. On pelvic exam, the patient has normal external female genitalia with no lesions or pain, but the cervix protrudes 2 cm past the hymenal ring, as do the anterior and posterior vaginal walls. You diagnose her with stage III uterovaginal prolapse.

BASIC SCIENCE PEARL   STEP 1

There are three levels of support to the vagina, the most important of which is the uterosacral/cardinal ligament complex (Level I), which supports the top, or "apex". Level II support is that of the lateral and anterior/posterior vaginal walls. The anterior vaginal tissue, separated from the bladder by the pubocervical muscularis, is attached laterally to the arcus tendineus fascia pelvic (ATFP), a condensation of the internal obturator fascia. Level III support is the support for the perineal body, the conjoined tendon of the bulbocavernosus muscles, external anal sphincter, superficial transverse perinei, and the rectovaginal septum.

CLINICAL PEARL   STEPS 2/3

During a hysterectomy, a surgeon should provide apical support to the vagina to prevent posthysterectomy prolapse because apical supports (the uterosacral ligaments and cardinal ligaments) are cut during a hysterectomy.

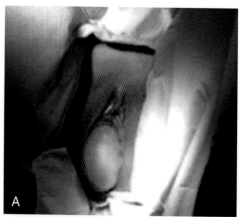

Fig. 63.1 Photograph of uterovaginal prolapse and depiction of pelvic organ quantification (POP-Q) measurements. Notice how the anterior vaginal wall and the vaginal apex protrude past the vaginal opening in the photograph, which would be depicted as positive numbers in the "C" point and Aa/Ba points in the POP-Q. (A is from Koski, ME, Chow D, Bedestani A, et al. 2012 Sep 1;80(3):542–6, fig 1; B is From Kobashi KC. Evaluation of patients with urinary Incontinence and pelvic prolapse. In: Wein AJ, Kavoussi LR, Novick AC, et al. Campbell-Walsh Urology. 10th ed. Philadelphia: Elsevier; 2012:1896-1908.e30)

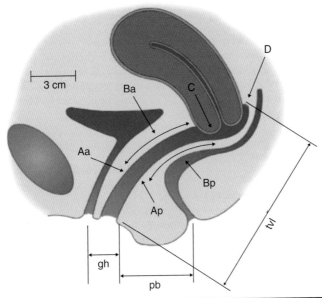

Point	Description	Range of values
Aa	Anterior vaginal wall 3 cm proximal to the hymen	−3 cm to +3 cm
Ba	Most distal position of remaining upper anterior vaginal wall	−3 cm to +tvl
C	Most distal edge of cervix or vaginal cuff scar	−
D	Posterior fornix (N/A if posthysterectomy)	−
Ap	Posterior vaginal wall 3 cm proximal to the hymen	−3 cm to +3 cm
Bp	Most distal position of remaining upper posterior vaginal wall	−3 cm to +tvl
gh (genital hiatus)	Measured from middle of external urethral meatus to posterior midline hymen	−
pb (perineal body)	Measured from posterior margin of gh to middle of anal opening	−
tvl (total vaginal length)	Depth of vagina when point D or C is reduced to normal position	−

B

Fig. 63.1, cont'd

TABLE 63.1 ■ **Stages of Pelvic Organ Prolapse**

Stage 0	No prolapse
Stage I	Leading edge descends to 2 cm above hymen
Stage II	Leading edge descends to within 1 cm of the hymen
Stage III	Leading edge extends greater than 1 cm past the hymen but not to total vaginal length minus 2 cm (TVL − 2 cm) past the hymen
Stage IV	Prolapse extends to TVL − 2 cm or greater ("complete" prolapse)

What additional workup should be performed for this patient?

Patients with POP often may have concomitant urinary incontinence, urinary frequency or urgency, urinary retention, and possibly fecal incontinence or constipation. At a minimum, a urinalysis should be obtained because patients with POP are prone to developing urinary tract infections (UTIs). Also, a postvoid residual (PVR) should be obtained by bladder ultrasound or catheter in order to rule out urinary retention.

> The patient states that, due to her upcoming vacation out of town, she does not desire surgical management at the moment.

What are the risks of not intervening?

The main detriment to health from POP is a decrease in comfort or quality of life; prolapse is rarely dangerous, although symptoms of prolapse may progress over time. In a study of women with prolapse observed without treatment for 2 years, only 19% of them had two or more further descents of the prolapse. There is rarely a need for emergent intervention. However, if the patient suffers from urinary retention or ureteral obstruction, which can occur secondary to severe prolapse (stage III or IV), or has severe ulcers or bleeding from prolapse friction, the prolapse may need to be more urgently managed.

What nonsurgical options can you offer to the patient?

Studies have demonstrated that physical therapy can improve symptoms and slightly improve anatomy. Physical therapy works on strengthening and coordinating the voluntary muscles of the pelvic floor (the levator ani muscles). A vaginal pessary provides another conservative option. A pessary is a soft, silicone device fitted to the patient and worn in the vagina to provide support to the vaginal walls.

> The patient decides that she would like to try a pessary for treatment at this time, and you schedule her for a pessary fitting in your office.

How should a pessary be fit and placed, and how would you counsel the patient about pessary use?

A pessary is placed inside the vagina, above the levator ani muscles, and the anterior aspect of the pessary usually sits behind the pubic bone. The pessary should be placed so the patient experiences no discomfort with it in place. Providers instruct the patient to perform Valsalva maneuvers in order to attempt to expel the device, and they may have the patients ambulate or void with the pessary in place to ensure comfort. The patient should be given precautions about the possibility of bleeding, vaginal discharge, and pain. Patients are instructed to remove the device every 1–2 weeks, if they are able, and perform self-cleaning. If the patient is unable to remove the device on her own, the patient can return to the doctor's office every 1–3 months for care.

> The patient is fitted with a #3 ring pessary with support, and she uses it and vaginal estrogen faithfully. After 3 months, she returns and complains that cleaning the pessary is burdensome, and she wants fewer visits to the doctor because she takes care of her grandchildren. She now desires surgical management.

What surgical modalities are available for her?

There are vaginal, laparoscopic, and robotic approaches to surgical management. Vaginal approaches to surgery often reattach the apex of the vagina to the uterosacral or sacrospinous ligaments, with or without the uterus left in place. In certain cases, some surgeons also use vaginal mesh to improve the strength of the repair. Repair of the anterior or posterior vaginal walls individually (colporrhaphy) can also be done at the time of surgery as needed. Open, laparoscopic, and robotic surgery can also be used to attach the vagina to the uterosacral ligaments or to perform a sacrocolpopexy, where mesh is used to attach the vagina to the anterior longitudinal ligament of the sacrum (Fig. 63.2). Sacrocolpopexy provides less chance of POP recurrence but more risk of complications (such as risks of bleeding, organ or blood vessel injury, and risks associated with mesh) than vaginal surgeries with natural tissue.

CLINICAL PEARL	**STEP 1**

Colpocleisis is sometimes offered to more elderly or less healthy patients to correct POP. Colpocleisis attaches the anterior and posterior vaginal walls to one another 1–2 cm inside the hymen. The resulting vagina is very short, and patients can no longer have sexual intercourse following this procedure. This surgery can be done in less time and with less risk than with other types of POP surgery, and the uterus can be left in place (Lefort's colpocleisis) or removed (colpectomy).

The patient would like to maintain her ability to have sexual activity and desires a very durable or long-lasting surgical repair. She is in good overall health and is a candidate for multiple types of surgery. After considering her options, she chooses an abdominal sacrocolpopexy.

How do you counsel her about the long-term durability of a POP surgery?

All patients who have had a prolapse surgery have some risk of prolapse recurrence. The colpocleisis has the lowest chance of recurrence (<1%), followed by vaginal mesh repairs and sacrocolpopexy, with a recurrence risk of 15%–25%, with the highest recurrence risk in vaginal native tissue repairs (20%–40%). She should be counseled about this before and after the surgery and told that she can decrease her risk for recurrence by avoiding certain modifiable risk factors, such as heavy lifting, smoking, obesity, and chronic constipation.

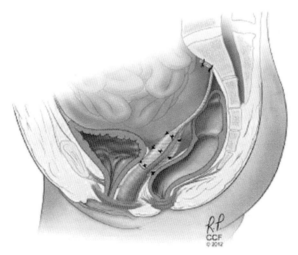

Fig. 63.2 Depiction of the sacrocolpopexy. The mesh is attached to the anterior and posterior vaginal walls and then to the anterior longitudinal ligament at the S1 level of the sacrum. *(From Clifton MM, Pizarro-Berdichevsky J,Goldman HB et al. Robotic female pelvic floor reconstruction: a review. Urology. 2016 May1;91:33–40, fig. 2.)*

The patient returns after her laparoscopic hysterectomy with bilateral salpingo-oophorectomy, sacrocolpopexy, and anterior and posterior repair. She reports no vaginal bulge, no urinary or fecal incontinence. She has been feeling well and has returned to daily physical activities. She wants to know "if this problem could ever come back."

BEYOND THE PEARLS

- When correcting for POP, studies have demonstrated that there is an increased possibility that the patient may suffer from de novo stress urinary incontinence after surgery because correction of prolapse straightens or "unkinks" the urethra. Some physicians will perform a concomitant midurethral sling or antiincontinence procedure at the same time as POP surgery to avoid this risk.
- Careful attention is needed to avoid the pudendal nerve and artery when performing the sacrospinous ligament suspension. Surgeons avoid this by placing sutures on the ligament 2 cm medial to the ischial spines.
- Cystourethroscopy is often performed at the end of surgery for POP, both to examine the bladder for any injuries and to ensure "jetting" of urine from the ureteral orifices in the bladder to rule out ureteral obstruction from the POP surgery.

Case Summary

- A 65-year-old woman presents with symptoms of "sitting on a ball." She is postmenopausal and reports increased pressure as the day progresses. History and physical exam reveal that the patient has Stage III uterovaginal prolapse, with defects of the apex (cervix) and anterior/posterior walls.
- The patient begins her management with a pessary device, but, due to the burden of pessary care, the patient later desires surgical management.
- The patient wants a more durable repair, and she opts for a laparoscopic hysterectomy, bilateral salpingo-oophorectomy, and mesh sacrocolpopexy with anterior and posterior repair, which resolves her symptoms.

References

Bump, R. C., & Norton, P. A. (1998). Epidemiology and natural history of pelvic floor dysfunction. *Obstetrics and Gynecology Clinics of North America, 25*, 723–746.

Cardozo, L., & Staskin, D. (Eds.). (2010). *Textbook of female urology and urogynaecology* (3rd ed) (pp. 457–463). London: Informa Healthcare.

DeLancey, J. O. L. (1992). Anatomic aspects of vaginal eversion after hysterectomy. *American Journal of Obstetrics and Gynecology, 166*, 1717.

Dooley, Y., Kenton, K., Cao, G., et al. (2008). Urinary incontinence prevalence; result from the National Health and Nutrition Examination Survey. *Journal of Urology, 179*(2), 656–661.

Fitzergald, M. P., Richter, H. E., Siddique, S., Thompson, P., & Zyczynski, H. (2006). Colpoclesisis: a review. *International Urogynecology Journal and Pelvic Floor Dysfunction, 17*(3), 261–271.

Gilchrist, A. S., Campbell, W., Steele, H., Brazell, H., Foote, J., & Swift, S. (2013). Outcomes of observation as therapy for pelvic organ prolapse: a study in the natural history of pelvic organ prolapse. *Neurourology and Urodynamics, 32*(4), 383–386.

Kwon, C. H., Golderbg, R. P., Koduri, S., & Sand, P. K. (2002). The use of intraoperative cystoscopy in major vaginal and urogynecologic surgeries. *American Journal of Obstetrics and Gynecology, 187*(6), 1466–1471.

Rogers, R. G., Sung, V. W., Iglesia, C. B., & Thakar, R. (2013). *Female pelvic medicine and reconstructive surgery*. New York, NY: McGraw-Hill.

Jennifer C. Thompson, MD ■ Gena C. Dunivan, MD

CASE 64

A 63-Year-Old Woman With Fecal Incontinence

A 63-year-old G3P3 presents with complaints of leakage of stool gradually worsening over 5 years. This is her first evaluation because she is highly embarrassed by this problem. She feels uncomfortable going on trips for fear of leaking stool and foul odor.

Why is it important to ask about fecal incontinence in women?

Fecal incontinence (FI) is common among women and severely affects their quality of life. FI is defined as the accidental loss of stool. Anal incontinence (AI) includes the loss of both stool and/or flatus. The prevalence of FI ranges from 7% to 15%, but is likely underestimated due to embarrassment and patient fear of discussing this condition. The effects on women's quality of life are significant and include emotional, social, and financial stress. Due to the unclear prevalence, limited self-disclosure rates, and strong impact on quality of life, health care providers should be proactive about screening women for FI. Most patients are highly ashamed and discouraged due to stool leakage, like this patient, so be empathic, use clear language, and emphasize that the problem is common and treatable.

When a woman presents with FI, what should you ask about her history?

The differential diagnosis for FI is broad (Table 64.1), so a comprehensive history should be obtained: frequency, timing, and consistency of bowel movements; associated symptoms (abdominal pain); incomplete emptying; and use of digital maneuvers to facilitate bowel movements. The mnemonic OLDCARTS—Onset, Location, Duration, Character, Aggravating factors, Relieving factors, Timing, Severity—can help guide your history.

TABLE 64.1 ■ Differential Diagnosis of Fecal Incontinence

Anatomic causes	Childbirth injury
	Fistula
	Rectal prolapse
	Surgery/Trauma
Skeletal muscle disease	Myasthenia gravis
	Myopathies
Smooth muscle dysfunction	Fecal impaction
	Scleroderma
Neurologic disease	Central: Stroke
	Spinal cord: Multiple sclerosis
	Peripheral: Cauda equine, diabetes mellitus
Miscellaneous	Irritable bowel syndrome
	Severe diarrhea
	Medications: Antacids, broad-spectrum antibiotics, proton pump inhibitors, diabetic medications, antidepressants, prostaglandins, laxatives

Specific events prior to onset of FI, such as recent birth or pelvic trauma/surgery, can narrow the differential. The patient's history of screening for colorectal cancer, such as past colonoscopy, should be discussed and screening ordered if not up to date.

> The patient describes leaking soft stool about two times each week. The leakage is worse with diarrhea, especially after eating spicy food. She leaks when she has a sudden urge to defecate and cannot make it to the bathroom in time.

What is the role of an obstetric history when evaluating a woman with FI?

Pregnancy, labor, and delivery all contribute to the development of FI. In particular, obstetric anal sphincter injury (OASI) is an important risk factor. Multiparity, operative vaginal delivery, episiotomy, and fetal macrosomia contribute to the risk of OASI. While some women notice an immediate change in bowel function after OASI, other women develop problems many years later due to loss of compensatory mechanisms over time.

In addition to obstetrical injuries, what are other risk factors associated with FI?

Other risk factors for FI are age, smoking, chronic diarrhea, previous anorectal surgery, obesity, urinary incontinence, neurologic disease, increased frequency of bowel movements, and fecal urgency. A thorough history will help the practitioner understand the problem.

> The patient has a history of hypertension, a bilateral tubal ligation, and takes no medications other than lisinopril. She has no allergies. She had three vaginal deliveries including one forceps delivery, her largest baby was 4.3 kg (9 lb 8 oz), and she recalls having "tears" with all her deliveries. She denies tobacco, alcohol, or drug use. Family history is negative for inflammatory bowel disease (IBD) or colon cancer. Although she has some risk factors for FI, you explain the exact cause is unclear. She wants to know why she could control her stool in the past, but not now.

What is the physiology of normal defecation?

Continence depends on the anal sphincter, pelvic floor musculature, stool consistency, rectal capacity/compliance, and neurologic function. Peristaltic colonic contractions move stool into the rectum, and sensory epithelium of the anal canal performs "rectal sampling" to determine if the contents are solid, liquid, or gas. If socially appropriate, the pelvic muscles relax and straighten the anorectal angle, rectosigmoid contractions are initiated, intraabdominal pressure increases voluntarily, and the rectal contents are expelled. When socially unacceptable, the anal sphincters contract, and the rectum accommodates to hold the contents until a later time.

What anatomic components are responsible for continence?

The rectum is a compliant reservoir for stool, and reduced compliance is associated with fecal urgency and incontinence. The puborectalis muscle, innervated by S2–S5 nerve roots, forms a sling around the anorectal junction and maintains the anorectal angle (Fig. 64.1). During rectal filling, sympathetic activation causes contraction of the internal anal sphincter (IAS) for defecation. The IAS is a continuation of the involuntary, circular smooth muscle of the rectum and contributes about 85% of resting anal sphincter pressure. The external anal sphincter (EAS), a striated muscle innervated by the S4 nerve root via the inferior rectal nerve, surrounds the IAS down to the anal verge. Its voluntary contraction provides the remainder of the resting pressure. The complexity and interdependence of these mechanisms explains why patients lose continence over time, any why a patient can develop incontinence years or decades after an OASI or an inciting event.

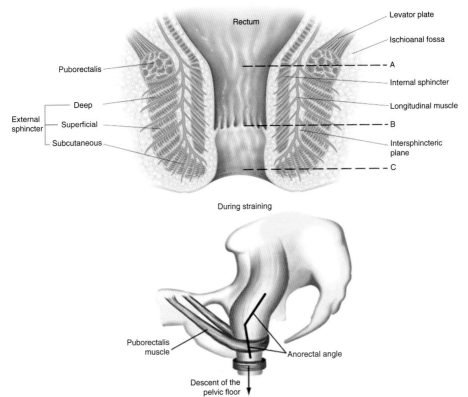

Fig. 64.1 Anatomy of the anal sphincter complex (*above*) showing planes through the proximal (A), mid (B), and distal (C) sphincter complex and another image demonstrating the rectal canal as related to the puborectalis muscle (*below*) that passes around the rectum and creates the anorectal angle and relaxes during straining. (*Above is from Halligan S. Endosonography.* Philadelphia, PA: Elsevier; 2015:269–81, fig. 20-2; *Below is from Lembo AJ,* Sleisenger and Fordtran's gastrointestinal and liver disease. Philadelphia, PA: Elsevier; 2016:270–96, fig. 19-1.)

What physical exam findings are important for the evaluation of FI?

The physical exam should focus on the abdomen and pelvis. The external genitalia and anus may show signs of prior obstetric injury as well as hemorrhoids, rectal prolapse, skin irritation around the anus, and scarring from prior obstetric trauma. The bulbocavernosus and anal wink reflexes verify S2–S4 neurological function. A vaginal exam evaluates the presence of stool, abnormal discharge, and vaginal prolapse. A rectal exam assesses for hemorrhoids, rectal prolapse, and anal sphincter strength.

The patient is afebrile with a heart rate of 82/min and blood pressure of 118/70 mm Hg. Her abdomen is soft and nontender. She has normal external female genitalia with intact reflexes. Speculum exam shows normal vaginal epithelium. On rectal exam, no masses or other lesions are palpated. She has normal sphincter resting tone, and a rectal squeeze strength scored 1/5 on a 5-point scale.

What studies are necessary for the workup of FI?

No specific tests are needed to evaluate FI; a thorough history and physical are all that are required to initiate treatment. Any "red flag" symptoms for colon cancer warrant a referral for a colonoscopy. Occasionally, after a patient sustains an anal sphincter disruption (i.e., traumatic delivery), endoanal ultrasound can be used to identify an anal sphincter laceration, but this is only merited if it will change treatment.

CLINICAL PEARL   **STEPS 2/3**

Red flags for colorectal cancer such as bloody stools, unexplained weight loss, and chronic anemia warrant further investigation and possible referral to gastroenterology, as does a significant family history for colon cancer.

The patient is discouraged because she has "tried a lot of things" already. She tried a fiber supplement and kept a food diary in the past. She noticed worsening of her symptoms with spicy and fried food and now avoids them. However, she is still very bothered by the FI.

What are other initial treatment options that should be offered to the patient?
First-line therapies include dietary changes, pelvic floor exercises, and medications. Food diaries are useful to help identify triggers for FI episodes or looser stools, such as greasy/fatty food, spicy food, lactose, gas-producing vegetables (i.e., broccoli), and artificial sweeteners. Fiber can help make stool more formed and easier to pass. The U.S. Department of Agriculture (USDA) recommends 22–28 g of fiber a day for women. Patients should be educated to increase fiber slowly and drink plenty of water. Scheduled toileting can also help improve FI because better emptying can help avoid accidents. The colon produces mass movements in the morning and after meals, so after breakfast is an ideal time to attempt a bowel movement. Elevating feet on a step stool while on the toilet may improve rectal emptying by straightening the puborectalis muscle to facilitate defecation. Agents such as loperamide or psyllium fiber can also help decrease FI.

BASIC SCIENCE/CLINICAL PEARL   **STEPS 1/2/3**

Loperamide acts on opioid receptors at the colonic smooth muscle and striated muscle of the anal sphincter. Increased transit time, reduced fecal volume, and limited fluid loss caused by loperamide all contribute to improving FI. However, loperamide may result in constipation. One study demonstrated that psyllium fiber and loperamide are equally effective in FI treatment.

The patient wants to know if there are "easy to do" therapies beyond what she has already tried. She wants to avoid surgery, if possible.

What other nonsurgical interventions are available to patients for FI?
Physical therapy (PT) treats FI by providing support with behavioral changes and strengthening the pelvic floor muscles. Many physical therapists who treat FI utilize biofeedback, audio and visual cues to enhance rectal sensation and train the sphincters to improve coordination of anal muscles.

The patient has made significant behavioral modifications, increased fiber and water intake, scheduled toileting, and undertook physical therapy. Her symptoms improved "for a while," but she is interested in "more permanent" options.

When should surgical options for FI be offered to patients, and what common surgical options are available?
Surgical therapies are reserved for patients with refractory FI who have failed conservative treatments because success rates vary and some surgeries for FI carry significant risk. Sacral neuromodulation (SNM) is often recommended. SNM involves the placement of an electrode into the S3 foramen to

stimulate the nerve complex innervating the rectum and anal sphincter complex. Success rates are as high as 63% at 12 months. Before SNM, the most commonly performed surgery for FI was the sphincteroplasty—surgical repair of the anal sphincters—but success was less than 50% at 5–10 years.

The patient opts to undergo implantation of a sacral neuromodulator, and she has great success when she follows-up 3 months later.

BEYOND THE PEARLS

- Assess patients complaining of FI for constipation because they may have overflow of looser fecal material that leaks around the harder, more distal stool.
- Anal receptive intercourse is a factor that contributes to FI in both men and women.
- Women with a prior fourth-degree laceration often want recommendations for future deliveries. Expert opinion recommends a repeat vaginal delivery if she does not have current symptoms of FI. It is reasonable to offer a Cesarean delivery if she is symptomatic.
- Although seemingly drastic, patients with FI who have failed multiple treatments report improved quality of life with an ostomy.
- Future treatment options in development for the treatment of FI include injection of stem cells into the anal sphincter muscle and magnetic beads.

Case Summary

- A 63-year-old woman has accidental stool leakage. She is embarrassed and hesitant to discuss it, but you carefully discuss her symptoms and risk factors.
- Her history and physical is consistent with idiopathic FI, and she attempts lifestyle measures such as fiber, toileting habits, and physical therapy with limited success.
- She undergoes a sacral neuromodulator implantation and has notable improvement in her symptoms.

References

Bharucha, A. E., Dunivan, G., Goode, P. S., et al. (2015). Epidemiology, pathophysiology, and classification of fecal incontinence: state of the science summary for the National Institute of Diabetes and Digestive and Kidney Diseases (NIDDK) workshop. *The American Journal of Gastroenterology, 110*(1), 127–136.

Frenckner, B., & Euler, C. V. (1975). Influence of pudendal block on the function of the anal sphincters. *Gut, 16,* 482.

Lamblin, G., Bouvier, P., Damon, H., et al. (2014). Long-term outcome after overlapping anterior anal sphincter repair for fecal incontinence. *International Journal of Colorectal Disease, 29*(11), 1377–1383.

Markland, A. D., Burgio, K. L., Whitehead, W. E., et al. (2015). Loperamide versus psyllium fiber for treatment of fecal incontinence: the fecal incontinence prescription (Rx) management (FIRM) randomized clinical trial. *Diseases of the Colon and Rectum, 58*(10), 963–993.

Miner, P. B., Jr. (2004). Economic and personal impact of fecal and urinary incontinence. *Gastroenterology, 126.*

Paquette, I. M., Madhulika, V. G., Kaiser, A. M., et al. (2015). The American Society of Colon and Rectal Surgeons' clinical practice guideline for the treatment of fecal incontinence. *Diseases of the Colon and Rectum, 58,* 7.

Salvioli, B., Barucha, A. E., Rath-Harvey, D., et al. (2001). Rectal compliance, capacity and rectoanal sensation in fecal incontinence. *The American Journal of Gastroenterology, 96,* 2158–2168.

Thin, N. N., Horrocks, E. J., Hotouras, A., et al. (2013). Systematic review of the clinical effectiveness of neuromodulation in the treatment of faecal incontinence. *The British Journal of Surgery, 100*(11), 1430–1447.

Wald, A. B., Cosman, B. C., & Whitehead, W. E. (2014). ACG clinical guidelines: management of benign anorectal disorders. *The American Journal of Gastroenterology, 109,* 1141–1157.

Wonderling, D., & Jones, C. (2007). Nice clinical guideline on managing faecal incontinence: evidence of the effectiveness and cost-effectiveness of surgical interventions. *Annals of the Royal College of Surgeons of England, 89*(6), 642–645.

INDEX

Note: Page numbers followed by *f* indicate figures, *t* indicate tables, and *b* indicate boxes.